Genetic Disorders Sourcebook,
  1st Edition
Genetic Disorders Sourcebook,
  2nd Edition
Head Trauma Sourcebook
Headache Sourcebook
Health Insurance Sourcebook
Health Reference Series Cumulative
  Index 1999
Healthy Aging Sourcebook
Healthy Children Sourcebook
Healthy Heart Sourcebook for Women
Heart Diseases & Disorders
  Sourcebook, 2nd Edition
Household Safety Sourcebook
Immune System Disorders Sourcebook
Infant & Toddler Health Sourcebook
Injury & Trauma Sourcebook
Kidney & Urinary Tract Diseases &
  Disorders Sourcebook
Learning Disabilities Sourcebook,
  1st Edition
Learning Disabilities Sourcebook,
  2nd Edition
Liver Disorders Sourcebook
Leukemia Sourcebook
Lung Disorders Sourcebook
Medical Tests Sourcebook
Men's Health Concerns Sourcebook
Mental Health Disorders Sourcebook,
  1st Edition
Mental Health Disorders Sourcebook,
  2nd Edition
Mental Retardation Sourcebook
Movement Disorders Sourcebook
Obesity Sourcebook
Ophthalmic Disorders Sourcebook,
  1st Edition
Oral Health Sourcebook
Osteoporosis Sourcebook
Pain Sourcebook, 1st Edition
Pain Sourcebook, 2nd Edition
Pediatric Cancer Sourcebook
Physical & Mental Issues in Aging
  Sourcebook

Podiatry Sourcebook
Pregnancy & Birth Sourcebook
Prostate Cancer
Public Health Sourcebook
Reconstructive & Cosmetic Surgery
  Sourcebook
Rehabilitation Sourcebook
Respiratory Diseases & Disorders
  Sourcebook
Sexually Transmitted Diseases
  Sourcebook, 1st Edition
Sexually Transmitted Diseases
  Sourcebook, 2nd Edition
Skin Disorders Sourcebook
Sleep Disorders Sourcebook
Sports Injuries Sourcebook, 1st Edition
Sports Injuries Sourcebook, 2nd Edition
Stress-Related Disorders Sourcebook
Stroke Sourcebook
Substance Abuse Sourcebook
Surgery Sourcebook
Transplantation Sourcebook
Traveler's Health Sourcebook
Vegetarian Sourcebook
Women's Health Concerns Sourcebook
Workplace Health & Safety Sourcebook
Worldwide Health Sourcebook

Teen Health Series

Diet Information for Teens
Drug Information for Teens
Mental Health Information
  for Teens
Sexual Health Information
  for Teens
Skin Health Information
  for Teens
Sports Injuries Information
  for Teens

AIDS
SOURCEBOOK

Third Edition

Health Reference Series

Third Edition

AIDS
SOURCEBOOK

*Basic Consumer Health Information about
Acquired Immune Deficiency Syndrome (AIDS)
and Human Immunodeficiency Virus (HIV) Infection,
Including Facts about Transmission, Prevention,
Diagnosis, Treatment, Opportunistic Infections,
and Other Complications, with a Section for
Women and Children, Including Details about
Associated Gynecological Concerns, Pregnancy,
and Pediatric Care*

*Along with Updated Statistical Information,
Reports on Current Research Initiatives, a Glossary,
and Directories of Internet, Hotline, and
Other Resources*

Edited by
Dawn D. Matthews

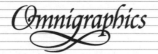

615 Griswold Street • Detroit, MI 48226

Bibliographic Note

Because this page cannot legibly accommodate all the copyright notices, the Bibliographic Note portion of the Preface constitutes an extension of the copyright notice.

Edited by Dawn D. Matthews

Health Reference Series

Karen Bellenir, *Managing Editor*
David A. Cooke, MD, *Medical Consultant*
Elizabeth Barbour, *Permissions Associate*
Dawn Matthews, *Verification Assistant*
Laura Pleva Nielsen, *Index Editor*
EdIndex, Services for Publishers, *Indexers*

* * *

Omnigraphics, Inc.

Matthew P. Barbour, *Senior Vice President*
Kay Gill, *Vice President—Directories*
Kevin Hayes, *Operations Manager*
Leif Gruenberg, *Development Manager*
David P. Bianco, *Marketing Consultant*

* * *

Peter E. Ruffner, *Publisher*

Frederick G. Ruffner, Jr., *Chairman*

Copyright © 2003 Omnigraphics, Inc.

ISBN 0-7808-0631-X

Library of Congress Cataloging-in-Publication Data

AIDS sourcebook : basic consumer health information about acquired immune deficiency
   syndrome (AIDS) and human immunodeficiency virus (HIV) infection, including facts
   about transmission, prevention, diagnosis, treatment, opportunistic infections, and other
   complications, with a section for women and children, including details about associated
   gynecological concerns, pregnancy, and pediatric care ; along with updated statistical
   informations, reports on current research initiatives, a glossary, and directories of
   Internet, Hotline, and other resources / edited by Dawn M. Matthews.--3rd ed.
      p. cm.-- (Health reference series)
      Includes index.
      ISBN 0-7808-0631-X
      1. AIDS (Disease)--Popular works. I. Matthews, Dawn D. II. Health reference series
   (Unnumbered)
   RC606.64.A337 2003
   362.1'969792--dc21   2003040531

Table of Contents

Preface ix

Part I: Understanding Acquired Immune Deficiency Syndrome (AIDS) and Human Immunodeficiency Virus (HIV)

Chapter 1—HIV Infection and AIDS: An Overview 3
Chapter 2—How HIV Causes AIDS 13
Chapter 3—Human Immunodeficiency Virus Type 2
            (HIV-2) 27
Chapter 4—HIV and Its Transmission 33
Chapter 5—HIV Transmission through Oral Sex 39
Chapter 6—Drug Use and Its Association to HIV
            Transmission 43
Chapter 7—Blood Safety 47
Chapter 8—Exposure to Blood: What Health-Care
            Workers Need to Know 53
Chapter 9—Living with AIDS—20 Years Later 61

Part II: Diagnosis and Treatment of AIDS

Chapter 10—HIV Testing: Overview 73
Chapter 11—Rapid HIV Tests: Questions and Answers 79
Chapter 12—Viral Load Tests 87

Chapter 13—Home Diagnostic Tests 91
Chapter 14—HIV Counseling, Testing, and Referral 97
Chapter 15—Treatment of HIV Infection: An Overview 113
Chapter 16—Approved Drugs for HIV Infection and
　　　　　　　AIDS-Related Conditions 119
Chapter 17—Protease Inhibitors 129
Chapter 18—Highly Active Antiretroviral Therapy
　　　　　　　(HAART) 133
Chapter 19—Attacking AIDS with Cocktail Therapy 141
Chapter 20—Pulsed Therapy and Structured
　　　　　　　Interruptions of AIDS Treatment 149
Chapter 21—Alternative and Complementary Treatments
　　　　　　　for AIDS 157
Chapter 22—Marijuana and AIDS Treatment 161

Part III: Complications Associated with AIDS

Chapter 23—Cryptosporidiosis (Crypto) 171
Chapter 24—Cytomegalovirus (CMV) 177
Chapter 25—Co-Infection with HIV and Hepatitis C Virus ... 179
Chapter 26—Lipodystrophy 185
Chapter 27—Disseminated Mycobacterium Avium
　　　　　　　Complex Disease (MAC) 193
Chapter 28—*Pneumocystis Carinii* Pneumonia (PCP) 197
Chapter 29—Tuberculosis and HIV 201
Chapter 30—AIDS-Related Kaposi's Sarcoma (KS) 207
Chapter 31—AIDS Dementia Complex (ADC) 211
Chapter 32—Peripheral Neuropathy 215
Chapter 33—Other Major Neurologic Complications in
　　　　　　　AIDS 217
Chapter 34—HIV Wasting Syndrome 221
Chapter 35—Drug Interactions in HIV Treatment 225

Part IV: Living with AIDS

Chapter 36—Living with HIV/AIDS: An Overview 237
Chapter 37—Depression and HIV/AIDS 245
Chapter 38—Nutrition Strategies for AIDS 251
Chapter 39—HIV and Preventing Infection from Unsafe
　　　　　　　Food and Water 257

Chapter 40—Traveling with AIDS: Protect Yourself from
Opportunistic Infections 261
Chapter 41—Household Pets: Special Precautions for
People with AIDS 265
Chapter 42—Caring for Someone with AIDS at Home 269
Chapter 43—Social Security Benefits for People Living
with AIDS 291

Part V: Issues for Women and Children with AIDS

Chapter 44—Women and AIDS................................... 305
Chapter 45—Gynecological Complications in Women
with HIV 311
Chapter 46—Women over 50 Living with HIV:
Menopause and Hormone Replacement
Therapy 327
Chapter 47—Gender Difference in Viral Load 339
Chapter 48—Pregnancy and HIV................................. 343
Chapter 49—Status of Perinatal HIV Prevention 347
Chapter 50—Pediatric AIDS 351
Chapter 51—Guidelines for the Use of Antiretroviral
Agents in Pediatric HIV Infection 357
Chapter 52—Preventing *Pneumocystis Carinii
Pneumonia* (PCP) in Children............................. 383

Part VI: Prevention and Research

Chapter 53—Combating Complacency in HIV Prevention 389
Chapter 54—Prevention and Treatment of Sexually
Transmitted Diseases as an HIV Prevention
Strategy 395
Chapter 55—Preventive Therapy for Non-Occupational
Exposure to HIV 399
Chapter 56—Prevention among Men Who Have Sex with
Men 403
Chapter 57—Prevention among Women Who Have Sex
with Women 407
Chapter 58—Condom Use and HIV Prevention...................... 411
Chapter 59—Centers for Disease Control and Prevention
(CDC) HIV/AIDS Prevention Activities 417

Chapter 60—HIV/AIDS Research: Successes Bring New
        Challenges 427
Chapter 61—Comprehensive International Program of
        Research on AIDS (CIPRA) 439
Chapter 62—The Thailand Phase III Vaccine Study 443
Chapter 63—HIV/AIDS Clinical Trials 451
Chapter 64—Taking Part in Research Studies: What
        Questions You Should Ask 465

Part VII: HIV/AIDS Statistical Information

Chapter 65—HIV/AIDS Statistics: An Overview...................... 471
Chapter 66—Surveillance of Health Care Workers with
        HIV/AIDS 475
Chapter 67—HIV/AIDS among African Americans................. 477
Chapter 68—HIV/AIDS among Hispanic Americans 481
Chapter 69—HIV/AIDS among U.S. Women 485
Chapter 70—HIV Prevalence among America's Youth 489

Part VIII: Additional Help and Information

Chapter 71—Glossary of AIDS-Related Terms 495
Chapter 72—Finding Reliable HIV/AIDS Information
        on the Internet 583
Chapter 73—National Organizations Providing
        HIV/AIDS Services 603
Chapter 74—National Religious AIDS Organizations
        and Hotlines 605
Chapter 75—CDC's National AIDS Hotline............................ 609

Index 613

Preface

About This Book

Evidence suggests that the human immunodeficiency virus (HIV) has been in the United States at least since 1978. HIV is the virus that causes AIDS (acquired immune deficiency syndrome). When AIDS first surfaced in the United States, there were no medicines to combat the underlying immune deficiency and few treatments existed for the opportunistic diseases that resulted. The situation now is more promising. Multiple drugs that act to slow HIV have been approved for use in the United States, and additional drugs are being tested. Because no vaccine for HIV is yet available, however, the only way to reduce the risk of infection by the virus is to avoid behaviors that are associated with HIV transmission.

AIDS Sourcebook, Third Edition, provides updated information about AIDS and its transmission, diagnosis, and treatment. It reports on new research and new strategies being used to help AIDS patients live longer, healthier lives. A special section focuses on the concerns of women and children with HIV/AIDS. This book also provides practical tips about such topics as nutrition, preventing opportunistic infections, and caring for someone with AIDS at home. Statistical data, updated information about prevention programs, a glossary of AIDS-related terms, and resource listings are also provided.

How to Use This Book

This book is divided into parts and chapters. Parts focus on broad areas of interest. Chapters are devoted to single topics within a part.

Part I: Understanding Acquired Immune Deficiency Syndrome (AIDS) and Human Immunodeficiency Virus (HIV) contains and overview of HIV/AIDS with specific information about how HIV causes AIDS and how the virus is transmitted. Other related topics, such as blood safety, occupational exposure, and risks associated with drug use, are also discussed.

Part II: Diagnosis and Treatment of AIDS provides information about HIV testing including rapid HIV testing, viral load tests, and home diagnostic tests. Treatment information about approved drugs, protease inhibitors, and highly active antiretroviral therapy (HAART) is included. Discussions about alternative and complementary therapies and the use of medical marijuana by AIDS patients are provided.

Part III: Complications Associated with AIDS describes some of the opportunistic infections and conditions that can occur in association with HIV/AIDS. Cryptosporidiosis (crypto), cytomegalovirus (CMV), AIDS-related Kaposi's sarcoma, AIDS dementia complex, and HIV wasting syndrome are among the topics included.

Part IV: Living with AIDS offers patients and caregivers updated information on coping with the day-to-day concerns surrounding AIDS management. Issues such as depression, nutrition, preventing opportunistic infections while traveling, and social security benefits are included. A chapter about caring for someone with AIDS at home contains additional information.

Part V: Issues for Women and Children with AIDS includes facts about gynecological complications, hormone replacement therapy, complications of pregnancy in women with HIV infection, and methods for preventing perinatal transmission of HIV to infants. It also provides information about pediatric AIDS and concerns related to the care of children with HIV/AIDS.

Part VI: Prevention and Research discusses strategies and governmental programs for preventing HIV transmission. Information about current research initiatives, including the Comprehensive International Program of Research on AIDS (CIPRA) and the Thailand Phase III Vaccine Study, is included. Chapters discussing clinical trials provide information for people interested in participating in research activities.

Part VII: HIV/AIDS Statistical Information reports on current demographic information about HIV/AIDS. Individual chapters report on various U.S. sub-populations, including African Americans, Hispanic Americans, women, and children.

Part VIII: Additional Help and Information includes a glossary of AIDS-related terms, information about finding reliable HIV/AIDS information on the internet, and resource lists of additional AIDS services and organizations.

Bibliographic Note

This volume contains documents and excerpts from publications issued by the following U.S. government agencies: AIDSinfo (formerly HIV/AIDS Clinical Trials Information Service [ACTIS] and HIV/AIDS Treatment Information Service [ATIS]); Centers for Disease Control and Prevention (CDC); ClinicalTrials.gov; National Cancer Institute (NCI); National HIV Testing Resources; National Institute of Allergy and Infectious Diseases (NIAID); National Institute of Mental Health (NIMH); Substance Abuse and Mental Health Services Administration (SAMHSA); the Social Security Administration (SSA); and the U.S. Food and Drug Administration (FDA).

In addition, this volume contains copyrighted documents from the following organizations and individuals: AIDS Nutrition Services Alliance; AIDS Treatment Data Network; InfoWeb (AEGIS); Healthcommunities.com; Kaiser Family Foundation; Neurologic AIDS Research Consortium/Washington University in St. Louis; New Mexico AIDS InfoNet; Project Inform; and the Seattle Treatment Education Project.

Acknowledgements

Special thanks go to the many organizations, agencies, and individuals who have contributed material for this *Sourcebook* and to the managing editor Karen Bellenir and permissions specialist Liz Barbour.

Note from the Editor

This book is part of Omnigraphics' *Health Reference Series*. The series provides basic information about a broad range of medical concerns. It is not intended to serve as a tool for diagnosing illness, in prescribing treatments, or as a substitute for the physician/patient relationship. All persons concerned about medical symptoms or the possibility of disease are encouraged to seek professional care from an appropriate health care provider.

Our Advisory Board

The *Health Reference Series* is reviewed by an Advisory Board comprised of librarians from public, academic, and medical libraries. We would like to thank the following board members for providing guidance to the development of this series:

Dr. Lynda Baker,
Associate Professor of Library and Information Science,
Wayne State University, Detroit, MI

Nancy Bulgarelli,
William Beaumont Hospital Library, Royal Oak, MI

Karen Imarisio,
Bloomfield Township Public Library, Bloomfield Township, MI

Karen Morgan,
Mardigian Library, University of Michigan-Dearborn,
Dearborn, MI

Rosemary Orlando,
St. Clair Shores Public Library, St. Clair Shores, MI

Medical Consultant

Medical consultation services are provided to the *Health Reference Series* editors by David A. Cooke, MD. Dr. Cooke is a graduate of Brandeis University, and he received his M.D. degree from the University of Michigan. He completed residency training at the University of Wisconsin Hospital and Clinics. He is board-certified in Internal Medicine. Dr. Cooke currently works as part of the University of Michigan Health System and practices in Brighton, MI. In his free time, he enjoys writing, science fiction, and spending time with his family.

Health Reference Series *Update Policy*

The inaugural book in the *Health Reference Series* was the first edition of *Cancer Sourcebook* published in 1989. Since then, the *Series* has been enthusiastically received by librarians and in the medical community. In order to maintain the standard of providing high-quality health information for the layperson the editorial staff at Omnigraphics felt it was necessary to implement a policy of updating volumes when warranted.

Medical researchers have been making tremendous strides, and it is the purpose of the *Health Reference Series* to stay current with the most recent advances. Each decision to update a volume will be made on an individual basis. Some of the considerations will include how much new information is available and the feedback we receive from people who use the books. If there is a topic you would like to see added to the update list, or an area of medical concern you feel has not been adequately addressed, please write to:

Editor
Health Reference Series
Omnigraphics, Inc.
615 Griswold Street
Detroit, MI 48226
E-mail: editorial@omnigraphics.com

Part One

Understanding Acquired Immune Deficiency Syndrome (AIDS) and Human Immuno-deficiency Virus (HIV)

Chapter 1

HIV Infection and AIDS: An Overview

AIDS—acquired immunodeficiency syndrome—was first reported in the United States in 1981 and has since become a major worldwide epidemic. AIDS is caused by the human immunodeficiency virus (HIV). By killing or damaging cells of the body's immune system, HIV progressively destroys the body's ability to fight infections and certain cancers. People diagnosed with AIDS may get life-threatening diseases called opportunistic infections, which are caused by microbes such as viruses or bacteria that usually do not make healthy people sick.

More than 700,000 cases of AIDS have been reported in the United States since 1981, and as many as 900,000 Americans may be infected with HIV. The epidemic is growing most rapidly among minority populations and is a leading killer of African-American males. According to the U.S. Centers for Disease Control and Prevention (CDC), AIDS affects nearly seven times more African Americans than whites and three times more Hispanics than whites (CDC *HIV/AIDS Surveillance Report,* Vol. 12, 2000).

How Is HIV Transmitted?

HIV is spread most commonly by having unprotected sex with an infected partner. The virus can enter the body through the lining of the vagina, vulva, penis, rectum, or mouth during sex.

A fact sheet from National Institute of Allergy and Infectious Disease (NIAID), dated May 2001; available online at http://www.niaid.nih.gov/factsheets/hivinf.htm.

HIV also is spread through contact with infected blood. Before donated blood was screened for evidence of HIV infection and before heat-treating techniques to destroy HIV in blood products were introduced, HIV was transmitted through transfusions of contaminated blood or blood components. Today, because of blood screening and heat treatment, the risk of getting HIV from such transfusions is extremely small.

HIV frequently is spread among injection drug users by the sharing of needles or syringes contaminated with very small quantities of blood from someone infected with the virus. It is rare, however, for a patient to give HIV to a health care worker or vice-versa by accidental sticks with contaminated needles or other medical instruments.

Women can transmit HIV to their babies during pregnancy or birth. Approximately one-quarter to one-third of all untreated pregnant women infected with HIV will pass the infection to their babies. HIV also can be spread to babies through the breast milk of mothers infected with the virus. If the mother takes the drug AZT during pregnancy, she can reduce significantly the chances that her baby will get be infected with HIV. If health care providers treat mothers with AZT and deliver their babies by cesarean section, the chances of the baby being infected can be reduced to a rate of 1 percent.

A study sponsored by the National Institute of Allergy and Infectious Diseases (NIAID) in Uganda found a highly effective and safe drug regimen for preventing transmission of HIV from an infected mother to her newborn that is more affordable and practical than any other examined to date. Interim results from the study show that a single oral dose of the antiretroviral drug nevirapine (NVP) given to an HIV-infected woman in labor and another to her baby within three days of birth reduces the transmission rate by half compared with a similar short course of AZT.

Although researchers have found HIV in the saliva of infected people, there is no evidence that the virus is spread by contact with saliva. Laboratory studies reveal that saliva has natural properties that limit the power of HIV to infect. Research studies of people infected with HIV have found no evidence that the virus is spread to others through saliva by kissing. No one knows, however, whether so-called deep kissing, involving the exchange of large amounts of saliva, or oral intercourse increase the risk of infection. Scientists also have found no evidence that HIV is spread through sweat, tears, urine, or feces.

Studies of families of HIV-infected people have shown clearly that HIV is not spread through casual contact such as the sharing of food utensils, towels and bedding, swimming pools, telephones, or toilet seats. HIV is not spread by biting insects such as mosquitoes or bedbugs.

HIV can infect anyone who practices risky behaviors such as:

- sharing drug needles or syringes

- having sexual contact with an infected person without using a condom

- having sexual contact with someone whose HIV status is unknown

Having a sexually transmitted disease such as syphilis, genital herpes, chlamydial infection, gonorrhea, or bacterial vaginosis appears to make people more susceptible to getting HIV infection during sex with infected partners.

What Are the Early Symptoms of HIV Infection?

Many people do not have any symptoms when they first become infected with HIV. Some people, however, have a flu-like illness within a month or two after exposure to the virus. This illness may include fever, headache, tiredness, and enlarged lymph nodes (glands of the immune system easily felt in the neck and groin). These symptoms usually disappear within a week to a month and are often mistaken for those of another viral infection. During this period, people are very infectious, and HIV is present in large quantities in genital fluids.

More persistent or severe symptoms may not surface for a decade or more after HIV first enters the body in adults, or within two years in children born with HIV infection. This period of asymptomatic infection is highly individual. Some people may begin to have symptoms within a few months, while others may be symptom-free for more than 10 years.

Even during the asymptomatic period, the virus is actively multiplying, infecting, and killing cells of the immune system. HIV's effect is seen most obviously in a decline in the blood levels of CD4+ T-cells (also called T4-cells)—the immune system's key infection fighters. At the beginning of its life in the human body, the virus disables or destroys these cells without causing symptoms.

As the immune system deteriorates, a variety of complications start to take over. For many people, their first sign of infection is large lymph nodes or swollen glands that may be enlarged for more than three months. Other symptoms often experienced months to years before the onset of AIDS include:

- lack of energy
- weight loss
- frequent fevers and sweats
- persistent or frequent yeast infections (oral or vaginal)
- persistent skin rashes or flaky skin
- pelvic inflammatory disease in women that does not respond to treatment
- short-term memory loss

Some people develop frequent and severe herpes infections that cause mouth, genital, or anal sores, or a painful nerve disease called shingles. Children may grow slowly or be sick a lot.

What Is AIDS?

The term AIDS applies to the most advanced stages of HIV infection. CDC developed official criteria for the definition of AIDS and is responsible for tracking the spread of AIDS in the United States.

CDC's definition of AIDS includes all HIV-infected people who have fewer than 200 CD4+ T-cells per cubic millimeter of blood. (Healthy adults usually have CD4+ T-cell counts of 1,000 or more.) In addition, the definition includes 26 clinical conditions that affect people with advanced HIV disease. Most of these conditions are opportunistic infections that generally do not affect healthy people. In people with AIDS, these infections are often severe and sometimes fatal because the immune system is so ravaged by HIV that the body cannot fight off certain bacteria, viruses, fungi, parasites, and other microbes.

Symptoms of opportunistic infections common in people with AIDS include:

- coughing and shortness of breath
- seizures and lack of coordination
- difficult or painful swallowing
- mental symptoms such as confusion and forgetfulness
- severe and persistent diarrhea
- fever

- vision loss
- nausea, abdominal cramps, and vomiting
- weight loss and extreme fatigue
- severe headaches
- coma

Children with AIDS may get the same opportunistic infections as do adults with the disease. In addition, they also have severe forms of the bacterial infections all children may get, such as conjunctivitis (pink eye), ear infections, and tonsillitis.

People with AIDS are particularly prone to developing various cancers, especially those caused by viruses such as Kaposi's sarcoma and cervical cancer, or cancers of the immune system known as lymphomas. These cancers are usually more aggressive and difficult to treat in people with AIDS. Signs of Kaposi's sarcoma in light-skinned people are round brown, reddish, or purple spots that develop in the skin or in the mouth. In dark-skinned people, the spots are more pigmented.

During the course of HIV infection, most people experience a gradual decline in the number of CD4+ T-cells, although some may have abrupt and dramatic drops in their CD4+ T-cell counts. A person with CD4+ T-cells above 200 may experience some of the early symptoms of HIV disease. Others may have no symptoms even though their CD4+ T-cell count is below 200.

Many people are so debilitated by the symptoms of AIDS that they cannot hold steady employment or do household chores. Other people with AIDS may experience phases of intense life-threatening illness followed by phases in which they function normally.

A small number of people (fewer than 50) first infected with HIV 10 or more years ago have not developed symptoms of AIDS. Scientists are trying to determine what factors may account for their lack of progression to AIDS, such as particular characteristics of their immune systems or whether they were infected with a less aggressive strain of the virus, or if their genes may protect them from the effects of HIV. Scientists hope that understanding the body's natural method of control may lead to ideas for protective HIV vaccines and use of vaccines to prevent the disease from progressing.

How Is HIV Infection Diagnosed?

Because early HIV infection often causes no symptoms, a doctor or other health care provider usually can diagnose it by testing a person's blood for the presence of antibodies (disease-fighting proteins) to HIV. HIV antibodies generally do not reach detectable levels in the blood for one to three months following infection. It may take the antibodies as long as six months to be produced in quantities large enough to show up in standard blood tests.

People exposed to the virus should get an HIV test as soon as they are likely to develop antibodies to the virus—within 6 weeks to 12 months after possible exposure to the virus. By getting tested early, people with HIV infection can discuss with a health care provider when they should start treatment to help their immune systems combat HIV and help prevent the emergence of certain opportunistic infections. Early testing also alerts HIV-infected people to avoid high-risk behaviors that could spread the virus to others.

Most health care providers can do HIV testing and will usually offer counseling to the patient at the same time. Of course, individuals can be tested anonymously at many sites if they are concerned about confidentiality.

Health care providers diagnose HIV infection by using two different types of antibody tests, ELISA and Western Blot. If a person is highly likely to be infected with HIV and yet both tests are negative, the health care provider may request additional tests. The person also may be told to repeat antibody testing at a later date, when antibodies to HIV are more likely to have developed.

Babies born to mothers infected with HIV may or may not be infected with the virus, but all carry their mothers' antibodies to HIV for several months. If these babies lack symptoms, a doctor cannot make a definitive diagnosis of HIV infection using standard antibody tests until after 15 months of age. By then, babies are unlikely to still carry their mothers' antibodies and will have produced their own, if they are infected. Health care experts are using new technologies to detect HIV itself to more accurately determine HIV infection in infants between ages 3 months and 15 months. They are evaluating a number of blood tests to determine if they can diagnose HIV infection in babies younger than 3 months.

How Is HIV Infection Treated?

When AIDS first surfaced in the United States, there were no medicines to combat the underlying immune deficiency and few treatments existed for the opportunistic diseases that resulted. Over the past 10 years, however, researchers have developed drugs to fight both HIV infection and its associated infections and cancers.

The U.S. Food and Drug Administration (FDA) has approved a number of drugs for treating HIV infection. The first group of drugs used to treat HIV infection, called nucleoside reverse transcriptase (RT) inhibitors, interrupts an early stage of the virus making copies of itself. Included in this class of drugs (called nucleoside analogs) are AZT (also known as zidovudine or ZDV), ddC (zalcitabine), ddI (dideoxyinosine), d4T (stavudine), and 3TC (lamivudine). These drugs may slow the spread of HIV in the body and delay the onset of opportunistic infections.

Health care providers can prescribe non-nucleoside reverse transcriptase inhibitors (NNRTIs), such as delavirdine (Rescriptor), nevirapine (Viramune), and efavirenz (Sustiva), in combination with other antiretroviral drugs.

More recently, FDA has approved a second class of drugs for treating HIV infection. These drugs, called protease inhibitors, interrupt virus replication at a later step in its life cycle. They include:

- ritonavir (Norvir)
- saquinavir (Invirase)
- indinavir (Crixivan)
- amprenavir (Agenerase)
- nelfinavir (Viracept)
- lopinavir (Kaletra)

Because HIV can become resistant to any of these drugs, health care providers must use a combination treatment to effectively suppress the virus.

Currently available antiretroviral drugs do not cure people of HIV infection or AIDS, however, and they all have side effects that can be severe. Some of the nucleoside RT inhibitors may cause a depletion of red or white blood cells, especially when taken in the later stages of the disease. Some may also cause an inflammation of the pancreas and painful nerve damage. There have been reports or complications and other severe reactions, including death, to some of the antiretroviral nucleoside analogs when used alone or in combination. Therefore, health care experts recommend that people on antiretroviral therapy be routinely seen and followed by their providers.

The most common side effects associated with protease inhibitors include nausea, diarrhea, and other gastrointestinal symptoms. In addition, protease inhibitors can interact with other drugs resulting in serious side effects.

Researchers have credited highly active antiretroviral therapy, or HAART, as being a major factor in reducing the number of deaths from AIDS in this country by 47 percent in 1997. HAART is a treatment regimen that uses a combination of reverse transcriptase inhibitors and protease inhibitors to treat patients. Patients who are newly infected with HIV as well as AIDS patients can take the combination.

While HAART is not a cure for AIDS, it has greatly improved the health of many people with AIDS and it reduces the amount of virus circulating in the blood to nearly undetectable levels. Researchers have shown that HAART cannot eradicate HIV entirely from the body. HIV remains present, lurking in hiding places such as the lymph nodes, the brain, testes, and the retina of the eye, even in patients who have been treated.

A number of drugs are available to help treat opportunistic infections to which people with HIV are especially prone. These drugs include:

- foscarnet and ganciclovir to treat cytomegalovirus eye infections
- fluconazole to treat yeast and other fungal infections
- trimethoprim/sulfamethoxazole (TMP/SMX) or pentamidine to treat *Pneumocystis carinii* pneumonia (PCP)

In addition to antiretroviral therapy, health care providers treat adults with HIV, whose CD4+ T-cell counts drop below 200, to prevent the occurrence of PCP, which is one of the most common and deadly opportunistic infections associated with HIV. They give children PCP preventive therapy when their CD4+ T-cell counts drop to levels considered below normal for their age group. Regardless of their CD4+ T-cell counts, HIV-infected children and adults who have survived an episode of PCP take drugs for the rest of their lives to prevent a recurrence of the pneumonia.

HIV-infected individuals who develop Kaposi's sarcoma or other cancers are treated with radiation, chemotherapy, or injections of alpha interferon, a genetically engineered naturally occurring protein.

How Can HIV Infection Be Prevented?

Because no vaccine for HIV is available, the only way to prevent infection by the virus is to avoid behaviors that put a person at risk of infection, such as sharing needles and having unprotected sex.

Many people infected with HIV have no symptoms. Therefore, there is no way of knowing with certainty whether a sexual partner is infected unless he or she has repeatedly tested negative for the virus and has not engaged in any risky behavior.

People should either abstain from having sex or use male latex condoms or female polyurethane condoms, which may offer partial protection, during oral, anal, or vaginal sex. Only water-based lubricants should be used with male latex condoms.

Although some laboratory evidence shows that spermicides can kill HIV, researchers have not found that these products can prevent a person from getting HIV.

The risk of HIV transmission from a pregnant woman to her baby is significantly reduced if she takes AZT during pregnancy, labor, and delivery, and her baby takes it for the first six weeks of life.

What Research Is Going on?

NIAID-supported investigators are conducting an abundance of research on HIV infection, including developing and testing HIV vaccines and new therapies for the disease and some of its associated conditions. Investigators are testing 29 HIV vaccines in people, and are developing or testing many drugs for HIV infection or AIDS-associated opportunistic infections. Researchers also are investigating exactly how HIV damages the immune system. This research is suggesting new and more effective targets for drugs and vaccines. NIAID-supported investigators also continue to trace how the disease progresses in different people.

Scientists are investigating and testing chemical barriers, such as topical microbicides, that people can use in the vagina or in the rectum during sex to prevent HIV transmission. They also are looking at other ways to prevent transmission, such as controlling sexually transmitted diseases and modifying people's behavior, as well as ways to prevent transmission from mother to child.

Chapter 2

How HIV Causes AIDS

A significant component of the research effort of the National Institute of Allergy and Infectious Diseases (NIAID) is devoted to the pathogenesis of human immunodeficiency virus (HIV) disease. Studies on pathogenesis address the complex mechanisms that result in the destruction of the immune system of an HIV-infected person. A detailed understanding of HIV and how it establishes infection and causes the acquired immunodeficiency syndrome (AIDS) is crucial to identifying and developing effective drugs and vaccines to fight HIV and AIDS. This chapter summarizes the state of knowledge in this area and provides a brief glossary of terms.

Overview

HIV disease is characterized by a gradual deterioration of immune function. Most notably, crucial immune cells called CD4+ T-cells are disabled and killed during the typical course of infection. These cells, sometimes called T-helper cells, play a central role in the immune response, signaling other cells in the immune system to perform their special functions.

A healthy, uninfected person usually has 800 to 1,200 CD4+ T-cells per cubic millimeter (mm3) of blood. During HIV infection, the number of these cells in a person's blood progressively declines. When a

A fact sheet from National Institute of Allergy and Infectious Disease (NIAID), dated October 2001; available online at http://www.niaid.nih.gov/factsheets/howhiv.htm.

person's CD4+ T-cell count falls below 200/mm3, he or she becomes particularly vulnerable to the opportunistic infections and cancers that typify AIDS, the end stage of HIV disease. People with AIDS often suffer infections of the lungs, intestinal tract, brain, eyes and other organs, as well as debilitating weight loss, diarrhea, neurologic conditions and cancers such as Kaposi's sarcoma and certain types of lymphomas.

Most scientists think that HIV causes AIDS by directly inducing the death of CD4+ T-cells or interfering with their normal function, and by triggering other events that weaken a person's immune function. For example, the network of signaling molecules that normally regulates a person's immune response is disrupted during HIV disease, impairing a person's ability to fight other infections. The HIV-mediated destruction of the lymph nodes and related immunologic organs also plays a major role in causing the immunosuppression seen in people with AIDS.

Scope of the HIV Epidemic

Although HIV was first identified in 1983, studies of previously stored blood samples indicate that the virus entered the U.S. population sometime in the late 1970s. In the United States, 774,467 cases of AIDS, and 448,060 deaths among people with AIDS had been reported to the Centers for Disease Control and Prevention (CDC) as of the end of 2000. Approximately 40,000 new HIV infections occur each year in the United States, 70 percent of them among men and 30 percent among women. Minority groups in the United States have been disproportionately affected by the epidemic.

Worldwide, an estimated 36.1 million people (47 percent of whom are female) were living with HIV/AIDS as of December 2000, according to the Joint United Nations Program on HIV/AIDS (UNAIDS). Through 2000, cumulative HIV/AIDS-associated deaths worldwide numbered approximately 21.8 million: 17.5 million adults and 4.3 million children younger than 15 years. Globally, approximately 5.3 million new HIV infections and 3.0 million HIV/AIDS-related deaths occurred in the year 2000 alone.

HIV Is a Retrovirus

HIV belongs to a class of viruses called retroviruses. Retroviruses are ribonucleic acid (RNA) viruses, and in order to replicate they must make a deoxyribonucleic acid (DNA) copy of their RNA. It is the DNA genes that allow the virus to replicate.

Like all viruses, HIV can replicate only inside cells, commandeering the cell's machinery to reproduce. However, only HIV and other retroviruses, once inside a cell, use an enzyme called reverse transcriptase to convert their RNA into DNA, which can be incorporated into the host cell's genes.

Slow viruses. HIV belongs to a subgroup of retroviruses known as lentiviruses, or slow viruses. The course of infection with these viruses is characterized by a long interval between initial infection and the onset of serious symptoms.

Other lentiviruses infect nonhuman species. For example, the feline immunodeficiency virus (FIV) infects cats and the simian immunodeficiency virus (SIV) infects monkeys and other nonhuman primates. Like HIV in humans, these animal viruses primarily infect immune system cells, often causing immunodeficiency and AIDS-like symptoms. These viruses and their hosts have provided researchers with useful, albeit imperfect, models of the HIV disease process in people.

Structure of HIV

The viral envelope. HIV has a diameter of 1/10,000 of a millimeter and is spherical in shape. The outer coat of the virus, known as the viral envelope, is composed of two layers of fatty molecules called lipids, taken from the membrane of a human cell when a newly formed virus particle buds from the cell. Recent evidence from NIAID-supported researchers indicates that HIV may enter and exit cells through special areas of the cell membrane known as lipid rafts. These rafts are high in cholesterol and glycolipids and may provide a new target for blocking HIV.

Embedded in the viral envelope are proteins from the host cell, as well as 72 copies (on average) of a complex HIV protein (frequently called spikes) that protrudes through the surface of the virus particle (virion). This protein, known as env, consists of a cap made of three molecules called glycoprotein (gp) 120, and a stem consisting of three gp41 molecules that anchor the structure in the viral envelope. Much of the research to develop a vaccine against HIV has focused on these envelope proteins.

The viral core. Within the envelope of a mature HIV particle is a bullet-shaped core or capsid, made of 2000 copies of another viral protein, p24. The capsid surrounds two single strands of HIV RNA, each of which has a copy of the virus's nine genes. Three of these, gag, pol, and env, contain information needed to make structural proteins for new virus particles. The env gene, for example, codes for a protein called gp160 that is broken down by a viral enzyme to form gp120 and gp41, the components of env.

Six regulatory genes, tat, rev, nef, vif, vpr, and vpu, contain information necessary for the production of proteins that control the ability of HIV to infect a cell, produce new copies of virus or cause disease. The protein encoded by nef, for instance, appears necessary for the virus to replicate efficiently, and the vpu-encoded protein influences the release of new virus particles from infected cells.

The ends of each strand of HIV RNA contain an RNA sequence called the long terminal repeat (LTR). Regions in the LTR act as switches to control production of new viruses and can be triggered by proteins from either HIV or the host cell.

The core of HIV also includes a protein called p7, the HIV nucleocapsid protein; and three enzymes that carry out later steps in the virus's life cycle: reverse transcriptase, integrase and protease. Another HIV protein called p17, or the HIV matrix protein, lies between the viral core and the viral envelope.

Replication Cycle of HIV

Entry of HIV into cells. Infection typically begins when an HIV particle, which contains two copies of the HIV RNA, encounters a cell with a surface molecule called cluster designation 4 (CD4). Cells carrying this molecule are known as CD4 positive (CD4+) cells.

One or more of the virus's gp120 molecules binds tightly to CD4 molecule(s) on the cell's surface. The binding of gp120 to CD4 results in a conformational change in the gp120 molecule allowing it to bind to a second molecule on the cell surface known as a coreceptor. The envelope of the virus and the cell membrane then fuse, leading to entry of the virus into the cell. The gp41 of the envelope is critical to the fusion process. Drugs that block either the binding or the fusion process are being developed and tested in clinical trials.

Studies have identified multiple coreceptors for different types of HIV strains; these coreceptors are promising targets for new anti-HIV drugs, some of which are now being tested in pre-clinical and clinical studies. In the early stage of HIV disease, most people harbor viruses that use, in addition to CD4, a receptor called CCR5 to enter their target cells. With disease progression, the spectrum of coreceptor usage expands in approximately 50 percent of patients to include other receptors, notably a molecule called CXCR4. Virus that utilizes CCR5 is called R5 HIV and virus that utilizes CXCR4 is called X4 HIV.

Although CD4+ T-cells appear to be the main targets of HIV, other immune system cells with and without CD4 molecules on their surfaces are infected as well. Among these are long-lived cells called monocytes and macrophages, which apparently can harbor large quantities of the virus without being killed, thus acting as reservoirs of HIV. CD4+ T-cells also serve as important reservoirs of HIV: a small proportion of these cells harbor HIV in a stable, inactive form. Normal immune processes may activate these cells, resulting in the production of new HIV virions. Cell-to-cell spread of HIV also can occur through the CD4-mediated fusion of an infected cell with an uninfected cell.

Reverse transcription. In the cytoplasm of the cell, HIV reverse transcriptase converts viral RNA into DNA, the nucleic acid form in which the cell carries its genes. Nine of the 15 antiviral drugs approved in the United States for the treatment of people with HIV infection—AZT, ddC, ddI, d4T, 3TC, nevirapine, delavirdine, abacavir and efavirenz—work by interfering with this stage of the viral life cycle.

Integration. The newly made HIV DNA moves to the cell's nucleus, where it is spliced into the host's DNA with the help of HIV integrase. HIV DNA that enters the DNA of the cell is called a provirus. Integrase is an important target for the development of new drugs.

Transcription. For a provirus to produce new viruses, RNA copies must be made that can be read by the host cell's protein-making machinery. These copies are called messenger RNA (mRNA), and production of mRNA is called transcription, a process that involves the host cell's own enzymes. Viral genes in concert with the cellular machinery control this process: the tat gene, for example, encodes a protein that accelerates transcription. Genomic RNA is also transcribed for later incorporation in the budding virion.

Cytokines, proteins involved in the normal regulation of the immune response, also may regulate transcription. Molecules such as tumor necrosis factor (TNF)-alpha and interleukin (IL)-6, secreted in elevated levels by the cells of HIV-infected people, may help to activate HIV proviruses. Other infections, by organisms such as Mycobacterium tuberculosis, may also enhance transcription by inducing the secretion of cytokines.

Translation. After HIV mRNA is processed in the cell's nucleus, it is transported to the cytoplasm. HIV proteins are critical to this process:

for example, a protein encoded by the rev gene allows mRNA encoding HIV structural proteins to be transferred from the nucleus to the cytoplasm. Without the rev protein, structural proteins are not made.

In the cytoplasm, the virus co-opts the cell's protein-making machinery—including structures called ribosomes—to make long chains of viral proteins and enzymes, using HIV mRNA as a template. This process is called translation.

Assembly and budding. Newly made HIV core proteins, enzymes and genomic RNA gather just inside the cell's membrane, while the viral envelope proteins aggregate within the membrane. An immature viral particle forms and buds off from the cell, acquiring an envelope that includes both cellular and HIV proteins from the cell membrane. During this part of the viral life cycle, the core of the virus is immature and the virus is not yet infectious. The long chains of proteins and enzymes that make up the immature viral core are now cleaved into smaller pieces by a viral enzyme called protease. This step results in infectious viral particles.

Drugs called protease inhibitors interfere with this step of the viral life cycle. Six such drugs—saquinavir, ritonavir, indinavir, amprenavir, nelfinavir, and lopinavir—have been approved for marketing in the United States.

Transmission of HIV

Among adults, HIV is spread most commonly during sexual intercourse with an infected partner. During sex, the virus can enter the body through the mucosal linings of the vagina, vulva, penis, or rectum after intercourse or, rarely, via the mouth and possibly the upper gastrointestinal tract after oral sex. The likelihood of transmission is increased by factors that may damage these linings, especially other sexually transmitted diseases that cause ulcers or inflammation.

Research suggests that immune system cells of the dendritic cell type, which reside in the mucosa, may begin the infection process after sexual exposure by binding to and carrying the virus from the site of infection to the lymph nodes where other immune system cells become infected. HIV also can be transmitted by contact with infected blood, most often by the sharing of needles or syringes contaminated with minute quantities of blood containing the virus. The risk of acquiring HIV from blood transfusions is now extremely small in the United States, as all blood products in this country are screened routinely for evidence of the virus.

Almost all HIV-infected children acquire the virus from their mothers before or during birth. In the United States, approximately 25 percent of pregnant HIV-infected women not receiving antiretroviral therapy have passed on the virus to their babies. In 1994, researchers demonstrated that a specific regimen of the drug zidovudine (AZT) can reduce the risk of transmission of HIV from mother to baby by two-thirds. The use of combinations of antiretroviral drugs has further reduced the rate of mother-to-child HIV transmission in the United States. In developing countries, cheap and simple antiviral drug regimens have been proven to significantly reduce mother-to-child transmission in resource-poor settings.

The virus also may be transmitted from an HIV-infected mother to her infant via breastfeeding.

Early Events in HIV Infection

Once it enters the body, HIV infects a large number of CD4+ cells and replicates rapidly. During this acute or primary phase of infection, the blood contains many viral particles that spread throughout the body, seeding various organs, particularly the lymphoid organs. Lymphoid organs include the lymph nodes, spleen, tonsils and adenoids.

Two to four weeks after exposure to the virus, up to 70 percent of HIV-infected persons suffer flu-like symptoms related to the acute infection. The patient's immune system fights back with killer T-cells (CD8+ T-cells) and B-cell-produced antibodies, which dramatically reduce HIV levels. A patient's CD4+ T-cell count may rebound somewhat and even approach its original level. A person may then remain free of HIV-related symptoms for years despite continuous replication of HIV in the lymphoid organs that had been seeded during the acute phase of infection.

One reason that HIV is unique is the fact that despite the body's aggressive immune responses, which are sufficient to clear most viral infections, some HIV invariably escapes. This is due in large part to the high rate of mutations that occur during the process of HIV replication. Even when the virus does not avoid the immune system by mutating, the body's best soldiers in the fight against HIV—certain subsets of killer T-cells that recognize HIV may be depleted or become dysfunctional.

In addition, early in the course of HIV infection, patients may lose HIV-specific CD4+ T-cell responses that normally slow the replication of viruses. Such responses include the secretion of interferons and other antiviral factors, and the orchestration of CD8+ T-cells.

Finally, the virus may hide within the chromosomes of an infected cell and be shielded from surveillance by the immune system. Such cells can be considered as a latent reservoir of the virus.

Course of HIV Infection

Among patients enrolled in large epidemiologic studies in western countries, the median time from infection with HIV to the development of AIDS-related symptoms has been approximately 10 to 12 years in the absence of antiretroviral therapy. However, researchers have observed a wide variation in disease progression. Approximately 10 percent of HIV-infected people in these studies have progressed to AIDS within the first two to three years following infection, while up to 5 percent of individuals in the studies have stable CD4+ T-cell counts and no symptoms even after 12 or more years.

Factors such as age or genetic differences among individuals, the level of virulence of an individual strain of virus, and co-infection with other microbes may influence the rate and severity of disease progression. Drugs that fight the infections associated with AIDS have improved and prolonged the lives of HIV-infected people by preventing or treating conditions such as *Pneumocystis carinii* pneumonia, cytomegalovirus disease, and diseases caused by a number of fungi.

HIV co-receptors and disease progression. Recent research has shown that most infecting strains of HIV use a co-receptor molecule called CCR5, in addition to the CD4 molecule, to enter certain of its target cells. HIV-infected people with a specific mutation in one of their two copies of the gene for this receptor may have a slower disease course than people with two normal copies of the gene. Rare individuals with two mutant copies of the CCR5 gene appear—in most cases—to be completely protected from HIV infection. Mutations in the gene for other HIV co-receptors also may influence the rate of disease progression.

Viral burden predicts disease progression. Numerous studies show that people with high levels of HIV in their bloodstream are more likely to develop new AIDS-related symptoms or die than individuals with lower levels of virus. For instance, in the Multicenter AIDS Cohort Study (MACS), investigators demonstrated that the level of HIV in an untreated individual's plasma 6 months to a year after infection—the so-called viral set point—is highly predictive of the rate of disease progression; that is, patients with high levels of virus are much more likely to get sicker, faster, than those with low levels of virus. The MACS and other studies have provided the rationale for providing aggressive antiretroviral therapy to HIV-infected people, as well as for routinely using newly available blood tests to measure viral load when initiating, monitoring and modifying anti-HIV therapy.

Potent combinations of three or more anti-HIV drugs known as highly active antiretroviral therapy or HAART can reduce a person's viral burden to very low levels and in many cases delay the progression of HIV disease for prolonged periods. However, antiretroviral regimens have yet to completely and permanently suppress the virus in HIV-infected people. Recent studies have shown that HIV persists in a replication-competent form in resting CD4+ T-cells even in patients receiving aggressive antiretroviral therapy who have no readily detectable HIV in their blood. Investigators around the world are working to develop the next generation of anti-HIV drugs.

HIV Is Active in the Lymph Nodes

Although HIV-infected individuals often exhibit an extended period of clinical latency with little evidence of disease, the virus is never truly completely latent although individual cells may be latently infected. Researchers have shown that even early in disease, HIV actively replicates within the lymph nodes and related organs, where large amounts of virus become trapped in networks of specialized cells with long, tentacle-like extensions. These cells are called follicular dendritic cells (FDCs).

FDCs are located in hot spots of immune activity in lymphoid tissue called germinal centers. They act like flypaper, trapping invading pathogens (including HIV) and holding them until B cells come along to initiate an immune response.

Close on the heels of B cells are CD4+ T-cells, which rush into the germinal centers to help B cells fight the invaders. CD4+ T-cells, the primary targets of HIV, may become infected as they encounter HIV trapped on FDCs. Research suggests that HIV trapped on FDCs remains infectious, even when coated with antibodies. Thus, FDCs are an important reservoir of HIV, and the large quantity of infectious HIV trapped on FDCs may explain in part how the momentum of HIV infection is maintained. Once infected, CD4+ T-cells may infect other CD4+ cells that congregate in the region of the lymph node surrounding the germinal center.

Over a period of years, even when little virus is readily detectable in the blood, significant amounts of virus accumulate in the lymphoid tissue, both within infected cells and bound to FDCs. In and around the germinal centers, numerous CD4+ T-cells are probably activated by the increased production of cytokines such as TNF-alpha and IL-6 by immune system cells within the lymphoid tissue. Activation allows uninfected cells to be more easily infected and increases replication of HIV in already infected cells.

While greater quantities of certain cytokines such as TNF-alpha and IL-6 are secreted during HIV infection, other cytokines with key roles in the regulation of normal immune function may be secreted in decreased amounts. For example, CD4+ T-cells may lose their capacity to produce interleukin 2 (IL-2), a cytokine that enhances the growth of other T-cells and helps to stimulate other cells' response to invaders. Infected cells also have low levels of receptors for IL-2, which may reduce their ability to respond to signals from other cells.

Breakdown of FDC networks. Ultimately, accumulated HIV overwhelms the FDC networks. As these networks break down, their trapping capacity is impaired, and large quantities of virus enter the bloodstream.

Although it remains unclear why FDCs die and the FDC networks dissolve, some scientists think that this process may be as important in HIV pathogenesis as the loss of CD4+ T-cells. The destruction of the lymphoid tissue structure seen late in HIV disease may preclude a successful immune response against not only HIV but other pathogens as well. This devastation heralds the onset of the opportunistic infections and cancers that characterize AIDS.

Role of CD8+ T-Cells

CD8+ T-cells are critically important in the immune response to HIV. These cells attack and kill infected cells that are producing virus. Thus, vaccine efforts are directed toward eliciting or enhancing these killer T-cells, as well as eliciting antibodies that will neutralize the infectivity of HIV.

CD8+ T-cells also appear to secrete soluble factors that suppress HIV replication. Several molecules, including RANTES, MIP-1alpha, MIP-1beta, and MDC appear to block HIV replication by occupying the co-receptors necessary for the entry of many strains of HIV into their target cells. There may be other immune system molecules—yet undiscovered—that can suppress HIV replication to some degree.

Rapid Replication and Mutation of HIV

HIV replicates rapidly; several billion new virus particles may be produced every day. In addition, the HIV reverse transcriptase enzyme makes many mistakes while making DNA copies from HIV RNA. As a consequence, many variants of HIV develop in an individual, some of which may escape destruction by antibodies or killer T-cells. Additionally, different strains of HIV can recombine to produce a wide range of variants or strains.

During the course of HIV disease, viral strains emerge in an infected individual that differ widely in their ability to infect and kill different cell types, as well as in their rate of replication. Scientists are investigating why strains of HIV from patients with advanced disease appear to be more virulent and infect more cell types than strains obtained earlier from the same individual.

Theories of Immune System Cell Loss in HIV Infection

Researchers around the world are studying how HIV destroys or disables CD4+ T-cells, and many think that a number of mechanisms may occur simultaneously in an HIV-infected individual. Recent data suggest that billions of CD4+ T-cells may be destroyed every day, eventually overwhelming the immune system's regenerative capacity.

Direct cell killing. Infected CD4+ T-cells may be killed directly when large amounts of virus are produced and bud off from the cell surface, disrupting the cell membrane, or when viral proteins and nucleic acids collect inside the cell, interfering with cellular machinery.

Apoptosis. Infected CD4+ T-cells may be killed when the regulation of cell function is distorted by HIV proteins, probably leading to cell suicide by a process known as programmed cell death or apoptosis. Recent reports indicate that apoptosis occurs to a greater extent in HIV-infected individuals, both in the bloodstream and lymph nodes. Apoptosis is closely correlated with the aberrant cellular activation seen in HIV disease.

Uninfected cells also may undergo apoptosis. Investigators have shown in cell cultures that the HIV envelope alone or bound to antibodies sends an inappropriate signal to CD4+ T-cells causing them to undergo apoptosis, even if not infected by HIV.

Innocent bystanders. Uninfected cells may die in an innocent bystander scenario: HIV particles may bind to the cell surface, giving them the appearance of an infected cell and marking them for destruction by killer T-cells after antibody attaches to the viral particle on the cell. This process is called antibody dependent cellular cytotoxicity.

Killer T-cells also may mistakenly destroy uninfected cells that have consumed HIV particles and that display HIV fragments on their surfaces. Alternatively, because HIV envelope proteins bear some resemblance to certain molecules that may appear on CD4+ T-cells, the body's immune responses may mistakenly damage such cells as well.

Anergy. Researchers have shown in cell cultures that CD4+ T-cells can be turned off by activation signals from HIV that leaves them unable to respond to further immune stimulation. This inactivated state is known as anergy.

Damage to Precursor Cells. Studies suggest that HIV also destroys precursor cells that mature to have special immune functions, as well as the microenvironment of the bone marrow and the thymus needed for the development of such cells. These organs probably lose the ability to regenerate, further compounding the suppression of the immune system.

Central Nervous System Damage

Although monocytes and macrophages can be infected by HIV, they appear to be relatively resistant to killing by the virus. However, these cells travel throughout the body and carry HIV to various organs, including the brain, which may serve as a hiding place or reservoir for the virus that may be relatively impervious to most anti-HIV drugs.

Neurologic manifestations of HIV disease are seen in up to 50 percent of HIV-infected people, to varying degrees of severity. People infected with HIV often experience cognitive symptoms, including impaired short-term memory, reduced concentration, and mental slowing; motor symptoms such as fine motor clumsiness or slowness, tremor, and leg weakness; and behavioral symptoms including apathy, social withdrawal, irritability, depression, and personality change. More serious neurologic manifestations in HIV disease typically occur in patients with high viral loads, generally when an individual has advanced HIV disease or AIDS.

Neurologic manifestations of HIV disease are the subject of many research projects. Current evidence suggests that although nerve cells do not become infected with HIV, supportive cells within the brain, such as astrocytes and microglia (as well as monocyte/macrophages that have migrated to the brain) can be infected with the virus. Researchers postulate that infection of these cells can cause a disruption of normal neurologic functions by altering cytokine levels, by delivering aberrant signals, and by causing the release of toxic products in the brain. The use of anti-HIV drugs frequently reduces the severity of neurologic symptoms, but in many cases does not, for reasons that are unclear.

Role of Immune Activation in HIV Disease

During a normal immune response, many components of the immune system are mobilized to fight an invader. CD4+ T-cells, for instance, may quickly proliferate and increase their cytokine secretion, thereby signaling other cells to perform their special functions. Scavenger cells called macrophages may double in size and develop numerous organelles, including lysosomes that contain digestive enzymes used to process ingested pathogens. Once the immune system clears the foreign antigen, it returns to a relative state of quiescence.

Paradoxically, although it ultimately causes immune deficiency, HIV disease for most of its course is characterized by immune system hyperactivation, which has negative consequences. As noted above, HIV replication and spread are much more efficient in activated CD4+ cells. Chronic immune system activation during HIV disease may also result in a massive stimulation of B cells, impairing the ability of these cells to make antibodies against other pathogens.

Chronic immune activation also can result in apoptosis, and an increased production of cytokines that may not only increase HIV replication but also have other deleterious effects. Increased levels of TNF-alpha, for example, may be at least partly responsible for the severe weight loss or wasting syndrome seen in many HIV-infected individuals.

The persistence of HIV and HIV replication plays an important role in the chronic state of immune activation seen in HIV-infected people. In addition, researchers have shown that infections with other organisms activate immune system cells and increase production of the virus in HIV-infected people. Chronic immune activation due to persistent infections, or the cumulative effects of multiple episodes of immune activation and bursts of virus production, likely contribute to the progression of HIV disease.

NIAID Research on the Pathogenesis of AIDS

NIAID-supported scientists conduct research on HIV pathogenesis in laboratories on the campus of the National Institutes of Health

(NIH) in Bethesda, Md., at the Institute's Rocky Mountain Laboratories in Hamilton, Montana, and at universities and medical centers in the United States and abroad.

An NIAID-supported resource, the NIH AIDS Research and Reference Reagent Program, in collaboration with the World Health Organization, provides critically needed AIDS-related research materials free to qualified researchers around the world.

In addition, the Institute convenes groups of investigators and advisory committees to exchange scientific information, clarify research priorities and bring research needs and opportunities to the attention of the scientific community.

Chapter 3

Human Immunodeficiency Virus Type 2 (HIV-2)

In 1984, 3 years after the first reports of a disease that was to become known as AIDS, researchers discovered the primary causative viral agent, the human immunodeficiency virus type 1 (HIV-1). In 1986, a second type of HIV, called HIV-2, was isolated from AIDS patients in West Africa, where it may have been present decades earlier. HIV-2 has many genetic similarities to HIV-1, but appears to be less efficient at replicating and spreading. Studies of the natural history of HIV-2 are limited, but to date comparisons with HIV-1 show some similarities while suggesting differences. Both HIV-1 and HIV-2 have the same modes of transmission and are associated with similar opportunistic infections and AIDS. In persons infected with HIV-2, immunodeficiency seems to develop more slowly and to be milder. Compared with persons infected with HIV-1, those with HIV-2 are less infectious early in the course of infection. As the disease advances, HIV-2 infectiousness seems to increase; however, compared with HIV-1, the duration of this increased infectiousness is shorter. HIV-1 and HIV-2 also differ in geographic patterns of infection; the United States has few reported cases. There have been reports of individuals infected simultaneously with both HIV-1 and HIV-2.

A fact sheet from the National Center for HIV, STD and TB Prevention, Centers for Disease Control and Prevention (CDC), 1998, updated in December 2002 by Dr. David A. Cooke, MD, Diplomate, American Board of Internal Medicine.

Which countries have a high prevalence* of HIV-2 infection?

HIV-2 infections are predominantly found in Africa. West African nations with a prevalence of HIV-2 of more than 1% in the general population are Cape Verde, Côte d'Ivoire (Ivory Coast), Gambia, Guinea-Bissau, Mali, Mauritania, Nigeria, and Sierra Leone. Other West African countries reporting HIV-2 are Benin, Burkina Faso, Ghana, Guinea, Liberia, Niger, Sao Tome, Senegal, and Togo. Angola and Mozambique are other African nations where the prevalence of HIV-2 is more than 1%. A significant proportion of all HIV cases in Portugal and Southern India are HIV-2.

*Prevalence is the proportion of cases present in a population at a given point in time.

What is known about HIV-2 in the United States?

The first case of HIV-2 infection in the United States was diagnosed in 1987. Since then, the Centers for Disease Control and Prevention (CDC) has worked with state and local health departments to collect demographic, clinical, and laboratory data on persons with HIV-2 infection. Of the 79 infected persons, 66 are black and 51 are male. Fifty-two were born in West Africa, 1 in Kenya, 7 in the United States, 2 in India, and 2 in Europe. The region of origin was not known for 15 of the persons, although 4 of them had a malaria-antibody profile consistent with residence in West Africa. AIDS-defining conditions have developed in 17, and 8 have died.

These case counts represent minimal estimates because completeness of reporting has not been assessed. Although AIDS is reported uniformly nationwide, the reporting of HIV infection, including HIV-2 infection, differs from state to state according to state policy.

Who should be tested for HIV-2?

Because epidemiologic data indicate that the prevalence of HIV-2 in the United States is very low, CDC does not recommend routine HIV-2 testing at U.S. HIV counseling and test sites or in settings other than blood centers. However, when HIV testing is to be performed, tests for antibodies to both HIV-1 and HIV-2 should be obtained if demographic or behavioral information suggests that HIV-2 infection might be present.

Persons at risk for HIV-2 infection include:

- Sex partners of a person from a country where HIV-2 is endemic (refer to countries listed earlier).

- Sex partners of a person known to be infected with HIV-2.

- People who received a blood transfusion or a nonsterile injection in a country where HIV-2 is endemic.

- People who shared needles with a person from a country where HIV-2 is endemic or with a person known to be infected with HIV-2.

- Children of women who have risk factors for HIV-2 infection or are known to be infected with HIV-2.

HIV-2 testing also is indicated for:

- People with an illness that suggests HIV infection (such as an HIV-associated opportunistic-infection) but whose HIV-1 test result is not positive.

- People for whom HIV-1 Western blot exhibits the unusual indeterminate test band pattern of gag (p55, p24, or p17) plus pol (p66, p51, or p32) in the absence of env (gp160, gp120, or gp41).

Among all HIV-infected people in North America, the prevalence of HIV-2 is very low compared with HIV-1. However, the potential risk for HIV-2 infection in some populations (such as those listed) may justify routine HIV-2 testing for all people for whom HIV-1 testing is warranted. The decision to implement routine HIV-2 testing requires consideration of the number of HIV-2-infected persons whose infection would remain undiagnosed without routine HIV-2 testing compared with the problems and costs associated with the implementation of HIV-2 testing.

The development of antibodies is similar in HIV-1 and HIV-2. Antibodies generally become detectable within 3 months of infection. Testing for HIV-2 antibodies is available through private physicians or state and local health departments.

Are blood donors tested for HIV-2?

- Since 1992, all U.S. blood donations have been tested with a combination HIV-1/HIV-2 enzyme immunoassay test kit that is sensitive to antibodies to both viruses. This testing has demonstrated that HIV-2 infection in blood donors is extremely rare. All donations detected with either HIV-1 or HIV-2 are excluded from any clinical use, and donors are deferred from further donations.

Is the clinical treatment of HIV-2 different from that of HIV-1?

Little is known about the best approach to the clinical treatment and care of patients infected with HIV-2. Given the slower development of immunodeficiency and the limited clinical experience with HIV-2, it is unclear whether antiretroviral therapy significantly slows progression. Not all of the drugs used to treat HIV-1 infection are as effective against HIV-2. In vitro (laboratory) studies suggest that nucleoside analogs are active against HIV-2, though not as active as against HIV-1. Protease inhibitors should be active against HIV-2. However, non-nucleoside reverse transcriptase inhibitors (NNRTIs) are not active against HIV-2. Whether any potential benefits would outweigh the possible adverse effects of treatment is unknown. Combination drug therapy is the standard of care for treatment of HIV-2, as it is with HIV-1. The specific drugs used may be somewhat different, however.

Monitoring the treatment response of patients infected with HIV-2 is more difficult than monitoring people infected with HIV-1. No FDA-licensed HIV-2 viral load assay is available yet. Viral load assays used for HIV-1 are not reliable for monitoring HIV-2. Response to treatment for HIV-2 infection may be monitored by following CD4+ T-cell counts and other indicators of immune system deterioration, such as weight loss, oral candidiasis, unexplained fever, and the appearance of a new AIDS-defining illness. More research and clinical experience is needed to determine the most effective treatment for HIV-2.

The optimal timing for antiretroviral therapy (i.e., soon after infection, when symptoms appear, or when CD4+ T-cell counts fall below a certain level) remains under review by clinical experts. *Guidelines for the Use of Antiretroviral Agents in HIV-Infected Adults and Adolescents*, by the Department of Health and Human Services Panel on Clinical Practices for Treatment of HIV Infection, may be helpful to the clinician who is caring for a patient infected with HIV-2; however, the recommendations on viral load monitoring and the use of NNRTIs would not apply to patients with HIV-2 infection.

What is known about HIV-2 infection in children?

HIV-2 infection in children is rare. Compared with HIV-1, HIV-2 seems to be less transmissible from an infected mother to her child.

However, cases of transmission from an infected woman to her fetus or newborn have been reported among women who had primary HIV-2 infection during their pregnancy. Zidovudine therapy has been demonstrated to reduce the risk for perinatal HIV-1 transmission and also might prove effective for reducing perinatal HIV-2 transmission. Zidovudine therapy should be considered for HIV-2-infected expectant mothers and their newborns, especially for women who become infected during pregnancy.

How should physicians and patients decide whether to start treatment for HIV-2?

Physicians caring for patients with HIV-2 infection should decide whether to initiate antiretroviral therapy after discussing with their patients what is known, what is not known, and the possible adverse effects of treatment. Given the rarity of HIV-2 infections, consultation with a specialist is recommended.

What can be done to control the spread of HIV-2?

Continued surveillance is needed to monitor HIV-2 in the U.S. population because the possibility for further spread of HIV-2 exists, especially among injecting drug users and people with multiple sex partners. Programs aimed at preventing the transmission of HIV-1 also can help to prevent and control the spread of HIV-2.

Chapter 4

HIV and Its Transmission

Research has revealed a great deal of valuable medical, scientific, and public health information about the human immunodeficiency virus (HIV) and acquired immunodeficiency syndrome (AIDS). The ways in which HIV can be transmitted have been clearly identified. Unfortunately, false information or statements that are not supported by scientific findings continue to be shared widely through the Internet or popular press. Therefore, the Centers for Disease Control and Prevention (CDC) has prepared this information to correct a few misperceptions about HIV.

How HIV Is Transmitted

HIV is spread by sexual contact with an infected person, by sharing needles and/or syringes (primarily for drug injection) with someone who is infected, or, less commonly (and now very rarely in countries where blood is screened for HIV antibodies), through transfusions of infected blood or blood clotting factors. Babies born to HIV-infected women may become infected before or during birth or through breast-feeding after birth.

In the health care setting, workers have been infected with HIV after being stuck with needles containing HIV-infected blood or, less frequently, after infected blood gets into a worker's open cut or a

A fact sheet from the National Center for HIV, STD and TB Prevention, Centers for Disease Control and Prevention (CDC), updated January 2001; available online at http://www.cdc.gov/hiv/pubs/facts/transmission.htm.

33

mucous membrane (for example, the eyes or inside of the nose). There has been only one instance of patients being infected by a health care worker in the United States; this involved HIV transmission from one infected dentist to six patients. Investigations have been completed involving more than 22,000 patients of 63 HIV-infected physicians, surgeons, and dentists, and no other cases of this type of transmission have been identified in the United States.

Some people fear that HIV might be transmitted in other ways; however, no scientific evidence to support any of these fears has been found. If HIV were being transmitted through other routes (such as through air, water, or insects), the pattern of reported AIDS cases would be much different from what has been observed. For example, if mosquitoes could transmit HIV infection, many more young children and preadolescents would have been diagnosed with AIDS.

All reported cases suggesting new or potentially unknown routes of transmission are thoroughly investigated by state and local health departments with the assistance, guidance, and laboratory support from CDC. No additional routes of transmission have been recorded, despite a national sentinel system designed to detect just such an occurrence.

The following paragraphs specifically address some of the common misperceptions about HIV transmission.

HIV in the Environment

Scientists and medical authorities agree that HIV does not survive well in the environment, making the possibility of environmental transmission remote. HIV is found in varying concentrations or amounts in blood, semen, vaginal fluid, breast milk, saliva, and tears. To obtain data on the survival of HIV, laboratory studies have required the use of artificially high concentrations of laboratory-grown virus. Although these unnatural concentrations of HIV can be kept alive for days or even weeks under precisely controlled and limited laboratory conditions, CDC studies have shown that drying of even these high concentrations of HIV reduces the amount of infectious virus by 90 to 99 percent within several hours. Since the HIV concentrations used in laboratory studies are much higher than those actually found in blood or other specimens, drying of HIV-infected human blood or other body fluids reduces the theoretical risk of environmental transmission to that which has been observed—essentially zero. Incorrect interpretation of conclusions drawn from laboratory studies have unnecessarily alarmed some people.

Results from laboratory studies should not be used to assess specific personal risk of infection because (1) the amount of virus studied is not found in human specimens or elsewhere in nature, and (2) no one has been identified as infected with HIV due to contact with an environmental surface. Additionally, HIV is unable to reproduce outside its living host (unlike many bacteria or fungi, which may do so under suitable conditions), except under laboratory conditions, therefore, it does not spread or maintain infectiousness outside its host.

Households

Although HIV has been transmitted between family members in a household setting, this type of transmission is very rare. These transmissions are believed to have resulted from contact between skin or mucous membranes and infected blood. To prevent even such rare occurrences, precautions, as described in previously published guidelines, should be taken in all settings—including the home—to prevent exposures to the blood of persons who are HIV infected, at risk for HIV infection, or whose infection and risk status are unknown. For example:

- Gloves should be worn during contact with blood or other body fluids that could possibly contain visible blood, such as urine, feces, or vomit.

- Cuts, sores, or breaks on both the care giver's and patient's exposed skin should be covered with bandages.

- Hands and other parts of the body should be washed immediately after contact with blood or other body fluids, and surfaces soiled with blood should be disinfected appropriately.

- Practices that increase the likelihood of blood contact, such as sharing of razors and toothbrushes, should be avoided.

- Needles and other sharp instruments should be used only when medically necessary and handled according to recommendations for health-care settings. (Do not put caps back on needles by hand or remove needles from syringes. Dispose of needles in puncture-proof containers.

Businesses and Other Settings

There is no known risk of HIV transmission to co-workers, clients, or consumers from contact in industries such as food-service establishments.

Food-service workers known to be infected with HIV need not be restricted from work unless they have other infections or illnesses (such as diarrhea or hepatitis A) for which any food-service worker, regardless of HIV infection status, should be restricted. CDC recommends that all food-service workers follow recommended standards and practices of good personal hygiene and food sanitation.

In 1985, CDC issued routine precautions that all personal-service workers (such as hairdressers, barbers, cosmetologists, and massage therapists) should follow, even though there is no evidence of transmission from a personal-service worker to a client or vice versa. Instruments that are intended to penetrate the skin (such as tattooing and acupuncture needles, ear piercing devices) should be used once and disposed of or thoroughly cleaned and sterilized. Instruments not intended to penetrate the skin but which may become contaminated with blood (for example, razors) should be used for only one client and disposed of or thoroughly cleaned and disinfected after each use. Personal-service workers can use the same cleaning procedures that are recommended for health care institutions.

CDC knows of no instances of HIV transmission through tattooing or body piercing, although hepatitis B virus has been transmitted during some of these practices. One case of HIV transmission from acupuncture has been documented. Body piercing (other than ear piercing) is relatively new in the United States, and the medical complications for body piercing appear to be greater than for tattoos. Healing of piercings generally will take weeks, and sometimes even months, and the pierced tissue could conceivably be abraded (torn or cut) or inflamed even after healing. Therefore, a theoretical HIV transmission risk does exist if the unhealed or abraded tissues come into contact with an infected person's blood or other infectious body fluid. Additionally, HIV could be transmitted if instruments contaminated with blood are not sterilized or disinfected between clients.

Kissing

Casual contact through closed-mouth or social kissing is not a risk for transmission of HIV. Because of the potential for contact with blood during "French" or open-mouth kissing, CDC recommends against engaging in this activity with a person known to be infected. However, the risk of acquiring HIV during open-mouth kissing is believed to be very low. CDC has investigated only one case of HIV infection that may be attributed to contact with blood during open-mouth kissing.

Biting

In 1997, CDC published findings from a state health department investigation of an incident that suggested blood-to-blood transmission of HIV by a human bite. There have been other reports in the medical literature in which HIV appeared to have been transmitted by a bite. Severe trauma with extensive tissue tearing and damage and presence of blood were reported in each of these instances. Biting is not a common way of transmitting HIV. In fact, there are numerous reports of bites that did not result in HIV infection.

Saliva, Tears, and Sweat

HIV has been found in saliva and tears in very low quantities from some AIDS patients. It is important to understand that finding a small amount of HIV in a body fluid does not necessarily mean that HIV can be transmitted by that body fluid. HIV has not been recovered from the sweat of HIV-infected persons. Contact with saliva, tears, or sweat has never been shown to result in transmission of HIV.

Insects

From the onset of the HIV epidemic, there has been concern about transmission of the virus by biting and bloodsucking insects. However, studies conducted by researchers at CDC and elsewhere have shown no evidence of HIV transmission through insects—even in areas where there are many cases of AIDS and large populations of insects such as mosquitoes. Lack of such outbreaks, despite intense efforts to detect them, supports the conclusion that HIV is not transmitted by insects.

The results of experiments and observations of insect biting behavior indicate that when an insect bites a person, it does not inject its own or a previously bitten person's or animal's blood into the next person bitten. Rather, it injects saliva, which acts as a lubricant or anticoagulant so the insect can feed efficiently. Such diseases as yellow fever and malaria are transmitted through the saliva of specific species of mosquitoes. However, HIV lives for only a short time inside an insect and, unlike organisms that are transmitted via insect bites, HIV does not reproduce (and does not survive) in insects. Thus, even if the virus enters a mosquito or another sucking or biting insect, the insect does not become infected and cannot transmit HIV to the next human it feeds on or bites. HIV is not found in insect feces.

There is also no reason to fear that a biting or bloodsucking insect, such as a mosquito, could transmit HIV from one person to another through HIV-infected blood left on its mouth parts. Two factors serve to explain why this is so—first, infected people do not have constant, high levels of HIV in their bloodstreams and, second, insect mouth parts do not retain large amounts of blood on their surfaces. Further, scientists who study insects have determined that biting insects normally do not travel from one person to the next immediately after ingesting blood. Rather, they fly to a resting place to digest this blood meal.

Effectiveness of Condoms

Condoms are classified as medical devices and are regulated by the Food and Drug Administration (FDA). Condom manufacturers in the United States test each latex condom for defects, including holes, before it is packaged. The proper and consistent use of latex or polyurethane (a type of plastic) condoms when engaging in sexual intercourse—vaginal, anal, or oral—can greatly reduce a person's risk of acquiring or transmitting sexually transmitted diseases, including HIV infection.

There are many different types and brands of condoms available—however, only latex or polyurethane condoms provide a highly effective mechanical barrier to HIV. In laboratories, viruses occasionally have been shown to pass through natural membrane (skin or lambskin) condoms, which may contain natural pores and are therefore not recommended for disease prevention (they are documented to be effective for contraception). Women may wish to consider using the female condom when a male condom cannot be used.

For condoms to provide maximum protection, they must be used consistently (every time) and correctly. Several studies of correct and consistent condom use clearly show that latex condom breakage rates in this country are less than 2 percent. Even when condoms do break, one study showed that more than half of such breaks occurred prior to ejaculation.

When condoms are used reliably, they have been shown to prevent pregnancy up to 98 percent of the time among couples using them as their only method of contraception. Similarly, numerous studies among sexually active people have demonstrated that a properly used latex condom provides a high degree of protection against a variety of sexually transmitted diseases, including HIV infection.

Chapter 5

HIV Transmission through Oral Sex

Oral Sex Is Not Considered Safe Sex

Like all sexual activity, oral sex carries some risk, particularly when one partner or the other is known to be infected with HIV, when either partner's HIV status is not known, and/or when one or the other partner is not monogamous or injects drugs. Numerous studies have demonstrated that oral sex can result in the transmission of HIV and other sexually transmitted diseases (STDs). Abstaining from oral, anal, and vaginal sex all together or having sex only with a mutually monogamous, uninfected partner are the only ways that individuals can be completely protected from the sexual transmission of HIV.

Oral Sex Is a Common Practice

Oral sex involves giving or receiving oral stimulation (i.e. sucking or licking) to the penis, the vagina, and/or the anus. Fellatio is the technical term used to describe oral contact with the penis. Cunnilingus is the technical term which describes oral-vaginal sex. Anilingus (sometimes called rimming) refers to oral-anal contact. Studies indicate that oral sex is commonly practiced by sexually active male-female and same-gender couples of various ages, including adolescents.

"Preventing the Sexual Transmission of HIV, the Virus that Causes AIDS: What You Should Know about Oral Sex," Centers for Disease Control and Prevention (CDC), 2000; available online at http://www.ftp.cdcnin.org/updates/oralsex.pdf.

39

Although there are only limited national data about how often adolescents engage in oral sex, some data suggest that many adolescents who engage in oral sex do not consider it to be sex; therefore they may use oral sex as an option to experience sex while still, in their minds, remaining abstinent. Moreover, many consider oral sex to be a safe or no risk sexual practice. In a recent national survey of teens conducted for The Kaiser Family Foundation, 26% of sexually active 15 to 17 year olds surveyed responded that one cannot become infected with HIV by having unprotected oral sex, and an additional 15% didn't know whether or not one could become infected in that manner.

Oral Sex and the Risk of HIV Transmission

The risk of HIV transmission from an infected partner through oral sex is much smaller than the risk of HIV transmission from anal or vaginal sex. Because of this, measuring the exact risk of HIV transmission as a result of oral sex is very difficult. In addition, since most sexually active individuals practice oral sex in addition to other forms of sex, such as vaginal and/or anal sex, when transmission occurs, it is difficult to determine whether or not it occurred as a result of oral sex or other more risky sexual activities. Finally, several co-factors can increase the risk of HIV transmission through oral sex, including: oral ulcers, bleeding gums, genital sores, and the presence of other STDs.

When scientists describe the risk of transmitting an infectious disease, like HIV, the term theoretical risk is often used. Very simply, theoretical risk means that passing an infection from one person to another is possible, even though there may not yet be any actual documented cases. Theoretical risk is not the same as likelihood. In other words, stating that HIV infection is theoretically possible does not necessarily mean it is likely to happen—only that it might. Documented risk, on the other hand, is used to describe transmission that has actually occurred, been investigated, and documented in the scientific literature.

Theoretical and Documented Risk of HIV Transmission during Oral-Penile Contact

Theoretical: In fellatio, there is a theoretical risk of transmission for the receptive partner (the person who is sucking) because infected pre-ejaculate (pre-cum) fluid or semen can get into the mouth. For the insertive partner (the person who is being sucked), there is a theoretical risk of infection because infected blood from a partner's bleeding gums or an open sore could come in contact with a scratch, cut, or sore on the penis.

Documented: Although the risk is many times smaller than anal or vaginal sex, HIV has been transmitted to receptive partners through fellatio, even in cases when insertive partners didn't ejaculate (cum).

Theoretical and Documented Risk of HIV Transmission during Oral-Vaginal Contact

Theoretical: Cunnilingus carries a theoretical risk of HIV transmission for the insertive partner (the person who is licking or sucking the vaginal area) because infected vaginal fluids and blood can get into the mouth. (This includes, but is not limited to, menstrual blood). Likewise, there is a theoretical risk of HIV transmission during cunnilingus for the receptive partner (the person who is having her vagina licked or sucked) if infected blood from oral sores or bleeding gums comes in contact with vulvar or vaginal cuts or sores.

Documented: The risk of HIV transmission during cunnilingus is extremely low compared to vaginal and anal sex. However, there have been a few cases of HIV transmission most likely resulting from oral-vaginal sex.

Theoretical and Documented Risk of HIV Transmission during Oral-Anal Contact

Theoretical: Anilingus carries a theoretical risk of transmission for the insertive partner (the person who is licking or sucking the anus) if there is exposure to infected blood, either through bloody fecal matter (bodily waste) or cuts/sores in the anal area. Anilingus carries a theoretical risk to the receptive partner (the person who is being licked/sucked) if infected blood in saliva comes in contact with anal/rectal lining.

Documented: There has been one published case of HIV transmission associated with oral-anal sexual contact.

41

Other STDs Can Also Be Transmitted from Oral Sex

Scientists have documented a number of other sexually transmitted diseases that have also been transmitted through oral sex. Herpes, syphilis, gonorrhea, genital warts (HPV), intestinal parasites (amebiasis), and hepatitis A are examples of STDs which can be transmitted during oral sex with an infected partner.

Reducing the Risk of HIV Transmission through Oral Sex

The consequences of HIV infection are life-long, life-threatening, and extremely serious. You can lower any already low risk of getting HIV from oral sex by using latex condoms each and every time. For cunnilingus or anilingus, plastic food wrap, a condom cut open, or a dental dam can serve as a physical barrier to prevent transmission of HIV and many other STDs. Because anal and vaginal sex are much riskier and because most individuals who engage in unprotected (i.e. without a condom) oral sex also engage in unprotected anal and/or vaginal sex, the exact proportion of HIV infections attributable to oral sex alone is unknown, but is likely to be very small. This has led some people to believe that oral sex is completely safe. It is not.

Chapter 6

Drug Use and Its Association to HIV Transmission

Sharing syringes and other equipment for drug injection is a well known route of HIV transmission, yet injection drug use contributes to the epidemic's spread far beyond the circle of those who inject. People who have sex with an injection drug user (IDU) also are at risk for infection through the sexual transmission of HIV. Children born to mothers who contracted HIV through sharing needles or having sex with an IDU may become infected as well.

Since the epidemic began, injection drug use has directly and indirectly accounted for more than one-third (36%) of AIDS cases in the United States. This disturbing trend appears to be continuing. Of the 42,156 new cases of AIDS reported in 2000, 11,635 (28%) were IDU-associated.

Racial and ethnic minority populations in the United States are most heavily affected by IDU-associated AIDS. In 2000, IDU-associated AIDS accounted for 26% of all AIDS cases among African American and 31% among Hispanic adults and adolescents, compared with 19% of all cases among white adults/adolescents.

IDU-associated AIDS accounts for a larger proportion of cases among adolescent and adult women than among men. Since the epidemic began, 57% of all AIDS cases among women have been attributed

"Drug-Associated HIV Transmission Continues in the United States," a fact sheet from the National Center for HIV, STD and TB Prevention, Centers for Disease Control and Prevention (CDC), updated March 2002; available online at http://www.cdc.gov/hiv/pubs/facts/idu.htm.

to injection drug use or sex with partners who inject drugs, compared with 31% of cases among men.

Noninjection drugs (such as crack cocaine) also contribute to the spread of the epidemic when users trade sex for drugs or money, or when they engage in risky sexual behaviors that they might not engage in when sober. One CDC study of more than 2,000 young adults in three inner-city neighborhoods found that crack smokers were three times more likely to be infected with HIV than non-smokers.

Strategies for HIV Prevention among IDUs

Comprehensive HIV prevention interventions for substance abusers must provide education on how to prevent transmission through sex. Numerous studies have documented that drug users are at risk for HIV through both drug-related and sexual behaviors, which places their partners at risk as well. Comprehensive programs must provide the information, skills, and support necessary to reduce both risks. Researchers have found that many interventions aimed at reducing sexual risk behaviors among drug users have significantly increased the practice of safer sex (e.g., using condoms, avoiding unprotected sex) among participants.

Drug abuse treatment is HIV prevention, but drug treatment slots are scarce. In the United States, drug use and dependence are widespread in the general population. Experts generally agree that there are about 1 million active IDUs in this country, as well as many others who use noninjection drugs or abuse alcohol. Clearly, the need for substance abuse treatment vastly exceeds our capacity to provide it. Effective substance abuse treatment that helps people stop using drugs not only eliminates the risk of HIV transmission from sharing contaminated syringes, but, for many, reduces the risk of engaging in risky behaviors that might result in sexual transmission. For injection drug users who cannot or will not stop injecting drugs, using sterile needles and syringes only once remains the safest, most effective approach for limiting HIV transmission.

To minimize the risk of HIV transmission, IDUs must have access to interventions that can help them protect their health. They must be advised to always use sterile injection equipment; warned never to reuse needles, syringes, and other injection equipment; and told that using syringes that have been cleaned with bleach or other disinfectants is not as safe as using new, sterile syringes.

Having access to sterile injection equipment is important, but it is not enough. Preventing the spread of HIV through injection drug use requires a comprehensive approach that incorporates several basic principles:

- ensure coordination and collaboration among all providers of services to IDUs, their sex partners, and their children
- ensure coverage, access to, and quality of interventions
- recognize and overcome stigma associated with injection drug use
- tailor services and programs to the diverse populations and characteristics of IDUs

Strategies for prevention should include:

- preventing initiation of drug injection
- using community outreach programs to reach drug users on the streets
- improving access to high quality substance abuse treatment programs
- instituting HIV prevention programs in jails and prisons
- providing health care for HIV-infected IDUs
- making HIV risk-reduction counseling and testing available for IDUs and their sex partners

HIV prevention and treatment, substance abuse prevention, and sexually transmitted disease treatment and prevention services must be better integrated to take advantage of the multiple opportunities for intervention—first, to help the uninfected stay that way; second, to help infected people stay healthy; and third, to help infected individuals initiate and sustain behaviors that will keep themselves safe and prevent transmission to others.

Chapter 7

Blood Safety

How Safe Is the Blood Supply in the United States?

The U.S. blood supply is among the safest in the world. Nearly all people infected with HIV through blood transfusions received those transfusions before 1985, the year HIV testing began for all donated blood.

The Public Health Service has recommended an approach to blood safety in the United States that includes stringent donor selection practices and the use of screening tests. U.S. blood donations have been screened for antibodies to HIV-1 since March 1985 and HIV-2 since June 1992. Blood and blood products that test positive for HIV are safely discarded and are not used for transfusions.

An estimated 1 in 450,000 to 1 in 660,000 donations per year are infectious for HIV but are not detected by current antibody screening tests. In August 1995, the FDA recommended that all donated blood and plasma also be screened for HIV-1 p24 antigen. The improvement of processing methods for blood products also has reduced

Text in this chapter is from the following: "How Safe Is the Blood Supply in the United States?" Centers for Disease Control and Prevention (CDC), 1998, available online at http://www.cdc.gov/hiv/pubs/faq/faq15.htm; "Blood Safety: The Importance of Donor Screening and Testing," an undated document from the Centers for Disease Control and Prevention (CDC) available online at http://www.cdc.gov/Washington/overview/bloodsaf.htm, cited December 2002; and "Global AIDS Program Technical Strategies Overview: 2.3 Blood Safety," 2001 Centers for Disease Control and Prevention (CDC), available online at http://www.cdc.gov/nchstp/od/gap/text/strategies/2_3_blood_safety.htm.

the number of infections resulting from the use of these products. Currently, the risk of infection with HIV in the United States through receiving a blood transfusion or blood products is extremely low and has become progressively lower, even in geographic areas with high HIV prevalence rates.

Blood Safety: The Importance of Donor Screening and Testing

In the context of other healthcare-related adverse events, the risks from blood transfusion are extremely small.

The current high level of safety is the result of continual refinement and improvements in several areas, including donor education and screening; testing by serologic, and most recently, by nucleic acid testing methods; and various treatment and inactivation procedures.

All blood donations are routinely tested for HIV, hepatitis B virus, hepatitis C virus, human T-lymphotropic virus, and syphilis. Use of nucleic acid testing techniques has reduced the risk of HIV transmission to about one per million units of blood transfused.

Continued vigilance is critical to protect the blood supply from known pathogens and to monitor for the emergence of new infectious agents.

Global Concerns about Blood Safety

Fifteen years after the development of a screening test for HIV, reducing transmission of HIV and other infectious diseases by blood transfusion remains a serious public health challenge in many developing countries. Throughout sub-Saharan Africa, blood transfusions are used primarily among young children for the treatment of malaria-associated anemia, among women for the treatment of anemia associated with pregnancy or complications of pregnancy, and to a lesser extent, for treatment of trauma and surgery patients. In many African countries, HIV and hepatitis infection among blood donors is extremely high. The high prevalence of infectious diseases among blood donors, coupled with the frequent use of transfusion, makes blood transfusion a serious, yet preventable, public health problem.

In the early stages of the epidemic, many countries strengthened their ability to improve blood safety with support from international organizations to cover the costs of HIV screening. Unfortunately, many international organizations have turned their focus to other prevention programs, leaving blood safety programs decidedly vulnerable.

Funding and infrastructure are needed to support recruitment and retention of low-risk volunteer donors. Blood shortages are prevalent and many countries are forced to rely on emergency donations from paid donors or family members. Blood collected from paid or family donors, however, is at increased risk for HIV and other infectious diseases and often does not reach patients quickly in emergency situations. A systematized blood transfusion service, that collects blood from low-risk donors, stores and tests blood in a standardized and unhurried fashion, using testing strategies that are appropriate for the local setting, with strong quality assurance, laboratory oversight, and management, are all needed if a safe blood supply is to be available and used appropriately.

Recognized Best Practices

A few countries in sub-Saharan Africa have developed blood programs that have improved the safety and availability of blood. These programs have increased the supply of blood from donors at low risk for infectious diseases, and improved the quality and safety of the blood supply through rigorous laboratory testing and quality control of the entire process from donor recruitment to transfusion. Through centralization of the blood transfusion service, cost savings have been achieved through improved efficiency, decreased waste, and economies of scale. These transfusion services have also addressed the key issues of preventing severe anemia and improving the appropriate use of blood.

CDC Experience and Capabilities

CDC has been involved in blood safety in the U.S. and internationally since the early days of the HIV/AIDS epidemic. CDC has strong experience in epidemiological research in blood safety, in evaluations of the clinical indications for transfusion, assessment of testing technologies and algorithms, strategies to prevent anemia, and identification of donor deferral criteria. CDC is well placed to provide state-of-the-art laboratory support both for blood screening and quality assurance.

CDC Approach

CDC is prepared to support a comprehensive approach to blood safety based on individual country needs. The comprehensive package is aimed at building or strengthening a national blood transfusion service, improving the safety and availability of blood, preventing severe anemia, improving the appropriate use of blood, and increasing the supply of blood from low-risk unremunerated volunteer blood donors.

Illustrative Activities

1. Strengthen blood transfusion service by supporting the following:

   > Training visits to countries with successful programs, such as Uganda and Zimbabwe.

   > Training in managing a national blood transfusion service.

   > Developing information management systems.

   > Developing national policies regarding blood transfusion.

2. Improve the safety and quality of the blood supply:

   > Evaluate screening tests; expand use of rapid tests in appropriate settings.

   > Strengthen capacity for pre- and post-screening counseling.

   > Support comprehensive quality assurance programs.

   > Assist procuring and distributing test kits and reagents for blood screening; provide training in management and forward planning to prevent stock interruptions.

   > Procure equipment and supplies for blood banks.

   > Train laboratory staff.

3. Improve the appropriate use of blood transfusion and prevent severe anemia:

   > Assist in developing clinical guidelines for blood transfusion.

   > Support training for clinicians in appropriate use of blood transfusion.

   > Promote access to and use of crystalloids as an alternative to blood transfusion for acute blood loss.

Assist in programs to prevent severe anemia in children and pregnant women through prevention, detection, and effective early treatment of malaria, nutritional deficiencies and complications of pregnancy.

Improve laboratory capacity for hemoglobin/hematocrit in outpatient and inpatient settings.

4. Increase the supply of blood from low risk donors:

Conduct epidemiological studies or obtain data from on-going surveillance programs to identify low risk groups to target for blood donor recruitment.

Assist in developing programs to educate and mobilize un-remunerated volunteer blood donors.

Assist in developing donor deferral strategies to prevent donations from those at high risk for transmitting HIV and other infectious diseases.

Technical Considerations

The key to a successful and sustainable blood safety program is to strengthen the infrastructure required to implement a comprehensive approach to blood safety. Supplying test kits alone is not sufficient to improve the safety, availability, and utilization of blood. Working with other donors to combine efforts for a comprehensive strategy will be necessary.

Operational Considerations

Fully functional blood banks with donor recruitment programs are essential to a safe and adequate blood supply that is used appropriately. Where these are not available, the use of rapid tests must be considered to ensure that safe blood can be supplied immediately on demand. Hospitals must have rapid test kits regularly available and ensure that they have been stored properly.

Resources

One important resource is exchange visits with blood transfusion services in other countries. Linking blood transfusion services with North American, European, African, and Asian partners may provide a valuable exchange mechanism.

Global AIDS Program (GAP) Support

National Center for HIV, STD, and TB Prevention (NCHSTP)
Internet: http://www.cdc.gov/nchstp

Public Health Practice Program Office (PHPPO)
Internet: http://www.phppo.cdc.gov

In-Country Support

Red Cross
Internet: http://www.ifrc.org

Key Partners

United States

American Red Cross
Internet: http://www.redcross.org

Fogarty International Foundation
Internet: http://www.nih.gov/fic

National Heart Lung and Blood Institute
Internet: http://www.nhlbi.nih.gov

American Association of Blood Banks
Internet: http://www.aabb.org

International

WHO Blood Safety Unit
Internet: http://www.who.int

Chapter 8

Exposure to Blood: What Health-Care Workers Need to Know

Health-care workers are at risk for occupational exposure to bloodborne pathogens, including hepatitis B virus (HBV), hepatitis C virus (HCV), and human immunodeficiency virus (HIV). Exposures occur through needlesticks or cuts from other sharp instruments contaminated with an infected patient's blood or through contact of the eye, nose, mouth, or skin with a patient's blood. Important factors that may determine the overall risk for occupational transmission of a bloodborne pathogen include the number of infected individuals in the patient population, the chance of becoming infected after a single blood contact from an infected patient, and the type and number of blood contacts.

Most exposures do not result in infection. Following a specific exposure, the risk of infection may vary with factors such as these:

- The pathogen involved

- The type of exposure

- The amount of blood involved in the exposure

- The amount of virus in the patient's blood at the time of exposure

Information from the Hospital Infections Program and the Division of Viral and Rickettsial Diseases, Centers for Disease Control and Prevention (CDC), 1999; available online at http://www.cdc.gov/ncidod/hip/blood/exp_to_blood.pdf.

Your employer should have in place a system for reporting exposures in order to quickly evaluate the risk of infection, inform you about treatments available to help prevent infection, monitor you for side effects of treatments, and to determine if infection occurs. This may involve testing your blood and that of the source patient and offering appropriate postexposure treatment.

How Can Occupational Exposures Be Prevented?

Many needlesticks and other cuts can be prevented by using safer techniques (e.g., not recapping needles by hand), disposing of used needles in appropriate sharps disposal containers, and using medical devices with safety features designed to prevent injuries. Many exposures to the eyes, nose, mouth, or skin can be prevented by using appropriate barriers (e.g., gloves, eye and face protection, gowns) when contact with blood is expected.

If an Exposure Occurs

What should I do if I am exposed to the blood of a patient?

1. Immediately following an exposure to blood:

    Wash needlesticks and cuts with soap and water

    Flush splashes to the nose, mouth, or skin with water

    Irrigate eyes with clean water, saline, or sterile irrigants

    No scientific evidence shows that using antiseptics or squeezing the wound will reduce the risk of transmission of a bloodborne pathogen. Using a caustic agent such as bleach is not recommended.

2. Following any blood exposure you should:

    Report the exposure to the department (e.g., occupational health, infection control) responsible for managing exposures. Prompt reporting is essential because, in some cases, postexposure treatment may be recommended and it should be started as soon as possible. Discuss the possible risks of acquiring HBV, HCV, and HIV and the need for postexposure treatment with the provider managing your exposure. You should have already received hepatitis

B vaccine, which is extremely safe and effective in preventing HBV infection.

Risk of Infection after Exposure

What is the risk of infection after an occupational expo-sure?

HBV: Health-care workers who have received hepatitis B vaccine
and have developed immunity to the virus are at virtually no risk for
infection. For an unvaccinated person, the risk from a single
needlestick or a cut exposure to HBV-infected blood ranges from 6-
30% and depends on the hepatitis B e antigen (HBeAg) status of the
source individual. Individuals who are both hepatitis B surface antigen (HBsAg) positive and HBeAg positive have more virus in their
blood and are more likely to transmit HBV.

HCV: Based on limited studies, the risk for infection after a
needlestick or cut exposure to HCV-infected blood is approximately
1.8%. The risk following a blood splash is unknown, but is believed to
be very small; however, HCV infection from such an exposure has been
reported.

HIV: The average risk of HIV infection after a needlestick or cut
exposure to HIV-infected blood is 0.3% (i.e., three-tenths of one percent, or about 1 in 300). Stated another way, 99.7% of needlestick/cut
exposures do not lead to infection. The risk after exposure of the eye,
nose, or mouth to HIV-infected blood is estimated to be, on average,
0.1% (1 in 1,000). The risk after exposure of the skin to HIV-infected
blood is estimated to be less than 0.1%. A small amount of blood on
intact skin probably poses no risk at all. There have been no documented cases of HIV transmission due to an exposure involving a
small amount of blood on intact skin (a few drops of blood on skin for
a short period of time). The risk may be higher if the skin is damaged
(for example, by a recent cut) or if the contact involves a large area of
skin or is prolonged (for example, being covered in blood for hours).

How many health-care workers have been infected with bloodborne pathogens?

HBV: The annual number of occupational infections has decreased
sharply since hepatitis B vaccine became available in 1982 (i.e., there

has been a 90% decrease in the number of estimated cases from 1985 to1996). Nonetheless, approximately 800 health-care workers become infected with HBV each year following an occupational exposure.

HCV: There are no exact estimates on the number of health-care workers occupationally infected with HCV. However, studies have shown that 1% of hospital health-care workers have evidence of HCV infection (about 1.8% of the U.S. population has evidence of infection). The number of these workers who may have been infected through an occupational exposure is unknown.

HIV: As of December 1998, CDC had received reports of 54 documented cases and 134 possible cases of occupationally acquired HIV infection among health-care workers in the United States since reporting began in 1985.

Treatment for the Exposure

Is vaccine or treatment available to prevent infections with bloodborne pathogens?

HBV: As mentioned above, hepatitis B vaccine has been available since 1982 to prevent HBV infection. All health-care workers who have a reasonable chance of exposure to blood or body fluids should receive hepatitis B vaccine. Vaccination ideally should occur during the health-care worker's training period. Workers should be tested 1-2 months after the vaccine series to make sure that vaccination has provided immunity to HBV infection.

Hepatitis B immune globulin (HBIG) is effective in preventing HBV infection after an exposure. The decision to begin treatment is based on several factors, such as:

- Whether the source individual is positive for hepatitis B surface antigen.
- Whether you have been vaccinated.
- Whether the vaccine provided you immunity.

HCV: There is no vaccine against hepatitis C, and no treatment after an exposure that will prevent infection. Immune globulin is not recommended. For these reasons, following recommended infection control practices is imperative.

HIV: There is no vaccine against HIV. However, results from a small number of studies suggest that the use of zidovudine after certain occupational exposures may reduce the chance of HIV transmission.

Postexposure treatment is not recommended for all occupational exposures to HIV because most exposures do not lead to HIV infection and because the drugs used to prevent infection may have serious side effects. Taking these drugs for exposures that pose a lower risk for infection may not be worth the risk of the side effects. You should discuss the risks and side effects with a health-care provider before starting postexposure treatment for HIV.

What about exposures to blood from an individual whose infection status is unknown?

HBV-HCV-HIV: If the source individual cannot be identified or tested, decisions regarding follow-up should be based on the exposure risk and whether the source is likely to be a person who is infected with a bloodborne pathogen. Follow-up testing should be available to all workers who are concerned about possible infection through occupational exposure.

What specific drugs are recommended for postexposure treatment?

HBV: If you have not been vaccinated, then hepatitis B vaccination is recommended for any exposure regardless of the source person's hepatitis B status. HBIG and/or hepatitis B vaccine may be recommended depending on your immunity to hepatitis B and the source person's infection status.

HCV: Currently there is no recommended postexposure treatment that will prevent HCV infection.

HIV: The Public Health Service recommends a 4-week course of two drugs (zidovudine and lamivudine) for most HIV exposures, or zidovudine and lamivudine plus a protease inhibitor (indinavir or nelfinavir) for exposures that may pose a greater risk for transmitting HIV (such as those involving a larger volume of blood with a larger amount of HIV or a concern about drug-resistant HIV). Differences in side effects associated with the use of these two drugs may influence which drug is selected in a specific situation.

These recommendations are intended to provide guidance to clinicians and may be modified on a case-by-case basis. Determining which drugs and how many drugs to use or when to change a treatment regimen is largely a matter of judgment. Whenever possible, consulting an expert with experience in the use of antiviral drugs is advised, especially if a recommended drug is not available, if the source patient's virus is likely to be resistant to one or more recommended drugs, or if the drugs are poorly tolerated.

How soon after exposure to a bloodborne pathogen should treatment start?

HBV: Postexposure treatment should begin as soon as possible after exposure, preferably within 24 hours, and no later than 7 days.

HIV: Treatment should be started promptly, preferably within hours as opposed to days, after the exposure. Although animal studies suggest that treatment is not effective when started more than 24-36 hours after exposure, it is not known if this time frame is the same for humans.

Starting treatment after a longer period (e.g., 1-2 weeks) may be considered for the highest risk exposures; even if HIV infection is not prevented, early treatment of initial HIV infection may lessen the severity of symptoms and delay the onset of AIDS.

Has the FDA approved these drugs to prevent bloodborne pathogen infection following an occupational exposure?

HBV: Yes. Both hepatitis B vaccine and HBIG are approved for this use.

HIV: No. The FDA has approved these drugs for the treatment of existing HIV infection, but not as a treatment to prevent infection. However, physicians may prescribe any approved drug when, in their professional judgment, the use of the drug is warranted.

What is known about the safety and side effects of these drugs?

HBV: Hepatitis B vaccine is very safe. There is no information that the vaccine causes any chronic illnesses. Most illnesses reported after an HBV vaccination are often related to other causes and not the vaccine. However, you should report any unusual reaction after a hepatitis B vaccination to your health-care provider.

HIV: All of the antiviral drugs for HIV have been associated with side effects. The most common side effects include upset stomach (nausea, vomiting, diarrhea), tiredness, or headache. The few serious side effects that have been reported in health-care workers using combination postexposure treatment have included kidney stones, hepatitis, and suppressed blood cell production. Protease inhibitors (indinavir and nelfinavir) may interact with other medicines and cause serious side effects and should not be used in combination with certain other drugs, such as prescription antihistamines. It is important to tell the health-care provider managing your exposure about any medications you are currently taking, if you need to take antiviral drugs for an HIV exposure.

Can pregnant health-care workers take the drugs recommended for postexposure treatment?

HBV: Yes. Women who are pregnant or breast feeding can be vaccinated against HBV infection and/or get HBIG. Pregnant women who are exposed to blood should be vaccinated against HBV infection, because infection during pregnancy can cause severe illness in the mother and a chronic infection in the newborn. The vaccine does not harm the fetus.

HIV: Pregnancy should not rule out the use of postexposure treatment when it is warranted. If you are pregnant you should understand what is known and not known regarding the potential benefits and risks associated with the use of antiviral drugs in order to make an informed decision about treatment.

Follow-Up after an Exposure

What follow-up should be done after an exposure?

HBV: Because postexposure treatment is highly effective in preventing HBV infection, CDC does not recommend routine follow-up after treatment. However, any symptoms suggesting hepatitis (e.g., yellow eyes or skin, loss of appetite, nausea, vomiting, fever, stomach or joint pain, extreme tiredness) should be reported to your health-care provider.

HCV: You should have an antibody test for hepatitis C virus and a liver enzyme test (alanine aminotransferase activity) as soon as possible after the exposure (baseline) and at 4-6 months after the exposure. Some clinicians may also recommend another test (HCV RNA) to detect HCV infection 4-6 weeks after the exposure. Report any symptoms suggesting hepatitis to your health-care provider.

HIV: You should be tested for HIV antibody as soon as possible after exposure (baseline) and periodically for at least 6 months after the exposure (e.g., at 6 weeks, 12 weeks, and 6 months). If you take antiviral drugs for postexposure treatment, you should be checked for drug toxicity by having a complete blood count and kidney and liver function tests just before starting treatment and 2 weeks after starting treatment. You should report any sudden or severe flu-like illness that occurs during the follow-up period, especially if it involves fever, rash, muscle aches, tiredness, malaise, or swollen glands. Any of these may suggest HIV infection, drug reaction, or other medical conditions.

You should contact the health-care provider managing your exposure if you have any questions or problems during the follow-up period.

What precautions should be taken during the follow-up period?

HBV: If you are exposed to HBV and receive postexposure treatment, it is unlikely that you will become infected and pass the infection on to others. No precautions are recommended.

HCV: Because the risk of becoming infected and passing the infection on to others after an exposure to HCV is low, no precautions are recommended.

HIV: During the follow-up period, especially the first 6-12 weeks when most infected persons are expected to show signs of infection, you should follow recommendations for preventing transmission of HIV. These include not donating blood, semen, or organs and not having sexual intercourse. If you choose to have sexual intercourse, using a condom consistently and correctly may reduce the risk of HIV transmission. In addition, women should consider not breast-feeding infants during the follow-up period to prevent exposing their infants to HIV in breast milk.

Chapter 9

Living with AIDS—
20 Years Later

One of the most devastating epidemics in human history began with little fanfare in 1981 when the U.S. Centers for Disease Control and Prevention quietly released a nine-paragraph report detailing five cases of an unusual disease in gay men.

The disease in the report, which came to be known as AIDS, soon would grab headlines nationwide. In the years since, it has never let go. Shortly after the report's release, doctors and scientists worldwide rapidly realized they were up against a new and little-understood viral foe with an almost sinister ability to outwit that most powerful of disease fighters—the human immune system. In turn, public fears mounted as news reports detailed the lack of medical weapons with which to assault this new, frightening disease and its potential to spread to those previously not thought to be at risk.

In the past two decades, many of these fears have been realized. AIDS has indeed become a 21st century plague. Fifty-eight million people worldwide have been infected with HIV, the virus that causes AIDS, according to the Joint United Nations Program on HIV/AIDS. Twenty-two million have died after the virus rendered their immune system nearly defenseless, leaving them open to some types of cancer, nerve degeneration and opportunistic infections such as tuberculosis and pneumonia that physicians once thought were under control.

"Living with AIDS—20 Years Later," by Anne Christiansen Bullers, U.S. Food and Drug Administration (FDA), *FDA Consumer* magazine, November-December 2001. And "AIDS: Activism and Advocacy," U.S. Food and Drug Administration (FDA), Publication No. (FDA) 01-1314, 2001.

Over the past 20 years, AIDS has become a part of life everywhere on the planet. Few people have been unaffected by its tragic toll, and it remains one of the most feared of all infections. That is not likely to change as the third decade of AIDS begins. Despite medical advances, a cure is elusive. AIDS is a serious, difficult-to-treat and ultimately fatal disease, though the outlook for those living with it has steadily improved in the United States as new drugs have gained approval from the Food and Drug Administration.

Twenty years of public discussion about AIDS has also yielded slow progress in the ongoing debate about how to fight the disease and care for those who have it. Today, the financial, political and social issues that stem from AIDS are discussed as much as its symptoms, and those issues grow more complex each year.

Simply put, "AIDS remains a challenge for us all," says Keith Henry, M.D., an internationally known researcher and clinician at the University of Minnesota and Hennepin County Medical Center in Minneapolis.

Understanding the Virus

Although AIDS was first recognized in 1981, HIV, the human immunodeficiency virus that causes AIDS, was not identified until 1983. Since then, researchers have been studying how the virus attacks and replicates itself inside cells of the immune system.

HIV is a virus—essentially a submicroscopic parasite consisting of a core of RNA wrapped in a protein coat—that cannot replicate without invading living cells. At its most basic level, a virus takes over the cell's mission control center to make the cell do HIV's bidding instead of functioning normally. Viruses responsible for influenza and the common cold operate similarly. However, while cold and flu viruses can make people miserable for a time, in healthy people they are usually defeated handily by the immune system.

HIV is different. It directly attacks the cells of the immune system, the body's defense system. Specifically, HIV goes after a type of immune cell called the CD4 lymphocyte. CD4 cells play a crucial role in the immune system because they coordinate the attack by white blood cells and antibodies on viruses and other body invaders.

HIV has a stealthy ability to escape detection as an enemy by CD4 cells. It then attaches to these cells and enters them. Once inside, the virus's genetic material takes command of the CD4 cell and forces it to make copies of the virus.

New copies of the virus burst forth from the cell, which then dies, and go in search of other cells to invade. The cycle continues again and again, with up to10 billion new HIV virus particles produced every day by the commandeered cells. About 2 billion new CD4 cells are needed each day if this process is to be kept in check.

But the body can't keep up. In fact, the number of CD4 cells drops off sharply as HIV's foothold in the body strengthens. The body becomes unable to protect itself not only from HIV, but also from other viruses, bacteria, fungi and parasites. This is when someone infected with HIV develops Acquired Immune Deficiency Syndrome, or AIDS.

Battling the Virus

These unique abilities of HIV have made the medical fight against it extremely challenging. Scientists and physicians had not seen anything like the virus before, and in the early 1980s there were no drugs to treat it. There also were few measures to combat the opportunistic infections that invaded the bodies of people whose immune systems had been decimated by HIV.

Prevention is the most effective weapon against HIV and AIDS. During the 1980s, gay rights organizations and public health professionals spearheaded campaigns to provide those most at risk for sexual transmission of the disease with some straightforward advice on how to prevent it—namely, the use of condoms.

Information aimed at intravenous drug users, who can acquire the virus by sharing needles with someone who is infected with HIV, also became available. The campaigns were often controversial, but AIDS researchers believe that they were effective, and helped to slow the spread of the disease both within at-risk communities and outside them.

"The message seemed to get through," says Tim Schacker, M.D., an AIDS researcher and clinician at the University of Minnesota in Minneapolis. AIDS advocacy organizations, now part of the landscape in every large city and a fixture during lobbying time at the state and federal level, also came into being. Their purpose was to seek support and money for prevention campaigns and also to direct public funds towards finding a cure.

"Education led to advocacy, that led to meetings with the FDA," said Martin Delaney, founding director of the AIDS advocacy group Project Inform in San Francisco. A corner seemed to be turned in the late 1980s and early 1990s. Public hysteria over the new virus began to recede. At the same time, prevention and lobbying campaigns matured, and medical research began bearing fruit in the form of new drugs.

The Golden Era

Despite their complex workings and complicated names, AIDS drugs are based on a relatively straightforward concept. By stopping or retarding the duplication of HIV inside the body's cells, the virus is prevented from overwhelming the immune system as it does when left unchecked. Researchers creating early HIV medicines followed this concept, and current medication has built on the theory.

The first drug to treat AIDS, the well-known AZT (zidovudine), was approved by the FDA in the United States in 1987. Initially created as a potential treatment for cancer, AZT was heralded as a wonder drug. Given the time and circumstances, it is understandable why. AZT was the first drug to show true promise in keeping the virus in check.

Consequently, AIDS patients and advocates began to demand access to the drug even while it was still in clinical trials. To accommodate patients' needs, the FDA streamlined the approval process to help get the drug to those who needed it while still ensuring its safety.

AZT belongs to a group of AIDS drugs known as nucleoside analogue reverse transcriptase inhibitors (NRTIs), which was the first group of drugs developed to fight the virus. These drugs work by interfering with an enzyme called reverse transcriptase that the virus needs to integrate itself into a human cell. In addition to AZT (Retrovir, zidovudine), NRTI drugs include Epivir (lamivudine, 3TC), Videx (didanosine, ddI), Hivid (zalcitabine, ddC), Zerit (stavudine, d4t), and one of the newest drugs on the market, Ziagen (abacavir).

However, AZT and the other NRTIs were no cure. While they seemed to lower the amount of virus in the blood—called the viral load—for a time or keep it in check, they didn't eradicate the virus from the body completely. Another troubling finding: AZT, which had held so much promise, began to lose its effectiveness as the virus began to change to overcome the drug's effect. Though inroads were being made, researchers knew there was still a long battle ahead.

"It was getting better, but people were still dying," says Jeffrey S. Murray, M.D., M.P.H., a veteran FDA researcher and clinician in the fight against AIDS. More weapons against HIV were needed. Gradually, the medical arsenal expanded. A major addition has been the protease inhibitors, which became widely available in 1995. Protease inhibitors include Crixivan (indinavir), Norvir (ritonavir), Viracept (nelfinavir), Fortovase (saquinavir), and Agenerase (amprenavir). Like NRTIs, these drugs interfere with the virus's ability to replicate in the body and inhibit the action of another key enzyme (protease). This enzyme is responsible for breaking apart large HIV proteins within the virus into smaller ones.

Another group of drugs to treat AIDS is the non-nucleoside reverse transcriptase inhibitors, or NNRTIs. Like AZT and other NRTIs, these drugs also interfere with the reverse transcriptase enzyme to prevent HIV from replicating in the body. NNRTI drugs include Viramune (nevirapine), Sustiva (efavirenz) and Rescriptor (delavirdine).

Combination Cocktails

None of these drugs proved to be a solution in and of themselves, particularly as the virus would again mutate to overcome the drug's effects. However, scientists began to realize that the drugs together packed a powerful punch against the virus. In 1995, the National Institute of Allergy and Infectious Diseases (NIAID) showed that combining these drugs slows the high rate of mutation, a characteristic of HIV.

The drug combinations became known as cocktails, a breezy name for a major advance in the battle against HIV. A new treatment era was born, accompanied by previously unknown levels of optimism.

Between 1996 and 1997, the number of AIDS-related deaths dropped 42 percent. Another decline, this time of 20 percent, followed between 1997 and 1998. In a report released by the Kaiser Family Foundation, AIDS-related deaths numbered 44,991 in 1993. Just five years later, the toll had dropped to only 17,171.

"That was the golden age," says the FDA's Murray. It was at this time when Ken Eppich of Minneapolis, then 53, was told he was HIV-positive. Eppich, who is gay, clearly remembers the sunny fall day in 1994 when he learned his diagnosis. Equally clear in his memory is the almost instant acceptance of his fate. Eppich believed that he would die soon, like so many of the friends and colleagues he had known with the disease. "I thought I had 18 months to live," Eppich says. Eppich set about making a will and making peace with himself. "I was OK with it. I'd had a good life."

Eppich's experience, however, epitomizes the changing expectations for AIDS patients brought on by this golden era. Having first learned of AIDS in the 1980s, he and his friends and family viewed AIDS as a death sentence. "I never asked for a prognosis and my doctor wisely didn't offer one. My friends were sure I was dying and my brother felt that the Thanksgiving of 1994 would be my last," Eppich says.

Instead, he was given a bunch of drugs he had never heard of. He took them, he read up on them—to the point that his doctor joked that the patient was the one really prescribing the medications—and made major changes in his life to stay healthy. And he lived.

Seven years later, in September 2001, Eppich found himself at a cabin in northern Minnesota on another clear, fall day with friends. They hoisted a toast to him and to his life. "(AIDS) is a part of me, but it doesn't define or control me," says Eppich. "I think of it as a manageable, chronic illness rather than a fatal disease."

Reality Check

Like Eppich, AIDS patients, today, can plan for their futures. But the optimism brought by the new drugs of the 1990s has dimmed as doctors and their patients have realized that the virus won't be vanquished so easily. Nor have the societal issues raised by the disease gone away.

The cocktails, the source of so much hope, have become less effective. As HIV replicates in the body, it is able to change ever so slightly. These changes have allowed it to steel itself against new drug enemies. Changing cocktail combinations has helped curb resistance, but researchers say there just aren't enough drugs or combinations to stay ahead of the constantly mutating virus. "It isn't even a question of when we're going to start losing people," says Murray. "We already have because we have run out of new effective drugs to try."

New drugs are currently in the pipeline and moving ahead at a rapid pace, according to Murray. Research on potential AIDS vaccines is underway, but progress has been slower. In fact, some have referred to the vaccine pipeline as a pipette. Since 1987, more than 40 different AIDS vaccines have been tested on a limited basis. Only one, AIDSVAX, has been thought promising enough to merit testing in humans in a large-scale study. Much of the research is being done in Thailand, though some of the work is also underway in the United States.

As the drug arsenal has expanded, so too has the debate about the disease, both within the medical community and outside it. In fact, the drugs that spawned the golden era of AIDS treatment have usually been at the heart of the discussion.

One major issue is that the drugs are expensive. Treatment for HIV and AIDS patients cost the United States government $6.9 billion in fiscal year 1999, up from $4.5 billion just two years before, according to the Kaiser Family Foundation.

The drugs also can be difficult to take. They must be taken on a strict schedule, and patients must remain on them for life. "Although some follow drug regimens nearly perfectly, perfect adherence is difficult," says Murray. "However, patients need to know that poor adherence to drugs may set them up for resistance."

Other pills prescribed to combat the side effects of anti-HIV drugs complicate the regimen. Eppich's day, for example, typically begins around 6:30 a.m. with a trip to the refrigerator, where one of his medications is kept. He then mixes the drug with a liquid and injects it into his side. Then he starts taking the first round of the 60-plus pills he takes every day. It's an hour and a half before he can start his day.

While the drugs keep the virus at bay, they often can make him feel less than healthy. He's nauseated sometimes and tired. Then there's another problem that he jokes about, but finds troublesome nonetheless. "I call it the eternal diarrhea," he says. "It's a part of life."

As more people have taken the drugs, more has become known about this side effect and others. Particularly troubling side effects include liver toxicity, nerve damage, diabetes, high cholesterol levels and unusual accumulations of fat in the neck and abdomen.

Physicians such as the University of Minnesota's Henry have monitored these effects and have listened to their patients. As a result, medical wisdom has changed. In February 2001, federal treatment guidelines changed significantly. Instead of recommending aggressively treating new AIDS patients with drugs, the guidelines now call for waiting until the immune system weakens significantly or until HIV in the blood reaches certain levels. The reason for this, says Henry, who was an international advocate for this change in philosophy, is that toxicities linked with the use of AIDS drugs appear to outweigh the benefits of early treatment with the drugs.

False Complacency

As the specter of AIDS receded, physicians, researchers and AIDS advocates began to notice that the effectiveness of the prevention message—the call for safe sex and drug practices made so stridently by AIDS advocates—also seemed to ebb. The incidence of HIV infections began to climb in the late 1990s. So did the incidence of some sexually transmitted diseases—such as gonorrhea—that are closely linked with the type of behavior associated with HIV transmission and are believed by some researchers to even play a role in HIV transmission.

Physicians and AIDS advocates believe these events may be linked to the development of the AIDS drugs. A new generation of people in AIDS risk groups, experts say, now appears to believe that the drugs will protect or cure them of the virus and that an AIDS diagnosis today isn't serious. "I hear about this all the time from patients," said Schacker, who sees patients at a Minneapolis clinic. "There is this belief that the drugs are so powerful that they can abandon safe sex practices. I am very concerned about it, and it's safe to say that [other researchers] are, too."

So are AIDS advocates such as Project Inform's Delaney. He says some of the problems are caused by unrealistic expectations created by pharmaceutical companies. "There were some overly cheery drug ads," Delaney says. "The message was, 'Don't worry about AIDS. It makes you prettier, it makes you sexier, it makes you stronger.'"

Researchers, physicians and advocates are beginning to target the issue and debate solutions. One researcher, Simon Rosser, Ph.D., M.P.H., of the University of Minnesota's Program in Human Sexuality, believes that an old tool, safe sex public health campaigns, needs to be dusted off and—more significantly—updated.

Rosser, who studies transmission of sexually transmitted diseases and the psychology involved, notes that dramatic advances have been made in treating AIDS. Yet little has been done, he says, to tailor public health messages and find ways to make them more effective. "Essentially, we are using the same techniques that were used in the 1980s," Rosser says.

Delaney echoes Rosser's concerns, but says that researchers also need to make sure they remain vigilant in their fight against the disease. In his opinion, some of the urgency to find new treatments for AIDS may have been lost. "The urgency of the old days is past, so the research is drifting in the doldrums of the past," Delaney says. "We're not going to let that happen."

What's Ahead?

As the third decade of AIDS begins, physicians, patients and advocates find themselves looking ahead while still dealing with issues like prevention that have been contended with since the historic CDC report in 1981. A cure, once thought to be imminent, is still years away. Despite this, those within the AIDS community of researchers, patients and advocates believe that progress has been made against the disease. Researchers know more than ever about the virus, experts say. That there are debates about treatment guidelines also is an advance, since once there were no treatments. The highly visible role in public debate played by AIDS patients and advocates has also helped to lift the stigma once associated with the disease, as well as helped ensure public funding for research and prevention.

The challenge now, experts say, is to bring the tools that have made progress against AIDS in the United States to other countries. High on the list are Africa and Asia, where lack of education and medicine have allowed the virus to spread and kill nearly unchecked.

Project Inform, for example, plans to help find cheaper tools for the diagnosis of HIV and effective ways to lobby the government for increased funding of the international AIDS effort. It may not seem like much, says Delaney and other experts, but perhaps the main lesson from the struggle against AIDS is that the fight will be a long one and that small advances add up. "We haven't lost hope," says Murray.

AIDS: Activism and Advocacy

During the late 1980s, some AIDS activists and others were critical of the FDA, saying the agency was holding up the availability of drugs for treatment. With a lack of effective therapies, people demanded government-sponsored research, large-scale Manhattan Project-style drug development, and the availability of a myriad of untested treatment approaches.

Unfortunately, many of the resulting efforts—often driven by sheer desperation—proved to be misguided. Some people mistakenly believed that the FDA's role was to develop new drugs. But even those who knew that the FDA's role is to review the results of drug research—not to develop and market new drugs—thought that the agency's approach was too conservative, given that people were dying from lack of treatment. In other words: How great a risk could even inadequate drugs pose when the inevitable outcome was death?

In 1988, the FDA created an AIDS coordination staff, now part of the agency's office of special health issues, to act as a bridge between the advocacy community and the agency. The two-way flow of information fostered by the office encouraged education and understanding on both sides. And the old adversarial relationship has given way to one that is more cooperative and constructive after more than a decade of working together.

The FDA has actively sought input on regulatory issues from AIDS patients. More than 45 patient representatives have participated on FDA advisory committees considering HIV/AIDS-related issues in recent years. The FDA realizes the value of the patient perspective. And the patient community has developed a better understanding and appreciation of the importance of regulatory oversight. The various benefits of this relationship have spilled into other areas well beyond HIV/AIDS.

Part Two

Diagnosis and Treatment of AIDS

Chapter 10

HIV Testing: Overview

Testing for HIV

Anyone who has unprotected sex with or shares a needle or syringe with someone who is HIV-positive, even once, is at risk for HIV infection. The ELISA and Western blot assay are the two most common ways to determine if a person is infected with HIV. In certain circumstances, PCR may be used. All three tests are performed on a small blood sample drawn from the arm.

Deciding to be tested for HIV can be difficult. Anyone who has questions or concerns should talk to a trained counselor at an HIV/AIDS testing center. People who want to be tested should look for a center that offers free, anonymous, confidential testing, and HIV counseling. People under the age 18 should find out if parental permission is required in their state.

For information on where to go for testing and HIV counseling, look under "Drug Abuse" in the yellow pages or call the CDC (Centers for Disease Control) National HIV/AIDS Hotline:

1-800-342-2437 (English)

1-800-344-7432 (Spanish)

1-800-243-7889 (TTY, for the hearing-impaired)

"Testing for HIV" and "Routine Testing." Reprinted with permission of Health communities.com from www.hivchannel.net © 2002 Healthcommunities.com, Inc. For further information contact Nancy Gable Lucas, Editor, at nlucas@health communities.com.

If someone is infected, the sooner they know, the better. They can stay healthy longer by seeking earlier treatment, and they can protect others by preventing transmission. Being tested too soon, however, (i.e., within 3 to 6 weeks of exposure) can result in unreliable test results. This is because the ELISA and Western blot do not test for the presence of the virus itself. They are used to test for proteins that the immune system produces to fight the virus. These proteins are known as antibodies and they usually do not show up in any of the tests until about 3 to 6 weeks after the initial infection.

ELISA

ELISA (enzyme-linked immunosorbent assay) is a quick and easy way to test for antibodies to HIV. The sensitivity (the percentage of positive results that are truly positive) and specificity (the percentage of negative results that are truly negative) of ELISA approach 100%, but false-positive and false-negative results do occur. A false-negative result is slightly more common, especially in women who have had multiple pregnancies or people who have received multiple blood transfusions.

If the result is positive or indeterminate, the test is repeated. If the second test is positive or indeterminate, a different test, usually the Western blot, is done to confirm the results.

What exactly is an enzyme-linked immunosorbent assay?

The blood sample is added to a plate that is coated with HIV antigens (HIV molecules that trigger an immune system response). A dye is then added that shows up only if HIV antibodies (proteins that the body produces in response to HIV infection) bind with the antigens.

Western Blot

The Western blot is generally used to confirm positive ELISA results, not to screen for infection. It produces more false positive results than ELISA (i.e., tests that show up positive even in HIV-negative people).

How does the Western blot work?

The test involves putting the blood sample on a strip of paper (made out of nitrocellulose), which is embedded with HIV antigens (HIV molecules that trigger an immune system response). The blood migrates along the paper, and a visible band shows up in places where HIV antibodies (proteins that the body produces in response to HIV infection) bind with the antigens.

PCR (Polymerase Chain Reaction)

Whereas ELISA and the Western blot detect the presence of antibodies to the virus, PCR looks for the virus itself, so it can detect HIV even in people who are not currently producing antibodies to the virus.

Specifically, PCR detects the presence of what is known as proviral DNA. Whereas humans and most other living beings are made up of DNA, HIV is made up of a slightly different type of genetic material known as RNA. Proviral DNA is a DNA copy of the virus's RNA. PCR is used:

- confirm the presence of HIV when the ELISA and Western blot are negative;

- in the first few weeks following infection, before antibodies are detectable;

- if the Western blot is indeterminate;

- in newborns for whom the presence of their mothers' antibodies complicates the other tests.

Routine Testing

HIV is a life-long infection that needs continuous monitoring and treatment. Monitoring HIV infection and its progression to AIDS involves the following types of tests:

- Viral load and T-cell/CD4+ counts measure how much HIV is in the blood and how quickly HIV/AIDS is progressing. They are used as guidelines for when to begin and change antiretroviral therapy.

- Resistance testing indicates if HIV has developed resistance to a particular antiretroviral drug. It helps the physician decide which antiretroviral medications to prescribe and when to change medication.

- Blood tests are done to evaluate the presence of HIV-related opportunistic infections.

Viral Load

A viral load test provides a measure of the amount of HIV in the blood, specifically the number of copies of viral RNA per one milliliter (ml or cc) of blood. Viral loads for HIV-infected people can range from undetectable to more than a million copies per ml. The tests are not sensitive enough yet to detect viral loads lower than about 25 copies per ml. So even though an undetectable viral load is a very good sign, it does not necessarily mean that the person is HIV-negative. It just means that there is not enough virus to be detected.

There are a variety of viral load tests available and patients should discuss with their health care provider the options. It is important that patients stick to one kind of test over time to be sure that changes in the viral load test reflect actual changes in the blood and not differences between the tests.

The American Medical Association guidelines for viral testing are as follows:

- Two tests should be performed within 1 or 2 weeks of each other to establish what is known as a baseline viral count. The baseline count provides an initial measure that the physician can use for monitoring the progression of HIV/AIDS. It is recommended that patients who have advanced HIV/AIDS disease be treated with antiretrovirals immediately after the first test in order to avoid potentially damaging delays.

- After the baseline viral count is measured, tests should be repeated every 3 to 6 months, along with T-cell/CD4 counts.

- Tests should be repeated 4 to 8 weeks after beginning or changing antiretroviral therapy.

Scientists have found a correlation between viral load and disease progression, that is the higher the viral load, the more the disease has progressed. Viral load provides an indication of how far the infection has progressed, even if there are no symptoms.

Viral load helps the physician determine when to start antiretroviral treatment and when to change medications. A higher viral load is an indication that treatment should be started or medications switched.

Viral load assay results may be thrown off if the patient has experienced any recent infection or immunization. Patients should wait several weeks after infection or immunization before having their viral load measured.

T-Cell Test, Also Known as CD4+ Count

The T-cell test is usually reported as the number of T-cells, also known as CD4+ cells, in one milliliter of blood. Healthy, uninfected people have between 500 and 1600 CD4+ cells per ml of blood. According to the Centers for Disease Control, a CD4+ cell count below 200/ml is a criterion for AIDS.

T-cell tests also provide a measure of a different kind of immune system cell known as a CD8+ cell. Sometimes the ratio of CD4+ to CD8+ cells is used to monitor HIV infection, since the ratio drops so dramatically in people with HIV/AIDS. In healthy people, there are normally about 1 to 2 CD4+ cells for every CD8+ cell. In people with HIV/AIDS, the ratio is reversed and there are many CD8+ cells for every CD4+ cell.

T-cell levels can change considerably throughout the day and depend on a variety of factors such as stress and fatigue. People should try to have the test at the same time of day. The number of CD4+ and CD8+ cells goes up during infection. So T-cell tests can vary depending on whether the patient has had any recent infections.

Chapter 11

Rapid HIV Tests:
Questions and Answers

Following are questions and answers regarding rapid HIV testing. The information will be useful to those seeking further understanding of this type of screening for HIV.

General Questions

What has been the routine test for HIV antibody testing?

The standard screening test for antibody to HIV is the enzyme immunoassay (EIA), which is widely used in the United States and around the world. This test requires serum or plasma, so a blood specimen must be drawn from a vein. Because EIA requires specialized equipment, the specimen must be sent to a laboratory, and test results are usually available several days to several weeks later. A negative screening test means a person is not infected with HIV, and does not require further testing. However, a diagnosis of HIV infection cannot be based on a reactive screening test alone. Thus, a reactive EIA is repeated, and repeatedly reactive EIA results are confirmed by a supplemental HIV antibody test—Western blot or immunofluorescence assay (IFA).

A fact sheet from the National Center for HIV, STD and TB Prevention, Centers for Disease Control and Prevention (CDC), 1998, updated in December 2002 by Dr. David A. Cooke, MD, Diplomate, American Board of Internal Medicine.

Until now, testing required two visits. During the first visit, a client receives pretest counseling, and blood is drawn for HIV testing. During the second visit, test results are communicated to the client, additional counseling is provided, and clients who need them are given referrals for additional services.

What is rapid HIV testing?

A rapid test for detecting antibody to HIV is a screening test that produces very quick results, usually in 10 to 30 minutes. Currently, two rapid HIV tests are licensed by the Food and Drug Administration (FDA) for use in the United States. The FDA has been prosecuting the manufacturers of several unapproved tests, which have been sold illegally on the Internet and elsewhere. The reliability of these unapproved kits is not known.

What is the difference between a rapid HIV test and an EIA?

The rapid HIV test is easier to use and produces results more quickly than the EIA does. The sensitivity and specificity of the rapid HIV test are just as good as those of the EIA.

What rapid HIV tests are available?

Currently, two rapid HIV tests are licensed by the FDA. These are the OraQuick Rapid HIV-1 Antibody Test, and the Murex Single Use Diagnostic System (SUDS) HIV-1 Test.

Will other rapid HIV tests be available in the future?

Several other rapid HIV tests are being used in many other countries. Still others, including one for use with oral fluids, are being developed. The new generation of rapid HIV tests may be quicker and easier to use.

Who can be tested with a rapid HIV test?

Rapid HIV testing is suitable for testing any person who would be eligible for HIV testing by EIA. However, the availability of rapid HIV tests may differ from one place to another.

Does the rapid HIV test cost more than the EIA?

Yes. The individual kit is more costly then the per-test cost of the EIA. EIA testing was designed for the automated processing of tests in batches (usually using a plate that can process 96 specimens at one time.) However, an analysis done in 1996 by Dr. Paul Farnham and his colleagues at CDC indicated that rapid HIV testing is more cost-effective than the current EIA-based system, because of the number of persons who actually learn their results. In other words, although EIA is less expensive, it is a waste of money to perform lab tests if the person tested never learns the test result, if two clinic visits are required to get test results, or if the clinic has to send field staff to locate people for test results. Since an EIA does not yield immediate results, most people must make a second visit to learn their results. Experience at publicly funded testing sites has shown that many persons (26% of those who tested positive for HIV and 33% of those who tested negative in 1996) do not return for their test results.

Are rapid HIV tests more accurate or less accurate than EIAs?

The rapid HIV test is just as accurate as an EIA. As is true of all screening tests (including the EIA), a reactive rapid HIV test result must be confirmed. Studies in countries where more than one type of rapid HIV test is available show that specific combinations of two or more different rapid HIV tests can provide results as reliable as those from an EIA and Western blot or IFA, the combination that is currently used in the United States. A second rapid HIV test for persons whose first rapid HIV test is reactive could significantly improve the predictive value of rapid HIV testing.

What is predictive value?

Predictive value is the calculated probability that a test result predicts whether a person is truly infected. This calculation produces a number that counselors can use in explaining HIV test results to their clients. For example, a higher predictive value means that a reactive test is more likely to indicate the person is truly infected.

If a person receives a negative rapid HIV test result, is a confirmatory test needed?

A negative antibody test result, whether it is from a rapid HIV test or an EIA, does not require a confirmatory test. However, a person may have been tested too soon, before antibodies developed. The average time between infection and the development of detectable antibodies is 25 days.

81

Does a negative rapid HIV test result mean that a person has nothing to worry about?

Not necessarily. For most people who are tested, a negative HIV antibody test result does mean that they are not infected. However, in some cases a person may have been tested too soon (before antibodies have developed, which requires an average of 25 days). That is why it is important to assess specific risk behaviors during counseling, and discuss ways to change risky behaviors.

What is a "reactive" HIV test result?

The term "reactive" is used to describe a test that has detected the presence of antibodies to HIV. It is recommended that all reactive tests be repeated immediately, by using the same test. Repeatedly reactive tests are then further confirmed, by using a different test on the same blood specimen.

After a reactive rapid HIV test result, how long does a person have to wait for the confirmatory test result?

The confirmatory tests are usually sent to a laboratory for processing; results are generally available in 1 to 2 weeks.

Technical, Counseling, and Implementation Questions

What is the cost of a rapid HIV test?

Prices may be different in different parts of the country. The test kit usually costs $6 to $10, which is more expensive than an EIA. However, the EIA requires expensive equipment and rapid HIV tests do not. Additional costs such as a laboratory or a laboratory technician's time for conducting the tests should also be considered. Rapid HIV tests are simpler to perform and require fewer specialized skills than does an EIA.

Can CDC HIV prevention funds be used to pay for rapid HIV tests?

Yes. CDC prevention funds can be used to support any FDA-approved HIV testing service.

If a confirmatory test is still needed, what is the advantage to sexually transmitted disease (STD) clinics of using rapid HIV testing?

The advantage to the clinic is that more people will receive their test results without expensive field visits. Most of the clients at all U.S. publicly funded testing sites, including STD clinics, test negative for HIV. For these persons (approximately 2.1 million in 1996), the need to make a second visit would be eliminated. Of all testing sites, STD clinics have had the lowest proportion of persons who return for HIV test results. Thus, rapid HIV tests have the potential to greatly increase the number of persons who learn their results. In addition, persons who test HIV-positive by the rapid HIV test can be advised immediately of their screening test result, and counseled about the need to take precautions to prevent the possibility of transmitting HIV. These persons of course need to return for their confirmatory test result.

What is the advantage to clients of using rapid HIV testing?

Interviews with persons being tested indicate that most persons prefer rapid HIV testing, and most persons who receive a positive HIV screening test result return on their own to learn the confirmed result (unlike the situation with current testing, in which many persons learn their test results only as a result of outreach). This also means that persons who are truly HIV-positive will learn of their infection sooner. This may help prevent infections that might otherwise have occurred between the time the person was tested and the time the person received results (sometimes as long as several weeks.)

Will people who have progressed to the late stages of AIDS continue to test positive on the rapid HIV tests?

Yes. The progression of HIV disease rarely affects the detection of HIV antibody.

Can rapid HIV tests be performed on infants?

The result of any HIV antibody test performed on an infant less than 15 months of age may reflect the mother's HIV status, because the antibodies are transferred from the mother to the baby. Until these antibodies disappear, only specific virus detection tests can determine the infection status of an infant.

Can clinic staff batch rapid HIV tests?

Yes. Batching, or collecting several specimens before testing all of them at the same time, can be done. This process can save money for a busy clinic, because fewer control test kits are required. However, accumulating a sufficient number of tests for a batch can result in excessive waiting time for the client, reducing the main benefit of the rapid HIV test—rapid results.

How long does the rapid HIV test take after the lab receives the specimen?

The rapid HIV test usually takes 10 to 30 minutes, depending on the test brand used. The waiting time depends on how many clients are being tested and whether the clinic is testing individual samples or batching them. Counseling can be performed while the test is being done.

What type of training will be available for HIV counselors at sites that use rapid HIV tests?

CDC is developing new guidance and training for counselors.

Are educational materials (e.g., handouts, videos) available for the clinics that want to use rapid HIV tests?

CDC will assist counselors and others who plan to develop such products. The manufacturers of rapid HIV tests usually have such materials as well.

Would telephoning clients to provide the results of a positive confirmatory HIV test be acceptable?

Current CDC counseling and testing guidelines state that positive HIV results should be communicated by personal contact. Whether this personal contact is established by phone or in person is a decision to be made at the local level.

What does the counselor tell a client who has a reactive rapid HIV test?

One of the more challenging counseling issues is how to communicate reactive rapid HIV test results to clients without the benefit of a same-day confirmatory test result. Counselors should be able to discuss with the client the likelihood of whether the rapid HIV test result means the client has HIV infection. This discussion should be based on the prevalence of HIV among persons tested at that clinic coupled with an assessment of the client's risk behaviors. In clinics that usually experience a high prevalence of HIV infection among their clients, a reactive rapid HIV test result is more likely to represent a true infection, especially in persons who report risk behaviors for HIV. Any person whose rapid HIV test is reactive should be counseled about the need to take precautions to prevent any possibility of transmitting HIV infection until their infection status has been determined by a confirmatory HIV test.

Do you start partner notification and referral services immediately upon receiving a reactive rapid HIV test result, or do you wait for the confirmatory test result?

Partner notification and referral services should not be initiated until the reactive rapid HIV test result has been confirmed.

Should a physician prescribe antiretroviral treatment for a pregnant woman on the basis of rapid HIV test results (per the PHS Guidelines)?

A negative rapid HIV test of course means that antiretroviral treatment is not necessary. Deciding what to do about therapy when the rapid HIV test is reactive is more complicated. If the circumstances are not urgent, it would be preferable to wait for the confirmatory test result. In other circumstances (such as a rapid HIV test result for a woman in labor, for whom no other result is available), physicians should base decisions about antiretroviral treatment on the predictive value of the preliminary rapid HIV test results and an assessment of the mother's HIV risk. (CDC. Public Health Service Task Force Recommendations for the Use of Antiretroviral Drugs in Pregnant Women Infected with HIV-1 for Maternal Health and for Reducing Perinatal HIV-1 Transmission in the United States. *MMWR* 1998;47(No. RR-2):1-31.)

Are confirmatory tests necessary for a rapid HIV test result to be considered a diagnosis of HIV infection?

As is true of current EIA antibody procedure, an initial reactive rapid HIV test result should be confirmed by Western blot or IFA. For persons who test positive by confirmatory testing, CDC and the Association of State and Territorial Public Health Laboratory Directors recommend that the test sequence be repeated, by using a different sample, to be absolutely certain of the results.

Chapter 12

Viral Load Tests

What Is Viral Load?

The viral load test measures the amount of HIV virus in your blood. There are different techniques for doing this:

- The PCR (polymerase chain reaction) test uses an enzyme to multiply the HIV in the blood sample. Then a chemical reaction marks the virus. The markers are measured and used to calculate the amount of virus. Roche produces this test.

- The bDNA (branched DNA) test combines a material that gives off light with the sample. This material connects with the HIV particles. The amount of light is measured and converted to a viral count. Chiron produces this test.

The PCR test results are often different from the bDNA results for the same sample. Because the tests are different, you should stick with the same kind of test (PCR or bDNA) to measure your viral load over time.

Viral loads are usually reported as copies of HIV in one milliliter of blood. The tests count up to about 1.5 million copies, and are always being improved to be more sensitive. The first bDNA test measured down to 10,000 copies. The second generation could detect as few as 500 copies. Now there are ultra sensitive tests that can detect less than 5 copies.

The best viral load test result is "undetectable." This does not mean that there is no virus in your blood; it just means that there is not enough for the test to find and count. With the first generation test, "undetectable" could mean 9,999 copies. "Undetectable" depends on the sensitivity of the test used on your blood sample.

How Is the Test Used?

The viral load test is helpful in several areas:

- In basic science, the test has been used to prove that HIV is never latent but is always multiplying. Many people with no symptoms of AIDS and high T-cell counts also had high viral loads. If the virus was latent, the test wouldn't have found any HIV in the blood.

- The test can be used for diagnosis, because it can detect a viral load at any time after HIV infection. This is better than the standard HIV (antibody) test, which can be negative after HIV infection and before the development of antibodies.

- For prognosis, viral load can help predict how long someone will stay healthy. The higher the viral load, the faster HIV disease progresses.

- Finally, the viral load test is valuable for managing therapy, to see if antiviral drugs are controlling the virus. Current guide-lines suggest measuring baseline (pre-treatment) viral load. A drug is working if it lowers viral load by at least 90% within 8 weeks. The viral load should continue to drop to less than 50 copies within 6 months. The viral load should be measured within 2 to 8 weeks after treatment is started or changed, and every 3 to 4 months after that.

How Are Changes in Viral Load Measured?

Repeat tests of the same blood sample can give results that vary by a factor of 3. This means that a meaningful change would be a drop to less than 1/3 or an increase to more than 3 times the previous test result. For example, a change from 200,000 to 600,000 is within the normal variability of the test. A drop from 50,000 to 10,000 would be significant. The most important change is to reach an undetectable viral load.

Viral load changes are often described as log changes. This refers to scientific notation, which uses powers of 10. For example, a 2-log drop is a drop of 102 or 100 times. A drop from 60,000 to 600 would be a 2-log drop.

What Do the Numbers Mean?

There are no magic numbers for viral loads. We don't know how long you'll stay healthy with any particular viral load. We don't know if 150,000 is twice as bad as 75,000. All we know so far is that lower is better and seems to mean a longer, healthier life.

U.S. treatment guidelines suggest that anyone with a viral load over 55,000 should be offered treatment.

Some people may think that if their viral load is undetectable, they can't pass the HIV virus to another person. THIS IS NOT TRUE. There is no safe level of viral load. Although the risk is less, you can pass HIV to another person even if your viral load is undetectable.

Are There Problems with the Viral Load Test?

There are some concerns with the viral load test:

- Only about 2% of the HIV in your body is in the blood. The viral load test does not measure how much HIV is in body tissues like the lymph nodes, spleen, or brain. HIV levels in lymph tissue and semen go down when blood levels go down, but not at the same time or the same rate.

- The viral load test results can be thrown off if your body is fighting an infection, or if you have just received an immunization (like a flu shot). You should not have blood taken for a viral load test within four weeks of any infection or immunization.

Chapter 13

Home Diagnostic Tests

More and more Americans are playing doctor in the privacy of their own bathrooms, using a few drops of blood or a urine sample to test for HIV, cholesterol, blood glucose, or evidence of colon or rectal cancer. In fact, a snippet of a child's hair now can confirm the use of illicit drugs.

Often seen as a less expensive and a more convenient alternative to a trip to the doctor's office, self-testing diagnostic and monitoring devices are booming in sales. Devices such as blood-glucose tests and blood-pressure kits make it easier for people to self-monitor conditions such as diabetes and hypertension. However, this technology-driven trend is not without limits and could result in serious problems for those who rely on the tests instead of on the expertise of their health-care provider. A recent shift in the home diagnostics market—from monitoring chronic illnesses to diagnosing serious or potentially fatal diseases—is raising red flags among health professionals.

For years, pregnancy tests and ovulation predictors dominated the home test kit market. While these devices still generate large numbers of self-care sales, other tools of the medical trade are fast becoming available outside the doctor's office—no prescription needed. Spiraling health-care costs, increased interest in preventive health care, and a desire for privacy are paving the way for products that

"Home Diagnostic Tests: The Ultimate House Call?" by Carol Lewis, U.S. Food and Drug Administration (FDA), *FDA Consumer* magazine, November-December 2001.

now include screening for the virus that causes AIDS and for drugs of abuse.

Screening tests often are used at home to check for symptoms of a disease when they may not be readily apparent. For example, people can measure their cholesterol and triglyceride levels—two types of fats in the blood—to help minimize the risk of cardiovascular disease.

Benefits and Limitations

Home test kits are, in many cases, as inexpensive as a co-payment to a doctor and a lot less time-consuming. Some can provide speedy results.

One sign of their overall increasing popularity is the fact that many pharmacists are moving home test kits from behind their counters onto free-standing displays. The lure of the Internet is also helping to make these devices more readily available.

Steven Gutman, M.D., director of the Food and Drug Administration's clinical laboratory devices division, says that consumers need to be wary about buying and using the kits on their own. "People need to carefully read the test-kit labeling and instructions, where important information and warnings about the product are listed," he says. Among other things, this information tells how a test works, and what to do when it doesn't. Home test kits are meant to be an adjunct to doctor visits, not a replacement for them. "Although the menu of home testing products has expanded," Gutman says, "the advice is still the same."

See Your Doctor, Too

While convenience, confidentiality, and the cost-saving benefits of home testing cannot be overlooked, doctors are concerned about the availability of medical tests that encourage self-diagnosis because of the possibility that the results could be misinterpreted and treatment might be delayed.

In addition, the diagnostic value of home test kits can be affected by users who don't follow instructions carefully. In an effort to conceive a child, Donna Trossevin of Frederick, Md., bought from a local pharmacy an ovulation predictor that uses body temperature to help pinpoint a woman's most fertile time. Although the kit consisted of only a thermometer and special paper to chart her daily temperatures, Trossevin says it was difficult to get accurate readings because "if you don't hold the instrument just so, you can easily misread the numbers."

And the half a degree increase from a person's normal temperature that a woman is looking for to predict ovulation "is such a small window of opportunity and easy to miss," says Trossevin. "I just never knew 100 percent whether I was ovulating or not."

Those who rely on home tests also miss out on pre- and post-test counseling, which offer information, support, competence, interpretation, and follow-up advice to consumers that only a health-care professional can give. The benefit of having a health-care professional involved in a test or screening procedure is that the results can be evaluated within the context of the whole health picture, not just one test. Furthermore, receiving news of potential pregnancy, illness, or infection over the phone, or from the color of a test strip, can be devastating.

"The first 72 hours following a positive result for an illness as serious as HIV is when people are most likely to hurt themselves," says Edward Geraty, a licensed clinical social worker with Behavioral Science Associates in Baltimore. Geraty says it's important to have a face-to-face relationship when delivering the news of a positive HIV test. Without it, he says, "there's a psychological component of the person's illness that is completely left out of the process." Bob Barret, Ph.D., agrees. A professor of counseling at the University of North Carolina at Charlotte, Barret believes that home test kits, particularly for HIV, "are best used only by those who are well-educated about the disease, and who are in touch with their emotions and have a good support system around them."

Find a Reputable Source

Accuracy, too, is an important consideration when it comes to home testing. False positive test results indicate that a condition is present when, in fact, it is not. False negatives are results that do not identify a condition that is present.

The Federal Trade Commission, which enforces consumer protection laws, recently reviewed results of several unapproved HIV test kits advertised and sold on the Internet for self-diagnosis at home. In every case, the kits showed a negative result when used on a known HIV-positive sample. Similarly, the FDA recently tested a number of unapproved home HIV test kits sold on the Internet that were confiscated during a criminal investigation. None produced accurate results. In reality, the outcome could have had grave consequences for a user in terms of mental and emotional stress, access to proper medical treatment, and transmission of the disease to others. The FDA's

Center for Biologics Evaluation and Research, which reviews all blood-related products, continues to investigate firms and people involved in the illegal sale of unapproved HIV home test kits in the United States.

Follow the Directions

Home test kits, for the most part, involve relatively simple procedures. Some are as straightforward as one pregnancy test in which chemically treated test strips dipped in urine produce colored indicator lines. Others require a finger prick and the placement of a blood sample onto a reagent strip. The strip is inserted into a machine that measures blood glucose levels. Still others, like the only FDA-cleared HIV home sample collection kit, consist of multiple components, ranging from pre-test counseling information to a personal identification number for obtaining the test's results. In any case, the FDA requires that the kits be simple enough for an average consumer to use at home without a doctor's supervision.

Some home tests give their results as positive or negative. Performance of these is described in terms of sensitivity—the probability that the results will be positive when a disease or condition is present; and specificity—the probability that the results will be negative when a disease or condition is not present. Other home tests give numerical results. Performance of these is described in terms of precision—how reproducible the results are when a test is run over and over; and accuracy—how well the results compare to a laboratory test. All diagnostic tests have limitations, and sometimes their use may produce erroneous or questionable results. Test results obtained at home can often be clarified by a physician, who may recommend another test that is handled by a laboratory.

Gutman, whose office is within CDRH, says that home test kits should not be stored in places where they might be exposed to extreme temperatures, since this may cause product deterioration over time. He also stresses the importance of checking test-kit expiration dates—chemicals in an outdated test may no longer work properly, so the results are not likely to be valid.

While manufacturers of professional test kits used in clinics and hospitals or doctor's offices are required to include sensitivity and specificity information in their labeling, the FDA does not make manufacturers of home test kits do so. But Lori Moore of Maysville, KY, thinks they should. "As a consumer, I want to see the data that supports this being a good brand," she says. "For the average person, this information truly lets them know what they're purchasing." But Moore happens to be more familiar with sensitivity and related product information than most people, since she has worked as a registered laboratory technician. Still, she insists that today's consumer wants more information visible on the product's label than is currently available.

Dave Lyle, a medical technologist in the FDA's clinical laboratory devices division, explains that "the decision was made several years ago to exclude this information from over-the-counter kits because it might confuse the consumer." However, Lyle agrees that "in today's world, most consumers are very sophisticated and want as much information as possible to make an informed decision."

Complications of home testing may interfere with obtaining accurate results. Consumers may not be able to follow the instructions. Proper collection, storage and shipment of specimens are all critical for accuracy. Samples held too long, for example, or subjected to severe temperature changes could generate false positive or negative readings. Urine samples taken too early or too late in the day or foods eaten that mimic the metabolites being measured also can produce inaccurate readings.

And people need to beware of bogus tests—those not cleared by the FDA. Unapproved home test kits do not come with any guarantee of accuracy or sensitivity, nor do they have a documented history of dependability. Proper training to interpret results is not provided with the kits, and they do not have a validated record of precision. This means that unapproved tests may be inconsistent and inaccurate.

Approved tests, on the other hand, have undergone extensive study and review by the manufacturer of the product to satisfy the FDA's requirement that they are as safe and accurate for consumer use as their laboratory counterparts are for professional use. For any in-home test, the manufacturer must convince the FDA that the results of a test will benefit consumers and that consumers have the knowledge necessary to decide whether testing themselves is appropriate. For example, Stewart says people purchasing blood pressure monitors should look for a statement in the label that says the device has been validated in a human study "where the statistics have been calculated to ensure that good accuracy can be demonstrated." Stewart says the label also should include a statement that says measurements obtained by the blood pressure monitor are equivalent to those obtained by a trained observer using a cuff and stethoscope.

"Indeed, reading the label is the most important thing," he says, "but it might also be useful to ask the pharmacist or one's doctor to get a recommendation."

Popular But Not Perfect

Amid sweeping changes in U.S. health care, the trend toward cost-effective self-care products used in the home emphasizes prevention and early intervention. The home test kit market is offering faster and easier products that lend themselves to being used in less-sophisticated environments to meet consumers' needs.

However, Gutman emphasizes, "even the best screening tests are occasionally wrong. No tests, whether performed at the lab or in the home, are perfect."

Buying Test Kits Online

The consequences of consumer health fraud range from significant financial loss to the failure to seek legitimate medical treatment. The Food and Drug Administration wants consumers to be aware that a number of unapproved test kits are being marketed on the Internet, as well as through magazine or newspaper promotions, for home use. Internet sites sell test kits that falsely claim everything from being FDA-approved to detecting illness within 15 minutes or less. Also, consumers may receive contaminated or counterfeit products, the wrong product, or no product at all. These elements "are complicated by the fact that with the Internet, you're not always sure you're in U.S. commerce," says Steven Gutman, M.D., director of the FDA's clinical laboratory devices division. Many home test kits not approved for use in the United States are available in other countries.

But Gutman adds that consumers can feel confident that home test kits purchased from a reputable drugstore or pharmacy have been cleared by the FDA. For peace of mind, he says people can log onto the agency's Web site at www.fda.gov/oc/buyonline/ for consumer tips and warnings for buying medical products online, and www.fda.gov/cdrh/ode/otclist.html for a regularly updated list of approved home test kits sold over the counter.

Gutman says that consumers should feel free to contact manufacturers of diagnostic devices intended for home use to determine if they have been reviewed by the FDA. The inability to reach a reliable party for this information, he says, "may in itself be a signal that the test may not be a wise purchase."

Chapter 14

HIV Counseling, Testing, and Referral

If you think you may have been infected with HIV and are unsure about getting a test to find out, the following information about HIV, testing, and counseling will help you decide.

HIV and AIDS Medical Care Offers Vital Benefits

Early medical attention can slow the growth of the human immunodeficiency virus (HIV), the virus that causes acquired immunodeficiency syndrome (AIDS). The slower the virus spreads, the longer an individual's body will be able to fight off the illnesses and life-threatening conditions that often accompany AIDS.

For example, some medicines can prevent the type of pneumonia that commonly strikes—and threatens the lives of—people who have HIV or AIDS. Doctors can also help stave off HIV-related illnesses by evaluating an individual's immune system on a regular basis. When the immune system begins to weaken, doctors can vaccinate a person against bacterial pneumonia and influenza, and treat those illnesses effectively if they occur. Without medical care, a person with HIV infection may quickly develop serious diseases. In addition, medical treatment with AZT (zidovudine), may reduce the risk of a pregnant woman infecting her unborn child with HIV.

From National HIV Testing Resources, Centers for Disease Control and Prevention (CDC), 2002; available online at http://www.hivtest.org/consumer/index.htm.

These and other medical options have increased the length and quality of life for those who have HIV. Keep this in mind as you decide whether or not to seek counseling and testing. Your decision can make the difference between staying well for a long time or becoming seriously ill more quickly. This chapter gives you the information you need to understand the benefits of counseling and testing. Use this information to make the choice that is right for you.

What Happens If I become Infected with HIV?

Being infected with HIV does not necessarily mean you have AIDS. It does mean you will carry the virus in your body for the rest of your life. It also means you can infect other people if you do things—such as have unprotected sex—that can transmit HIV. You can infect others even if you feel fine and have no symptoms of illness. Perhaps more importantly, you can infect others when you don't know you carry HIV.

The Best Way to Know Whether You Are Infected: HIV-Antibody Counseling and Testing

The HIV-antibody test is the only way to tell if you are infected. You cannot tell by looking at someone if he or she carries HIV. Someone can look and feel perfectly healthy and still be infected. In fact, an estimated one-third of those who are HIV-positive do not know it. Neither do their sex partners.

When HIV enters the bloodstream, it begins to attack certain white blood cells called T4 lymphocyte cells (helper cells). The immune system then produces antibodies to fight off the infection. Although these antibodies are ineffective in destroying HIV, their presence in the blood is used to confirm HIV infection. Testing can tell you whether or not you have developed antibodies to HIV.

You should receive counseling before and after taking the HIV-antibody test. This counseling will help you understand the results of your test, learn how to protect your health, and (if you are infected) gain the knowledge of how to prevent passing the virus to others. Regardless of your HIV status, counseling should be a central part of the testing process.

Should I Seek HIV Counseling and Testing?

If you have engaged in behavior that can transmit HIV, it is very important that you consider counseling and testing. The following checklist will help you assess your degree of risk.

If I think I have been exposed to HIV, how soon can I get tested?

To find out when you should be tested, discuss it with your testing site staff or personal physician. The tests commonly used to detect HIV infection actually look for antibodies produced by your body to fight HIV. Most people will develop detectable antibodies within 3 months after infection, the average being 20 days. In rare cases, it can take up to 6 months. It would be extremely uncommon to take longer than 6 months to develop detectable antibodies. For this reason, the Centers for Disease Control and Prevention currently recommends getting tested 6 months after the last possible exposure to the virus. (It is possible to be exposed during unprotected vaginal, anal, or oral sex; as well as when sharing needles). It is important, during the 6 months between exposure and the test, to protect yourself and others from further possible exposures to HIV.

Who should get an HIV test?

Counseling and early diagnosis of HIV infection are recommended for:

- persons attending sexually-transmitted disease clinics and drug-treatment clinics;

- persons who have had multiple partners and had unprotected anal, oral or vaginal sex;

- partners of injection drug users (either spouses, sex partners, or needle-sharing partners);

- women of childbearing age;

- TB patients; and

- patients who received transfusions of blood or blood components between early 1978 and mid-1985.

- In addition, people considering marriage should seek information about AIDS, as well as voluntary counseling and testing.

- The President also has mandated the screening of immigrants entering the United States, foreign service personnel, and inmates of Federal prisons.

Why is the Centers for Disease Control and Prevention (CDC) recommending that all pregnant women be tested for HIV?

CDC recommends that pregnant women be tested for HIV for two reasons. First, if HIV positive, a woman can take medications that lower the chance of passing HIV to her infant before, during, or after birth. Second, HIV testing and counseling provides an opportunity for a woman to find out if she is infected and, if so, to receive medical treatment that may help delay the progression of HIV. For women who are not infected, counseling provides an opportunity to learn important information about how to avoid being exposed to HIV.

Without medical treatment, an infected woman's child has about a one in four chance of being born with HIV. Medical treatment with zidovudine (ZDV, also known as AZT or Retrovir) during pregnancy and labor has dramatically reduced the risk of transmission of HIV from mother to baby, with an over 75% decrease in pediatric AIDS cases in 1998. An HIV-positive woman should not breast-feed her baby and the infant should be given AZT for the first several weeks of life. Even then, the risk of infecting the child cannot be totally eliminated. In 1999, 300-400 babies were born with HIV. In 1998, the U.S. Public Health Services released updated recommendations for offering antiretroviral therapy to HIV-positive pregnant women.

Am I at Risk?

Evidence suggests that HIV, the virus that causes AIDS, has been in the United States at least since 1978. The following are known risk factors for HIV infection. If you answer yes to any of these questions, you should definitely seek counseling and testing. You may be at increased risk of infection if any of the following apply to you since 1978.

- Have you shared needles or syringes to inject drugs or steroids?

- If you are a male, have you had unprotected sex with other males?

- Have you had unprotected sex with someone who you know or suspect was infected with HIV?

- Have you had a sexually transmitted disease (STD)?

- Have you received a blood transfusion or clotting factor between 1978 and 1985?

- Have you had unprotected sex with someone who would answer yes to any of the above questions?

If you have had sex with someone whose history of risk-taking behavior is unknown to you or if you or they may have had many sex partners, then you have increased the chances that you might be HIV infected.

If you plan to become pregnant, counseling and testing is even more important. Without treatment, an HIV-infected woman has about an 1-in-4 chance of infecting her baby during pregnancy or delivery. Medical treatment can reduce this to about a 1-in-12 chance.

Reasons for Seeking Counseling and Testing

People consider counseling and testing for a number of reasons, some of which may apply to you:

- Knowing whether or not you have HIV infection would alert you to your need to seek medical care to prevent or delay life-threatening illnesses. Your test result (positive or negative) would also help your doctor determine the cause and best treatment of the various illnesses you may have now or in the future. For example, if you are HIV-positive, tuberculosis (TB) and syphilis are treated differently than if you are HIV-negative.

- If you find out you are infected, knowing your result would help you protect your sex partner(s) from infection and illness. If they are not infected, you can avoid infecting them.

- Knowing your result would help you assess the safety of having a child.

- Knowing your result, even if you are infected (positive test result), may be less stressful than the anxiety of thinking you might be infected but not knowing. If your result indicates you are not infected (negative), you can take action to be sure you don't become infected in the future.

Understanding the HIV Counseling and Testing Process

It is very important that you understand the confidentiality policies of the testing center. Ask your testing counselor how the center will protect your test results. Most counseling and testing centers follow one of two policies:

Confidential Testing

The confidential testing site records your name with the test result. Your record will be kept secret from everybody except medical personnel, or in some states, the state health department. You should ask who will know the result and how it will be stored. If you have your HIV antibody test done confidentially, you can sign a release form to have your test result sent to your doctor.

Anonymous Testing (Not Available in All States)

No one asks your name. You are the only one who can tell anyone else your result. If you wish to be tested, ask your health department, doctor, or the CDC National STD and AIDS Hotlines (1-800-342-AIDS) about the location of facilities near you.

Where can I get tested for HIV infection?

Many places offer HIV testing including local health departments, private doctors' offices, hospitals, and sites specifically set up to provide HIV testing. It is important to get tested at a place that also provides counseling about HIV and AIDS. Counselors can answer any questions you might have about risky behavior and ways you can protect yourself and others in the future. In addition, counselors can help you understand the meaning of the test results and tell you about AIDS-related resources in your area.

The CDC National STD and AIDS Hotlines can answer questions about testing and can refer you to testing sites in your area. You can also go to the HIV Testing Sites database for a list of sites in your area. You may call the CDC National STD and AIDS Hotlines 24 hours a day, 365 days a year at:

1-800-342-AIDS (1-800-342-2437)
1-800-AIDS-TTY (1-800-243-7889) TTY
1-800-344-SIDA (1-800-344-7432) Spanish

What about home test kits?

Home test kits are also available as a way to test for HIV infection. Although home HIV tests are sometimes advertised through the Internet, currently only the Home Access test is approved by the Food and Drug Administration. The Home Access test kit can be found at most drug stores. The testing procedure involves pricking your finger, placing drops of blood on a specially treated card, and then mailing the card in for testing at a licensed laboratory. Customers are given an identification number to use when phoning for the test results. Callers may speak to a counselor before taking the test, while waiting for the test result, and when getting the result.

Deciding Where to Go for Counseling and Testing

Depending on where you live, you may have several different counseling and testing options. These options include publicly funded HIV testing centers, community health clinics, sexually transmitted disease (STD) clinics, family planning clinics, hospital clinics, drug treatment facilities, TB clinics, and your doctor's office. In making your choice, you may want to consider these factors:

- If you have been to a particular place for health care before, you may feel more comfortable receiving counseling and testing from staff you know than strangers.

- If the center can provide immune system monitoring and medical care if you are infected with HIV, it might speed up the beginning of your medical treatment.

- Some counseling and testing centers offer special features. For instance, if you use drugs, you can receive counseling, testing and help for addiction at a drug treatment facility.

At some centers, such as doctor's offices or clinics, information about your test result may become part of your medical record and may be seen by healthcare workers, insurers, or employers. Your status may become known to your insurance company if you make a claim for health insurance benefits or apply for life insurance or disability insurance. If any healthcare provider suggests testing you for HIV antibodies, discuss the reasons and the potential benefits before deciding whether or not to take the test.

You can search online or call the CDC National STD and AIDS Hotlines (1-800-342-AIDS) to get the address of places where you can get counseling and testing. Do not go to a hospital emergency room to be counseled and tested. You should go to an emergency room only if you have a health problem that demands urgent attention. Also, do not give blood at a blood donation center as a way to get tested for HIV antibodies. Blood donation centers are not HIV-antibody counseling and testing centers and should not be used as such.

The Process of Counseling and Testing Counseling

You should receive reading materials before you enter a group or private session with a counselor or doctor. He or she might ask why you want to be tested. Your counselor should also ask about your behavior and that of your sex partner(s). This will help you and your counselor determine if testing is appropriate for you. If testing is appropriate, your counselor or doctor should:

- Describe the test and how is done.

- Explain AIDS and the ways HIV infection is spread.

- Discuss ways to prevent the spread of HIV.

- Explain the confidentiality of the test results.

- Discuss the meaning of possible test results.

- Ask what impact you think the test result will have on you.

- Address the question of whom you might tell about your result.

- Discuss the importance of telling your sex and/or drug-using partner(s) if the result indicates HIV infection.

If these questions are not covered, or if you have any other questions, ask them. You should come prepared with questions that have been on your mind. Also ask your doctor or counselor how you will be told of the test result. If your test result is negative, the post-test counselor will talk to you about how to avoid behaviors that will put you at risk for infection.

Informed Consent

You have the right to be fully informed about any medical procedure, to refuse it, or to agree to it. You should be asked to read a statement saying that you have been informed about the HIV-antibody testing procedure, you understand it, and you consent to have it done.

The Blood Test

A small amount of blood will be drawn from your arm, taken to a lab, and tested. The time it takes to get your test results varies in different areas. It can take anywhere from a few days to a few weeks.

The Waiting Period

This period of days or weeks can produce anxiety and tension. Some people decide during this time that they do not want to know their test result and never return to receive it. It is very important that you finish the process and find out the test result in spite of your anxiety.

It is also important that until you return for your result and post-test counseling you act as if you were infected and could transmit the virus. In other words, don't have unprotected sex or don't have sex at all, and don't share needles.

When your result arrives, you may be asked to return to the counseling and testing center to receive the information in person. Everyone tested should receive counseling, whether the result is positive or negative.

Counseling after the Test

Your counselor should tell you your result and, regardless of whether it is positive or negative, how to protect your health and the health of others. He or she will review methods to prevent the spread of HIV.

Type of Tests

The ELISA (Enzyme-Linked Immunosorbent Assay) is a commonly used screening test. It can be performed relatively quickly and easily. If a reactive (so called positive) result occurs, the test is repeated to check the result.

If an ELISA test yields two or more positive results, a different test such as the Western blot is used to confirm these results. The Western blot is more specific and takes longer to perform than the ELISA. Together, the two tests are more than 99.9 percent accurate. Further evaluation can be done if results of repeated ELISA and Western blot tests are unclear.

The Meaning of Your Test Result

Negative Result

A negative result means that no HIV antibodies were found in your blood. Your condition is called seronegative. This usually means you are not infected.

A negative test result does not mean you are immune to HIV. No one is immune to HIV. Even if you test negative, you should take steps to protect your health and the health of your sex and/or drug-using partner(s). Do not engage in behaviors that can transmit HIV. These behaviors include having unprotected sexual intercourse with an infected person or sharing needles or syringes with an infected person. Your post-test counselor will discuss these behaviors with you.

There is a small chance that you may be infected, even though you tested negative. It takes time for the body to develop HIV antibodies after infection. Almost all people develop HIV antibodies within 3 months, but it can take up to 6 months after infection for some persons. If you engaged in behavior that can transmit the virus during the 6 months just before your test, you may be infected but still test negative because your body may not yet have produced antibodies. To be sure, you must be retested at least 6 months after you last engaged in behavior that can transmit HIV.

Indeterminate Result

Once in a while, test results are unclear. The lab cannot tell whether they are positive or negative, even if the test has been performed correctly. If this happens to you, it is important that you discuss this with your counselor or doctor, and, if appropriate, be tested again. A very small number of people may test positive even though they are not infected. These are called false positive results. If you do test positive, you should discuss with your counselor or doctor whether or not retesting a new blood sample is appropriate.

Positive Result

A positive result means antibodies to HIV were found in your blood. This means you have HIV infection. Your condition is called HIV-positive or seropositive. You will most likely develop AIDS, but no one can know when you will get sick. Within 10 years after infection, about half of untreated people have developed AIDS. However, prompt medical care may delay the onset of AIDS and prevent some life-threatening conditions.

If your test result is positive, you should immediately take a number of important steps to protect your health.

- See a doctor, even if you don't feel sick. Ask if this doctor has experience treating people with HIV infection and is familiar with

AIDS and HIV-related issues. Tell the doctor your test result and discuss immune system monitoring and treatment. Monitoring and appropriate medical action are the ways to slow the growth of HIV and to delay the onset of AIDS.

- Take a tuberculosis (TB) test. You may be unknowingly infected with TB. You could become seriously ill if your TB goes undetected. TB can be treated successfully if detected early in your HIV infection.

- Ask your doctor if you should get a flu or other vaccine.

- Enroll in a program to help you stop using drugs, drinking a lot of alcoholic beverages, or smoking. This will help you reduce or stop engaging in behaviors that can weaken your body.

- Consider joining a support group for people with HIV infection. Such support can help you cope with being HIV infected.

You should tell anyone with whom you have had unprotected sex (vaginal, anal, or oral) or shared needles since 1978 that you are (and they may be) infected with HIV. It is especially important that you tell current and recent partners. Health professionals can tell your sex and/or drug-using partner(s) for you or help you tell them yourself. All of your present and past partners should be referred for counseling and testing. If they are HIV positive, prompt medical care may delay the onset of AIDS and prevent some life-threatening conditions. Also, they may unknowingly infect others. You have an important role to play in helping stop the spread of HIV infection.

Telling people about your test result can be a very sensitive matter. You may want to discuss it with your testing counselor. They can assist you in telling your sex or drug-using partners. If you choose to tell your partners yourself, do not make accusations. Be prepared for partners to become upset or hostile. Urge them to be counseled and tested as soon as possible.

What if I test positive for HIV?

If you test positive for HIV, immediate medical treatment and a healthy lifestyle can help you stay well. There are now many drugs that treat HIV infection and AIDS-related illnesses. Prompt medical care may help delay the onset of AIDS and prevent some life-threatening conditions.

You can immediately take a number of important steps to protect your health:

- See a doctor, even if you do not feel sick. Try to find a doctor who has experience in treating HIV.

- Have a TB (tuberculosis) test done. You may be infected with TB and not know it. Undetected TB can cause serious illness, but it can be successfully treated if caught early.

- Smoking cigarettes, drinking too much alcohol, or using illegal drugs (such as cocaine) can weaken your immune system. Cessation programs are available that can help you reduce or stop using these substances.

- Have a screening test for sexually transmitted diseases (STDs). Undetected STDs can cause serious health problems. It is also important to practice safe-sex behaviors so you can avoid getting STDs.

How a Positive Test Result Might Affect Your Life

Being infected with HIV is not only a health matter. It raises financial and social issues as well. One of these issues is insurance. Discuss these issues with a qualified counselor.

Your ability to pay for health care can effect your access to monitoring and treatment. If you do not have health insurance or if you depend upon Medicaid, you may need special assistance to get treatment.

As of 2000, multiple drugs that act to slow HIV have been approved for use in the United States. More drugs are being tested. To find out about experimental treatments, call the AIDS Clinical Trials Information Service (1-800-TRIALS-A, that is, 1-800-874-2572), Monday through Friday between 9 a.m. and 7 p.m. Eastern time. Centers that offer experimental drug treatments for AIDS-related illnesses may not be available everywhere.

Some people who do not understand AIDS may avoid persons who they know are infected with HIV. Some people who are infected have been targets of discrimination in employment, housing, and insurance. Some have been deeply hurt by the reactions of friends and family members. You should be prepared to encounter uncomfortable reactions and to deal with these issues. However, the Americans with Disabilities Act (ADA) can protect you from many forms of discrimination, especially on the job and where you live, and ensure you receive services available to the public. A support group can help you cope with any fears or discrimination.

If I test HIV negative, does that mean that my partner is HIV negative also?

No. Your HIV test result reveals only your HIV status. Your negative test result does not tell you whether your partner has HIV.

HIV is not necessarily transmitted every time a person is exposed to the virus. Therefore, your taking an HIV test should not be seen as a method to find out if your partner is infected. Testing should never take the place of protecting yourself from HIV infection. If your behaviors are putting you at risk for exposure to HIV, it is important to reduce your risks.

Following are answers to some questions you may have about HIV-antibody counseling and testing.

Does it take long to get an appointment to be counseled and tested?

It depends on where you live. Some counseling and testing facilities can schedule appointments very quickly. Others may take a few weeks. Call your local health department to find out.

How much does HIV counseling and testing cost?

Most publicly funded testing sites are free or require only a minimum fee. If you go to your doctor for counseling and testing, the cost may vary. In some areas, it can be more than $200. Ask about the cost beforehand.

When I had a blood test done for my annual physical, to get a marriage license, or to qualify for insurance, was I tested for HIV antibodies?

You should not assume that your blood was tested for HIV antibodies. If you are concerned, ask your healthcare provider specifically if your blood was or will be tested for HIV antibodies.

What if an insurance company wants me to take the test?

An insurance company may require that you be tested for HIV infection if you apply for a health or life policy. The test may be required either to determine if you will be covered or to set up the rate of coverage. You have the right not to take the test. You must choose whether to take the test or find an insurer who will not ask you to do so. If the test is required, you may wish to be tested anonymously or confidentially first.

Will my insurer find out if I test positive?

Your insurer will know you took the test if you pay for the test through insurance. Insurers can find out your test result only if you release it. On some insurance forms, your signature authorizes release of medical records. If you are concerned, do not sign medical release forms unless you know their purpose. You may also choose to be counseled and tested at a facility separate from your health care provider. These facilities include publicly funded testing sites, sexually transmitted disease clinics, and family planning clinics. Search on-line or call your health department or the CDC National STD and AIDS Hotlines (1-800-342-AIDS) to find out the nearest facility that offers confidential counseling and testing.

Does the government keep track of those who test positive?

The U.S. Public Health Services does not record or collect names of people who test positive. The state health departments that do collect names treat this information as highly confidential. Most states have laws against releasing confidential information without permission. Call your state or local health department to find out what the laws are in your state.

My partner tested negative. That means I'm not infected, right?

Your partner's test does not always tell your status. The only way to know whether or not you are infected is to have your blood tested for HIV infection.

Even though I tested negative, why do I have symptoms?

See a doctor about your symptoms. They are most likely caused by something other than HIV infection. Early symptoms of HIV infection can be similar to the symptoms of many other diseases that occur in people who are not infected with HIV. If you test negative and still think you might be infected, consider retesting. If you test negative again, and you have not engaged in behavior that can transmit HIV in the past 6 months, you are probably not infected with HIV.

Can I continue to work if I have HIV infection?

Yes, you can continue to work if you have HIV infection. HIV cannot be spread by contact that does not involve blood, semen, or vaginal secretions. Many years after infection, some people still have no symptoms and continue to work productively. In the later stages of HIV infection, illness may make you too sick to work. It depends on your health and your job duties.

How can I find a doctor who will treat me?

Call your local medical society. They should be able to refer you to a doctor who will help you. For additional help, you can contact a local AIDS organization. The people there may be able to help you find a doctor who is experienced with HIV and AIDS-related issues. For the telephone numbers of these organizations, you can search the online NPIN Resources and Services database or call the CDC National STD and AIDS Hotlines 1-800-342-AIDS; Spanish 1-800-344-7432; Deaf access 1-800-243-7889 (TTY).

Chapter 15

Treatment of HIV Infection: An Overview

When AIDS was first recognized in 1981, patients with the disease were unlikely to live longer than a year or two. Since then, scientists have developed an effective arsenal of drugs that can help many people infected with HIV (human immunodeficiency virus) live longer and healthier lives. The treatment and prevention of HIV is a high priority for the National Institute of Allergy and Infectious Diseases (NIAID). Research supported by NIAID has greatly advanced our understanding of HIV and how it causes AIDS. This knowledge provides the foundation for NIAID's AIDS research effort and continues to support studies designed to further extend and improve the quality of life of those infected with HIV.

What drugs have been developed for HIV infection?

Sixteen drugs have been approved for treating HIV infection. They are called antiretroviral drugs because they attack HIV, which is a retrovirus. Once inside the cell, HIV uses specific enzymes to survive. Antiretroviral drugs work by interfering with the virus' ability to use these enzymes. They fall into two categories.

- **Reverse transcriptase inhibitors** interfere with an enzyme called reverse transcriptase or RT that HIV needs to make

A fact sheet from National Institute of Allergy and Infectious Disease (NIAID), dated January 2002; available online at http://www.niaid.nih.gov/factsheets/treat-hiv.htm.

copies of itself. There are two main types of RT inhibitors and they each work differently.

> *Nucleoside / nucleotide drugs* provide faulty DNA building blocks, halting the DNA chain that the virus uses to make copies of itself.
> *Non-nucleoside RT inhibitors* bind RT so the virus cannot carry out its copying function.

- **Protease inhibitors** interfere with the protease enzyme that HIV uses to produce infectious viral particles.

Table 15.1. Drugs Approved for HIV Infection

Nucleoside/ Nucleotide RT Inhibitors	Non-Nucleoside RT Inhibitors	Protease Inhibitors
abacavir	delavirdine	ritonavir
ddC	nevirapine	saquinavir
ddI	efavirenz	indinavir
d4T		amprenavir
3TC		nelfinavir
ZDV		lopinavir
tenofovir		

Do antiretroviral drugs cure HIV infection?

No, the currently available drugs cannot cure HIV infection. This is because HIV can become resistant to any one drug. Researchers initially attacked this problem by using a combination of antiretroviral drugs to suppress the virus. By combining both RT inhibitors and protease inhibitors, NIAID-supported research groups and drug companies developed the potent and effective combination therapy called highly active antiretroviral therapy or HAART.

Although the use of HAART has greatly reduced the number of deaths due to AIDS, this powerful combination of drugs cannot suppress the virus indefinitely. In addition, while people with HIV are living longer, new medical problems are surfacing. These new problems have not been seen before in people who have been infected with the virus for a long time.

What kind of problems do antiretroviral drugs cause?

People with HIV must take complicated treatment regimens, often taking several drugs on a daily basis. Patients may forget to take their medicine, find the food restrictions difficult to deal with, and may experience unpleasant side effects.

Aside from the complicated dosing regimens, antiretroviral drugs themselves may cause serious medical problems. Metabolic changes are occurring in people with chronic HIV infection. One of these changes causes HIV-associated lipodystrophy syndrome (HIV-LS). This condition results in abnormal fat distribution and cholesterol and glucose abnormalities. Gender and HIV infection itself can influence cell metabolism, making it difficult to distinguish adverse drug effects from the natural progression of the disease.

Some anti-HIV drugs are toxic to mitochondria, the energy-producers in cells. Tissues that require high levels of energy, like muscles and nerves, are most susceptible to the affects of damaged mitochondria. A disrupted mitochondrial energy supply can result in muscle wasting, heart failure, peripheral nerve damage causing numbness and pain, low blood cell counts, swelling and fatty degeneration of the liver, and inflammation of the pancreas. Other more general signs include fatigue, depression, and high lactic acid levels in the blood.

Osteonecrosis, or weakened bones, is another condition that is being seen more frequently in persons with HIV infection that may be a side effect of anti-HIV drugs.

What is NIAID doing to prevent complications from anti-HIV drugs?

To determine which drugs are responsible for HAART-associated toxicities, NIAID supports studies comparing the various drugs, alone and in combination. Strategies to reduce dependence on toxic drug regimens include:

• Using structured treatment interruption (STI) protocols

• Combining immune-based therapies with HAART

• Using studies to compare different dosing schedules, as well as early versus delayed treatment

Researchers also are evaluating combining, switching or avoiding regimens containing agents known to cause specific metabolic toxicities.

Other strategies to minimize toxicity include specific interventions to treat HAART-associated complications. Such interventions include lipid-lowering agents for treatment of blood lipid abnormalities and testosterone supplementation for abdominal obesity in men.

In addition, researchers are following the metabolic effects of various antiretroviral regimens in pregnant women and their infants and in HIV-infected children and adolescents, and include long-term follow up of such patients.

How does research ensure safety?

NIAID supports the development and testing of new classes of antiretroviral compounds or combinations that will be able to continuously suppress the virus with few side effects. Such studies will provide accurate and extensive information about the safety of the new agents and combinations. They will identify potential uncommon, but important, toxicities of newly approved agents. Studies are also underway to assess rare toxicities of older approved agents, especially the results of long-term use.

Through its Multi-center AIDS Cohort Study (MACS) program and the Women's Interagency HIV Study (WIHS), NIAID supports long-term studies of HIV disease in both men and women. Since their inception, these cohort studies have enrolled and collected data on more than 8,000 people. In addition to the information gleaned from this epidemiological gold mine, other studies on the specific metabolic complications of HIV treatment are supported through both the adult and pediatric AIDS Clinical Trials Groups (AACTG and PACTG) as well as through the Terry Beirn Community Programs for Clinical Research on AIDS (CPCRA) program.

Are any new drugs in the pipeline?

The Pharmaceutical Research and Manufacturers Association lists nearly two dozen new anti-HIV drugs now in development. They include new protease inhibitors and more potent, less toxic RT inhibitors, as well as drugs that interfere with entirely different steps in the virus' lifecycle. These new categories of drugs include:

- Fusion inhibitors—drugs that interfere with HIV's ability to enter a cell.

- Integrase inhibitors—drugs that interfere with HIV's ability to insert its genes into a cell's normal DNA.

116

In addition, scientists are learning how immune modulators help boost the immune system's response to the virus and may make the existing anti-HIV drugs more effective. Therapeutic vaccines are also being evaluated for this purpose and could help reduce the number of anti-HIV drugs needed or the duration of treatment.

Chapter 16

Approved Drugs for HIV Infection and AIDS-Related Conditions

This chapter contains a list of drugs approved by the U.S. Food and Drug Administration (FDA) for treatment of HIV infection and AIDS-related conditions. The list contains the name of the company that produces this drug, and the date of approval. More information about HIV/AIDS-related drugs can be found on the FDA's website at http://www.fda.gov.

Approved Drugs

Abacavir (Ziagen)

Glaxo Wellcome

Approved December 17, 1998 to treat HIV-1 in adults and children.

Agenerase (Amprenavir)

Glaxo Wellcome

Approved April 15, 1999 to treat HIV-1 in adults and children.

Alitretinoin (Panretin) gel 0.1%

Ligand Pharmaceuticals

Approved on February 2, 1999 for the topical treatment of cutaneous lesions in patients with AIDS-related Kaposi's sarcoma.

Food and Drug Administration (FDA), February 19, 2002; available online at http://www.fda.gov/oashi/aids/stat_app.html.

Amphotericin B Liquid Complex (Abelcet, ABLC, AmBisome)

The Liposome Company

Approved November 20, 1995 for the treatment of aspergillosis.

Atovaquone (Mepron, 566C80)

Glaxo Wellcome

Approved November 25, 1992 for the treatment of mild to moderate *Pneumocystis carinii* pneumonia (PCP) in patients who are intolerant to Bactrim or Septra.

Approved February 8, 1995 for the treatment of mild to moderate PCP in patients who are intolerant of Trimethoprim-Sulfamethoxazole (TMP-SMX).

Approved January 5, 1999 for the prevention of PCP.

Azithromycin (Zithromax)

Pfizer, Inc.

Approved June 14, 1996 for the prevention of *Mycobacterium avium* complex in persons with advanced HIV infection.

Cidofovir (Vistide, HPMPC)

Gilead Sciences, Inc.

Approved June 27, 1996 for the treatment of AIDS-related cytomegalovirus retinitis.

Clarithromycin (Biaxin, Klacid)

Abbott Laboratories

Approved December 23, 1993 for the treatment of disseminated mycobacterial infections due to *Mycobacterium avium*-intracellulare complex (MAC).

Approved October 12, 1995 for prophylaxis of disseminated MAC in patients with advanced HIV infection.

Daunorubicin-liposomal (DaunoXome)

Nexstar

Approved April 8, 1996 for the treatment of advanced HIV-related Kaposi's sarcoma.

Delavirdine mesylate (DLV, Rescriptor)

Pharmacia & Upjohn

Approved April 4, 1997 for use in combination with appropriate antiretrovirals when therapy is warranted for treatment of HIV infection.

Didanosine (ddI, Dideoxyinosine, Videx)

Bristol Myers-Squibb

Approved October 9, 1991 for treatment of adult and pediatric patients with advanced HIV who are intolerant to or deteriorating on AZT.

September 1992 expanded indication and dosage recommendations reduced.

Approved July 17, 1996 for treatment of HIV infection when antiretroviral therapy is warranted.

Approved October 31, 2000, Videx EC, enteric coated capsule, approved for combination with other antiretroviral agents, as indicated for the treatment of HIV-1 infection in adults whose management requires once-daily administration of didanosine or an alternative didanosine formulation.

Doxorubicin hydrochloride-liposomal (Doxil)

Sequus Pharmaceuticals, Inc.

Approved November 17, 1995 for the treatment of Kaposi's sarcoma in AIDS patients who are intolerant to or have disease progression on prior combination chemotherapy.

Dronabinol (Marinol)

Roxane Laboratories

Approved December 23, 1992 for the treatment of anorexia associated with weight loss in patients with AIDS.

Efavirenz (Sustiva)

DuPont Pharmaceuticals

Approved September 17, 1998 for the treatment of HIV-1 infection, in combination with other antiretroviral agent(s).

Erythropoietin (EPO, Epogen, Procrit)

Amgen

Approved December 31, 1990 for the treatment of anemia related to AZT therapy in HIV infection.

Famciclovir (Famvir)

SmithKline Beecham

Approved June 12, 1998 for the treatment of recurrent mucocutaneous herpes simplex infections in HIV-infected patients.

Fluconazole (Diflucan)

Pfizer, Inc.

Approved January 29, 1990 for the treatment of oropharyngeal and esophageal candidiasis and for the treatment of cryptococcal meningitis.

Approved November 13, 1994 for the treatment of pediatric patients with cryptococcal meningitis and candida infections.

Fomivirsen Sodium Injection (Vitravene intravitreal injectable)

Isis Pharmaceuticals

Approved on August 26, 1998 for the local treatment of cytomegalovirus (CMV) retinitis in patients with acquired immunodeficiency syndrome (AIDS) who are intolerant of or have a contraindication to other treatment(s) for CMV retinitis or who were insufficiently responsive to previous treatment(s) for CMV retinitis.

Foscarnet (Foscavir)

Astra Pharmaceuticals

Approved September 27, 1991 for the treatment of cytomegalovirus (CMV) retinitis in patients with AIDS.

Approved June 16, 1995 for the treatment of acyclovir-resistant mucocutaneous herpes simplex virus infections in immunocompromised patients.

Approved February 1997 for combination therapy with Foscavir and ganciclovir of patients who have relapsed after monotherapy with either drug.

Ganciclovir (IV, Oral)(Cytovene, DHPG)

Syntex

Approved June 23, 1989 (IV) for treatment of cytomegalovirus (CMV) retinitis in immunocompromised patients.

Approved December 22, 1994 (oral) for maintenance therapy for CMV retinitis in some patients.

Approved October 31, 1995 (oral) for prophylaxis of CMV disease.

Ganciclovir (Implant) (Vitrasert)

Chiron Corporation

Approved March 5, 1996 for the treatment of cytomegalovirus retinitis in patients with AIDS.

Immune globulin (IV) (Gamimune N, Gamma Globulin, IGIV)

Bayer Pharmaceutical Division

Approved December 27, 1993 for prevention of bacterial infections in pediatric HIV infection.

Indinavir sulfate (Crixivan, IDV, MK-639)

Merck & Co.

Approved March 14, 1996 for use alone or in combination with nucleoside analogues for the treatment of HIV infection in adults.

Approved December 17, 1998 new 333 mg capsule formulation.

Interferon Alfa-2a (Roferon-A)

Hoffman-La Roche

Approved November 21, 1988 for the treatment of AIDS-related Kaposi's sarcoma in selected patients.

Interferon Alfa2b (Intron-A)

Schering-Plough

Approved November 21, 1988 for the treatment of adult AIDS-related Kaposi's sarcoma.

Approved February 22, 1991 for the treatment of chronic hepatitis C (Non-A, Non-B hepatitis or HCV).

Itraconazole (Sporanox)

Janssen Pharmaceutical

Approved September 11, 1992 for the treatment of histoplasmosis, blastomycosis, and aspergillosis in immunocompromised and non-immunocompromised patients.

Approved March 29, 1994 for the treatment of pulmonary and extra pulmonary aspergillosis in patients who are intolerant of or refractory to amphotericin B.

Approved February 1997 (oral solution) for the treatment of oropharyngeal and esophageal candidiasis.

Kaletra (lopinavir and ritonavir)

Abbott Laboratories

Approved September 15, 2000 for combination with other anti-retroviral agents for the treatment of HIV-1 infection in adults and pediatric patients age six months and older.

Lamivudine (Epivir, 3TC)

Glaxo Wellcome

Approved November 17, 1995 for combination use with AZT as a treatment option for HIV infection in adults and pediatrics patients greater than or equal to 3 months old.

Lamivudine/Zidovudine (Combivir)

Glaxo Wellcome

Approved September 27, 1997 for the treatment of HIV infection in adults and adolescents greater than or equal to12 years old.

Megestrol acetate (Megace, Ovarian)

Mead Johnson Laboratories

Approved September 10, 1993 for the treatment of anorexia, cachexia, or unexplained, significant weight loss in patients with AIDS.

Nelfinavir mesylate (NFV, Viracept)

Agouron Pharmaceuticals

Approved March 14, 1997 for the treatment of HIV infection when antiretroviral therapy is warranted in adults and pediatrics greater than or equal to 2 years old.

Nevirapine (Viramune, BI-RG-587)

Boehringer Ingelheim Pharmaceuticals, Inc.

Approved June 24, 1996 for use in combination with nucleoside analogues for the treatment of HIV-infected adults experiencing clinical and/or immunologic deterioration.

Paclitaxel (Taxol)

Bristol Myers-Squibb Pharmaceutical Research Institute

Approved August 4, 1997 for the second-line treatment of AIDS-related Kaposi's sarcoma.

Pentamidine (aerosolized) (NebuPent)

Fujisawa

Approved June 15, 1989 for the prevention of *Pneumocystis carinii* pneumonia.

Rifabutin (Ansamycin, Mycobutin)

Adria Laboratories

Approved December 23, 1992 for the prevention of *Mycobacterium avium* complex in patients with advanced HIV.

Ritonavir (Norvir, ABT-538)

Abbott Laboratories

Approved March 1, 1996 for use alone or in combination with nucleoside analogues for the treatment of HIV infection.

Approved March 14, 1997 for the use of alone or in combination with nucleoside analogues for the treatment of HIV infection in selected patients.

Approved June 29, 1999 soft gelatin, 100 mg capsule.

Saquinavir mesylate (Invirase [hard gel capsule], SQV)

Hoffmann-La Roche

Approved December 7, 1995 for combination use with nucleoside analogues for the treatment of advanced HIV infection in selected patients.

Approved November 7, 1997, Fortovase, soft gel capsule.

Somatropin rDNA (Serostim)

Serono Laboratories

Approved August 23, 1996 for the treatment of AIDS-wasting and cachexia.

Stavudine (d4T, Zerit)

Bristol Myers-Squibb

Approved June 17, 1994 for the treatment of adults with advanced HIV infection who are intolerant to or deteriorating on approved therapies.

Approved January 4, 1996 for the treatment of adults with HIV infection who have undergone prolonged treatment with AZT.

Approved September 6, 1996 for the treatment of pediatrics with HIV infection who have undergone prolonged prior AZT therapy.

Sulfamethoxazole/Trimethoprim (Bactrim when combined with Trimethoprim; Septra when combined with Trimethoprim; SMX)

Glaxo Wellcome

Approved June 23,1981 for the treatment of *Pneumocystis carinii* pneumonia (PCP).

Approved January 7,1994 for the prevention of PCP.

Trimethoprim/Sulfamethoxazole (Bactrim when combined with Sulfamethoxazole; Septra when combined with Sulfamethoxazole; SMX)

Hoffmann La-Roche

Approved June 23, 1981 for the treatment of *Pneumocystis carinii* pneumonia (PCP).

Approved January 7, 1994 for the prevention of PCP.

Trimetrexate glucuronate (with Leucovorin)(Neutrexin, TMTX)

U.S. Bioscience

Approved December 17, 1993 for the treatment of moderate to severe *Pneumocystis carinii* pneumonia when intolerant or refractory to TMP/SMX or when TMP/SMX is contraindicated.

Trizivir (fixed-dose combination of Ziagen (abacavir/ABC), Retrovir (zidovudine/AZT), and Epivir (lamivudine/3TC))

Glaxo Wellcome

Approved November 14, 2000 for the treatment of HIV in adults and adolescents. Trizivir is not recommended for treatment in adults or adolescents who weigh less than 40 kilograms because it is a fixed-dose tablet.

Valcyte (oral valganciclovir HCL)

Roche Laboratories

Approved March 29, 2001 for the treatment of cytomegalovirus (CMV) retinitis in patients with acquired immunodeficiency syndrome (AIDS).

Viread (tenofovir disoproxil fumarate)

Gilead Sciences

Approved (accelerated) October 26, 2001 for treatment of HIV-1 infection in combination with other antiretroviral medicines. Viread is the first nucleotide analog approved for HIV-1 treatment. Nucleotides are similar to nucleoside analogs, and block HIV replication in the same manner.

Zalcitabine (ddC, Dideoxycytidine, HIVID)

Hoffmann-La Roche

Approved June 19, 1992 for combination use with AZT for the treatment of selected patients with advanced HIV disease. This approval was based on the accelerated approval regulations.

Approved August 5, 1994 for monotherapy treatment of advanced HIV for those aged more than 13 years who are intolerant to or have disease progression on AZT.

Zidovudine (Azidothymidine, AZT, Retrovir, ZDV)

Glaxo Wellcome

Approved March 19, 1987 for the treatment of adult AIDS, or symptomatic HIV and CD4 less than or equal to 200.

September 28, 1989 in syrup formulation

January 1990, decreased recommended dosage.

February 2,1990 in intravenous dosage form.

March 1990 for use in early symptomatic HIV disease and in asymptomatic HIV infection where there is evidence of impaired immunity.

May 3, 1990 for the treatment of pediatric HIV infection (ages 3 months to 12 years).

August 8, 1994 for the prevention of perinatal transmission in HIV+ pregnant women between 14 and 34 weeks gestation and for newborns of HIV+ mothers.

Chapter 17

Protease Inhibitors

HIV is a virus that goes through many steps during its life cycle. Once HIV infects a human cell, the virus uses proteins and chemicals inside that cell to make more copies of itself. Protease is a chemical, known as an enzyme, that HIV needs in order to make new viruses. Protease inhibitors (PIs) block the protease enzyme. When protease is blocked, HIV makes copies of itself that can't infect new cells. Studies have shown that protease inhibitors can reduce the amount of virus in the blood and increase CD4 cell counts. In some cases these drugs have improved CD4 cell counts, even when they were very low or zero.

The biggest news and the greatest benefits to people with HIV came when protease inhibitors (PIs) were discovered and made into anti-HIV treatments. When people started taking them in combination with other drugs, the number of people who became ill from opportunistic infections, or died from AIDS, dropped by about 70%.

However, studies have also shown that these effects can wear off over time. This happens because HIV makes more of itself all the time. Each new HIV virus that gets made may be slightly different than the one it made before. The new protease that the virus has made may resist the drugs that worked for viruses with the older type of protease. This is what scientists call drug resistance.

A Simple FactSheet from the Simple Facts Project, a program of the AIDS Treatment Data Network, © 2002 AIDS Treatment Data Network, reprinted with permission. Available online at http://www.atdn.org/simple/protease.html.

When this happens, other protease inhibitors usually become less effective as well.

The best way to avoid drug resistance is to stop or reduce HIV production in the body. The less HIV made in the body, the less chance of a virus created that's resistant to anti-HIV drugs. To keep HIV levels as low as possible, it's recommended that protease inhibitors be taken in combination with at least two other anti-HIV drugs. This is called Highly Active Anti-Retroviral Therapy or HAART. Studies have shown that when certain protease inhibitors are combined, the anti-HIV effect is increased, which can help prevent or overcome resistance. This is called protease boosting. Some doctors will order a drug resistance test to determine a patient's resistance profile, in order to decide the best drug combination to use.

There are six FDA approved protease inhibitors so far, they are: amprenavir (Agenerase), indinavir (Crixivan), lopinavir/ritonavir (Kaletra), ritonavir (Norvir), saquinavir (Fortovase), and nelfinavir (Viracept). Atazanavir (Zrivada) is the seventh protease inhibitor still under development. It is expected to be approved soon.

How Are They Taken?

Protease inhibitors are pills that need to be taken at least twice a day. It's very important to stick to the exact dose and schedule for taking a protease inhibitor. That way, you keep enough protease inhibitor in your body to block HIV. Make sure to find out how the protease inhibitor should be taken, for example, on an empty or full stomach. For anyone with HIV, a thorough medical check-up is a good idea before starting protease inhibitor treatment.

What Are the Side Effects?

Five years of HAART did not produce the hoped for cure, but these drugs have helped many people to greatly improve their health. Unfortunately, long-term side effects have become an especially difficult problem. Every PI has a common menu of possible side effects that you may experience. Some people experience none of them. Others have a very hard time tolerating the drugs.

Diabetes: There is a government warning about protease inhibitors causing high blood sugar and diabetes. Symptoms to watch out for include increased thirst and hunger, unexplained weight loss, increased urination, fatigue, and dry, itchy skin. These symptoms usually show up 10-11 weeks after starting the protease inhibitor.

Lipodystrophy: Another side effect being reported with HAART combinations are problems with how your body absorbs fats and other nutrients. The symptoms can include high levels of a type of fat called cholesterol, and other fats known as triglycerides. High blood fat levels can make you feel very tired, and generally ill. Other symptoms are a swollen belly, big breasts, loss of weight in the face so you look very thin, and loss of muscle in the arms and legs. These side effects have been given the name lipodystrophy. One of the most serious lipodystrophy-related problems is high level of fats (cholesterol and triglycerides) in the blood. High levels of fats in the blood can increase the risk of heart attacks and pancreatitis. Due to these risks, it's important to have your cholesterol and triglyceride levels checked regularly if you're taking protease inhibitors.

Many doctors now recommend you be given another test that measures how much fat is in your blood. The test should be done before starting HIV treatment, and at least every three months afterwards. The test is called a fasting lipid test. The fasting part means you don't eat about 12 hours before you take the test. You should keep to a low fat diet if the results of the test are high. A nutritionist can help make sure there's very little fat in your diet. If you're at serious risk for heart disease because of things like smoking or existing heart problems, you may have to stop taking the HIV drugs you're on. After a while of not taking any anti-HIV drugs, your doctor may want you to try a different combination.

Liver Toxicity: Other less common side effects caused by protease inhibitors include increases in liver function tests, which can indicate toxicity to the liver. Anyone taking a protease inhibitor should have his or her liver function closely monitored. Blood tests can be done that check the health of the liver and other organs. These tests look for problems, such as hepatitis infections, that could effect how the protease inhibitors work, or increase the chance of side effects. Protease inhibitors can make hepatitis worse, so it's important to know if you have hepatitis B and/or C before starting a protease inhibitor.

Keep in mind that in order for protease inhibitors to be effective, they need to be taken on time, and at the right dose. It is important to tell your doctor if you are having trouble sticking to schedule because of side effects. There are ways to manage these side effects. Your doctor may reduce the dose, or switch you to another drug.

Drug Interactions

Protease inhibitors can affect the absorption of other drugs by the body. These are called drug interactions. Your health care provider should go over any potential drug interactions with you when starting a protease inhibitor. It may be necessary to change or alter the dose of certain medications to make sure that the protease inhibitor can work properly. Some herbs and supplements, such as St. John's Wort and garlic supplements, can affect the level of protease inhibitors in your blood. You should always tell your health care provider if you are taking herbs and supplements.

The Simple Facts Project is a program of The Network. If you need help finding out whether or not a specific drug or therapy is covered by private or public insurance, contact The Network at 212-260-8868 or 800-734-7104 (In New York). This information does not intend to promote or endorse any specific treatment for any health related condition.

Chapter 18

Highly Active Antiretroviral Therapy (HAART)

HIV drugs are used to slow the reproduction of the virus, thus slowing the progression of HIV disease to AIDS.

There are three classes of FDA-approved antiretroviral drugs: Nucleoside/Nucleotide Reverse Transcriptase Inhibitors (NRTIs), Protease Inhibitors (PIs), and Non-Nucleoside Reverse Transcriptase Inhibitors (NNRTIs).

The recommended treatment for HIV is a combination drug treatment called Highly Active Anti-Retroviral Therapy, or HAART. HAART combines three or more HIV drugs.

The recommended HAART regimens are efavirenz plus two NRTIs, indinavir plus two NRTIs, nelfinavir plus two NRTIs, ritonavir and indinavir plus two NRTIs, ritonavir and lopinavir plus two NRTIs, or ritonavir and saquinavir plus two NRTIs.

In general, taking only two drugs is not recommended, because the resulting decrease in viral load is temporary for most people. For most people, taking only one antiretroviral drug is also not recommended (the exception is pregnant women, who may be offered zidovudine alone or with other drugs to reduce the risk of passing HIV to their infants).

If you are pregnant or considering becoming pregnant, there are additional drug considerations.

Excerpted from "HIV and Its Treatment: What You Should Know," 2nd Edition, 2002 HIV/AIDS Treatment Information Service (ATIS), now part of AIDSinfo; available online at http://aidsinfo.nih.gov/other/hivtr.pdf.

You may experience negative side effects (drug toxicities) when you take HIV drugs. Some of these side effects are serious, even life threatening, so you may have to change drugs.

Possible side effects of HAART:

- liver problems

- diabetes

- fat maldistribution (lipodystrophy syndrome)

- high cholesterol

- increased bleeding in patients with hemophilia

- decreased bone density

- skin rash

Side effects that may seem minor, such as fever, nausea, and fatigue, can mean there are serious problems. You should always discuss any side effects you are having with your doctor.

What are some of the negative side effects of HAART?

In general, your viral load is the most important indicator that your treatment is working. Other important factors are:

- your CD4+ T-cell count,

- your recent health history, and

- results of physical examinations.

Your viral load should be tested 2-8 weeks after you start treatment. If your drugs are working, your viral load should decrease. It should continue to decrease as you continue to take your medication.

Throughout HIV treatment, your viral load should be tested every 3-4 months to make sure your drugs are still working. If your viral load is still detectable within 4-6 months after starting treatment, you should talk to your doctor about possibly changing your HIV drugs.

How fast, or how much, your viral load decreases may depend on other factors as well. These factors can include your baseline viral load and CD4+ T-cell count (before starting therapy), whether you have used HIV drugs before, whether you have any AIDS-related illnesses, and how closely you have followed (adhered to) your therapy. Talk to your doctor if you are concerned about the results of your viral load tests.

CD4+ T-cell counts may also help show how well your medications are working. After starting HIV treatment, your CD4+ T-cell count should be tested every 3-6 months. Talk to your doctor if you are concerned about your CD4+ T-cell counts.

How will I know if my treatment is working?

There are several reasons for this. Two of the more important reasons are drug intolerance and drug failure. Drug intolerance means that there are side effects that make it difficult to take the drugs as directed. Drug failure means that the drugs are not working well enough to decrease your viral load. You should ask your doctor to explain why any changes are needed in your treatment.

If the reason is drug intolerance, your doctor may change the drug(s). He or she may replace one or more of your current drugs with different ones of the same strength and class. If the reason is drug failure, your doctor should change all your drugs to new ones you have never taken. If you have been taking three drugs, and all three drugs cannot be changed, then at least two drugs should be changed. Using new drugs will reduce the risk of developing drug resistance.

Before changing HIV drugs, you should talk to your doctor about:

- all HIV drugs you have taken before,

- the strength of the new drugs your doctor recommends,

- possible side effects of the new drugs,

- how well you will be able to follow (adhere to) the new treatment, and

- the number of HIV drugs remaining that you have not yet used.

You may be eligible to participate in a clinical trial using new drugs or treatment strategies. For more information about participating in a clinical trial, ask your doctor, or visit the National Library of Medicine's ClinicalTrials.gov web site at: http://www.ClinicalTrials.gov.

My doctor wants to change my drug therapy. Why would this be recommended?

If you are pregnant or want to become pregnant, you must consider the general risks and benefits of drug treatment to both you and your child. Some of the drugs (such as efavirenz and hydroxyurea) should be avoided, because they may cause birth defects if taken early in pregnancy.

The effects of other drugs are not yet known. It is important for you to talk with your doctor before and during your pregnancy so that you can decide together on the best treatment for you and your baby.

If you are already taking HIV drugs, talk to your doctor about the potential risks and known benefits to your baby if you continue drug treatment during your pregnancy. No one can tell you for sure if your baby will be born HIV-infected. But there are steps you can take to reduce the risk of transmitting HIV to your baby. Talk to your doctor. He or she should offer you zidovudine (AZT) therapy by itself or with other HIV drugs. AZT has been shown to reduce the risk of passing HIV to your baby by almost 70%. The additional HIV drugs will treat your infection and may provide extra protection for your baby.

However, the possible side effects for you and your baby of using multiple drugs during pregnancy are not well understood. Other actions to help protect your baby include getting regular prenatal care and adhering to your HIV drug treatment plan.

Adherence

Adherence refers to how closely you follow—or adhere to—a prescribed drug treatment plan. It includes your willingness to begin treatment and your ability to take medications (antiretroviral drugs) as directed. Studies have shown that adherence may be difficult for many patients, including people who are HIV-infected as well as those who take daily medications for other diseases. Adherence is a major issue in HIV treatment for two reasons.

First, adherence affects how well the HIV drugs decrease viral load. When you skip medication doses even once, the virus has the opportunity to make copies of itself more rapidly. This makes it difficult for the drugs to be effective. Other factors that may affect treatment effectiveness include your baseline viral load and CD4+ T-cell count, whether you have any AIDS-related illnesses, and whether you have used HIV drugs before.

Second, adherence to HIV treatment is very important to prevent drug resistance. Studies have shown that when you skip doses, you may develop strains of HIV that are drug-resistant. This may leave you with fewer treatment options if your viral load does not decrease. Because drug-resistant strains can be transmitted to others, it has serious consequences for anyone with whom you engage in risky behavior.

Is adherence important for HIV treatment?

There are several reasons why many patients have difficulty adhering to an HIV treatment plan. One reason is that HIV treatment plans are very complicated. Studies have shown that many people may have difficulty adhering to even simple treatment plans. Yet HIV treatment may involve taking 25 or more pills each day. In addition, some HIV drugs must be taken on an empty stomach, while others must be taken with meals. This can be difficult for many people, especially those who are sick or experiencing HIV symptoms. Also, HIV-infected patients may need to continue their treatment regimens for a long time, perhaps for their entire lives.

HIV-infected patients have reported other reasons for poor adherence, including unpleasant side effects (like nausea), sleeping through doses, traveling away from home, being too busy, feeling sick or depressed, or simply forgetting to take their medications.

If you are considering HIV treatment, there are several steps you can take before starting treatment to help adherence:

1. Play an active role in your treatment plan. Ask your doctor to describe all your treatment options, including known benefits and potential risks of starting treatment. Also ask your doctor to explain any side effects or other problems that may result from the drugs. It is important for you to understand the goals of treatment and to be fully committed to the treatment plan.

2. Talk to your doctor about personal issues that may affect your adherence. Studies have shown that adherence may be harder for people dealing with substance abuse or alcoholism, unstable housing, mental illness, or major life crises. Adherence also may be harder for other patients who:

    do not have advanced HIV disease,

    must follow very complex treatment regimens, and

    have had problems taking medications in the past.

    Talk to your doctor about these or any other issues that you feel may affect your adherence to a treatment plan.

3. Consider a dry run—practice your treatment plan using vitamins, jelly beans, or mints. This will help you determine ahead of time which doses might be difficult.

4. After you and your doctor decide on a treatment plan, ask for a written copy. This should list each medication, when and how much to take, and if it must be taken with food or on an empty stomach. It also should include your doctor's name and phone number and the date of your next visit.

5. Most important, talk to your doctor about how to tailor your treatment plan to your lifestyle. For example, many patients find it helpful to identify things they normally do at the times they will be taking their medication. Studies have shown that patients who arrange their medication schedule around their daily routines adhere to their treatment plans better than those who do not. Activities that may be helpful in remembering your medication schedule include getting out of bed in the morning, taking a child to school, leaving work, or watching a TV show. If you decide take medicine as part of your regular activities, make sure you take it before the activity, not after.

Your commitment to a treatment plan is critical. Talk to your doctor about any concerns you may have about starting—and adhering to—your treatment plan. For many people, it takes two or three office visits to feel comfortable about starting HIV treatment.

I've started HIV treatment. What can I do to help my treatment work?

As described previously, the effectiveness of your treatment will depend on several factors. One of the most important things you can do is find a strategy that works for you. This will help you adhere to your treatment plan as closely as possible. Here are some other ways to improve your adherence:

1. Use daily or weekly pill boxes or egg cartons to organize your medications. Some people find it helpful to count and set out a week's worth of medications at a time, with one space of the pill box or egg carton for each part of the day. Try to do this at the same time each week, for example, every Sunday night at bedtime.

2. Use timers, alarm clocks, or pagers to remind you when to take your medication. For each dose, try to take your medication at the same time each day.

3. Try keeping your medications where you will take them. Some patients find it helpful to keep their first morning dose next to the alarm clock or coffee pot. Others like to keep backup supplies of their medications at their workplace or in their briefcase.

4. Keep a medication diary. Try writing the names of your drugs on a 3 x 5 card or in your daily planner, and then check off each dose as you take it. You might want to try write yourself a reminder in your calendar or planner to take any doses that are difficult to remember.

5. Plan ahead for weekends, holidays, and changes in routine. Many studies have shown that weekends are a serious problem for adherence. Decide ahead of time how you will remember to take all of your doses. Also, if you are going on vacation, traveling on business, or changing jobs, write out a plan for remembering your medications.

6. Develop a support network. This may include family members, friends, or coworkers who can remind you to take your medication. Some patients also find it helpful to join a support group for people living with HIV infection.

7. Don't run out of your medication. Contact your doctor or clinic if your supply will not last until your next visit. Tell your doctor if you are having any problems related to your medication, including those below:

    Side effects. If you are experiencing any side effects, tell your doctor what they are, and when you notice them.

    Skipped doses. Do not be afraid to admit to skipped doses. Your doctor knows that some people do have difficulty taking each dose as prescribed. If you have skipped doses, tell your doctor which medication(s) you skipped, and when.

    Difficulty taking your medication as directed. If you are supposed to take medications on an empty stomach, or with food, and this is difficult for you, tell your doctor. If there is a time of day that is difficult for you to take your dose, tell your doctor this.

    Your treatment plan interferes with your lifestyle. If you feel your treatment plan is too complicated or unrealistic for you to follow, talk to your doctor about other options you may have. It is important that you tell your doctor right away about any problems you are having with your treatment plan. Your doctor needs this information to help you get the most out of your treatment plan and provide workable options, if necessary.

Summary

Managing HIV infection is complicated, but new treatments can both improve the quality of your life and extend your life. To help you successfully manage your health, remember these tips:

- See your doctor regularly (every 3-6 months or as advised) to check your CD4+ T-cell count, viral load, and general health, and to discuss treatment and prevention strategies.

- Be an active part of your health care team. Tell your doctor about any problems, and be sure your doctor explains concepts to you in such a way that you clearly understand your options.

- Educate yourself. The more you know about HIV infection and HIV treatment, the better you will be able to judge the risks and benefits of your options.

Chapter 19

Attacking AIDS with Cocktail Therapy

It was spring of 1996 when Beth Bye says she returned from the dead. The Wisconsin woman hadn't actually died, but with her body ravaged in the late stages of AIDS infection, she had run out of options, and death was, indeed, near. AIDS-related dementia and blindness had crept in—signs that her doctor told her meant time was short. She made funeral arrangements and considered moving to a hospice for her remaining days.

Then, as if to say not so fast, medical science handed her another option. New drugs called protease inhibitors, first approved in 1995, were about to revolutionize the treatment of patients infected with the AIDS virus. These drugs usually are taken with two other drugs called reverse transcriptase inhibitors. The combined drug cocktail has helped change AIDS in the last three years from being an automatic death sentence to what is now often a chronic, but manageable, disease.

Within two months of beginning the triple cocktail treatment, also known as highly active antiretroviral therapy (HAART), Bye's viral load—a measure of new AIDS virus produced in the body—dropped to undetectable levels. Her red and white blood cell counts normalized, an important sign that the immune system was starting to work again. Suddenly she could do simple things she had long given up,

"Attacking AIDS with a 'Cocktail' Therapy: Drug Combo Sends Deaths Plummeting," by John Henkel, *FDA Consumer* magazine, July-August 1999; available online at http://www.fda.gov/fdac/features/1999/499_aids.html.

such as walk the dog for 2 miles. Bye, now 40, was even able to return to her teaching job and currently works 30 hours a week. "My recovery was like being on death row and getting that last minute pardon from the governor," she says.

This so-called "Lazarus Effect," named for the biblical figure who was raised from the dead, has occurred with many AIDS patients who take the triple therapy. "It returns many who were debilitated and dying to relatively healthy and productive life," says Richard Klein, HIV/AIDS coordinator for the Food and Drug Administration's Office of Special Health Issues.

Many health experts, in fact, credit the powerful HAART therapy with helping the domestic AIDS death rate to drop by 47 percent in 1997, the last year for which figures are available. Other factors have contributed as well, says Anthony Fauci, M.D., director of the National Institute of Allergy and Infectious Diseases. "It is also likely that increased access to care, our growing expertise and experience in caring for HIV-infected people, and the decrease in new HIV infections in the late 1980s due to prevention efforts are partly responsible for the reduction in HIV-related deaths we are seeing today."

In 1997, for the first time since 1990, AIDS fell out of the top 10 causes of death in the United States, dropping from 8th to 14th place, according to the national Centers for Disease Control and Prevention. By 1998, about 16,000 people were still alive who would have died the previous year if AIDS mortality had continued at its former rate. Still, about 40,000 new infections occur yearly.

A One-Two Punch

So far, the combination HAART treatment is the closest thing medical science has to an effective therapy. The key to its success in some patients lies in the drug combination's ability to disrupt HIV at different stages in its replication. Reverse transcriptase inhibitors, which usually make up two drugs in the HAART regimen, restrain an enzyme crucial to an early stage of HIV duplication. Protease inhibitors hold back another enzyme that functions near the end of the HIV replication process. The combination can be prescribed to those newly infected with the virus, as well as AIDS patients.

FDA approved the first drug specifically to combat HIV and AIDS in 1987. Commonly known as AZT (zidovudine), it is in the family of reverse transcriptase inhibitors called nucleoside analogs. Others in this class include ddI (didanosine), ddC (zalcitabine), D4T (stavudine), 3TC (lamivudine), and most recently Ziagen (abacavir). In 1997, FDA approved Combivir, a mixture of AZT and 3TC that allows patients to reduce the number of pills needed, which can be upwards of 20 a day for certain drug combinations.

Viramune (nevirapine), the first reverse transcriptase inhibitor in a class called non-nucleoside analogs, was approved in 1996. The following year, FDA approved a related drug, Rescriptor (delavirdine). In 1998, a third drug in this class, Sustiva (efavirenz) was approved.

Protease inhibitors, the last part of the triple cocktail, have only been on the market about three years. FDA approved the first one, Invirase (saquinavir), in late 1995. Others approved since include Norvir (ritonavir), Crixivan (indinavir), Viracept (nelfinavir), and Agenerase (amprenavir). Viracept was the first of its class to be labeled for use in children and adults. Norvir and Agenerase are now approved for children as well. FDA also has approved Fortovase, a new formulation of saquinavir that comes in a soft gelatin capsule that allows more drug to be absorbed into the body than the earlier version.

Regimen Has Drawbacks

Though the use of protease inhibitors with other AIDS drugs has had a drastic impact on the health of HIV and AIDS patients, there are drawbacks. For example, the HAART treatment is not an AIDS cure, says FDA's Klein. Though HIV, the virus that causes AIDS, may not be detectable in the blood following successful HAART treatment, experts generally feel that the virus is still present, lurking in hiding spots such as the lymph nodes, the brain, testes, and the retina.

"The improved sense of well-being, and the belief that lower viral load means they will not transmit the virus, has translated, in some communities, to a lapse in certain prevention practices," Klein says. He adds that this is dangerous because infected people, even with diminished viral counts, can spread the virus.

Another concern is that the combination therapy, besides being very expensive, requires a much more complicated treatment regimen. "Patients need to stay aware of and adhere to their dosing schedule," says Klein. "If not taken on a strict regimen, protease inhibitors can result in the emergence of HIV strains that are resistant to treatment." Numerous studies also have shown that viral load can rapidly rebound to high levels if patients discontinue part or all of the triple therapy regimen.

AIDS treatments may interact with many commonly prescribed drugs. For example, Pfizer Inc. plans to label its impotence drug Viagra to warn of possible interactions with certain protease inhibitors, which appear to raise levels of Viagra in the blood.

AIDS drugs also may prompt onset of diabetes or a worsening of existing diabetes and hyperglycemia (high blood sugar), along with increased bleeding in people with hemophilia types A or B.

Some patients on triple therapy have experienced a type of weight redistribution where face and limbs become thin while breasts, stomach or neck enlarges. Some have nicknamed the appearance of fat deposits at the back of the shoulders buffalo hump. Fat deposits in the midsection are sometimes called Crix belly, after the drug Crixivan, "although it has been seen in people taking all approved protease inhibitors," says Klein.

Research is currently under way to determine if protease inhibitors cause a permanent change in fat metabolism. "There is considerable concern over the long-term effects for patients," says Klein, including the possibility that the cholesterol increases in some patients who experience fat redistribution could increase the risk for cardiovascular complications such as strokes or heart attacks. FDA has asked each of the makers of protease inhibitors to study these abnormalities.

AIDS-Related Illnesses

Because AIDS patients have suppressed immune systems, they can fall prey to certain illnesses that people with healthy immune responses don't get, or get only very rarely. One common such illness is *Pneumocystis carinii* pneumonia (PCP), which can be life-threatening. Treatments to prevent PCP are NebuPent (aerosolized pentamidine), a fine mist inhaler, and drugs such as Bactrim and Septra that contain both trimethoprim and sulfa. Mepron (atovaquone) is approved for treating mild-to-moderate PCP in pregnant women and patients who cannot tolerate standard treatment. Neutrexin (trimexetrate glucoronate) also is approved for pregnant women and for moderate-to-severe PCP when given with leucovorin (folinic acid).

Cytomegalovirus retinitis is a potentially severe AIDS-related eye infection that can lead to blindness. Approved treatments include ganciclovir, marketed as Cytovene in oral dosage and as Vitrasert as an implant, Foscavir (foscarnet), and Vistide (cidofovir).

For *mycobacterium avium*, an infection that before AIDS was almost always confined to patients with severe chronic lung diseases such as emphysema, FDA has approved Biaxin (clarithromycin), Mycobutin (rifabutin), and Zithromax (azithromycin).

Kaposi's sarcoma (KS) is a type of AIDS-related cancer that causes characteristic purple or pink skin tumors that are flat or slightly raised. Intron A (human interferon-alpha), doxorubicin liposome injection, or daunorubicin citrate liposome injection can be used to treat KS. Panretin, a topical gel, also is approved for treating certain types of KS lesions.

AIDS wasting syndrome involves major weight loss, chronic diarrhea or weakness, and constant or intermittent fever for at least 30 days. Approved treatments include Marinol (dronabinol), Megace (megestrol), and Serostim (somatropin rDNA for injection).

Pregnant Women and Children

In 1998 recommendations, the Public Health Service Task Force stated that the decision to take anti-HIV drugs during pregnancy should be made by the pregnant woman after her health care-provider has explained benefits and risks. There are some compelling reasons to take the drugs. For example, an HIV-positive pregnant woman who takes AZT after the first trimester decreases the chance of the baby being born with HIV. Studies show that AZT taken according to a strict regimen decreases by nearly 66 percent the odds of infecting the newborn.

The task force says women should consider delaying therapy until after the 10th to 12th week of pregnancy, after the fetus's organs have gone through their most rapid development. This delay may minimize any adverse effects of AZT on fetal development, but it needs to be balanced with the health of the mother and possible transmission of HIV to the fetus.

Most children with HIV became infected from their mothers near the time of birth. This means that for many babies, treatment can be started soon after birth. Federal guidelines recommend that all HIV-infected children younger than 1 year and all HIV-infected children of any age with symptoms of HIV infection or evidence of immune suppression be treated with anti-HIV drugs. For HIV-infected children with no symptoms, therapy can be deferred if risk of disease is considered low based on viral load and immune status.

Triple combination therapy can be used for all HIV-infected infants, children and adolescents treated with HIV drugs. Infants during the first six weeks of life who have been exposed to HIV but whose HIV status is unknown can be treated with AZT as sole therapy. Infants diagnosed with HIV while receiving AZT alone should be switched to combination therapy.

In the Future

Though the AIDS death rate has dropped drastically, and educational efforts aimed at curbing the number of new HIV infections have had a small impact, experts say the next hurdles are to develop an AIDS-preventive vaccine and to create new therapies, such as ones that would effectively treat AIDS patients when drug-resistant strains of HIV develop. On both fronts, promising efforts are in progress.

For example, NIAID is conducting trials of three novel HIV vaccine approaches. One trial is testing a vaccine applied to spots such as the moist tissues lining the urinary and reproductive tracts. This is because most HIV infections, such as those acquired through sexual exposure, are transmitted across these mucosal sites. Researchers theorize that a vaccine that prompts the body to produce antibodies at these sites may have a protective effect against the AIDS virus.

Another vaccine approach is using common *Salmonella* bacteria to deliver HIV proteins in a way that may trigger the body to produce a better immune response. A third study is examining a cancer drug, GM-CSF, to determine its effect on stimulating immunity. NIAID also is experimenting with a vaccine approach that neutralizes antibodies to HIV, which then bind to the virus in a way that may prevent it from infecting cells.

A new class of drugs called fusion inhibitors has been shown in early trials to block HIV's entry into cells, which may keep the virus from reproducing. These drugs hold particular promise for patients whose HIV viral loads have rebounded to elevated levels because the virus strains they carry have become resistant to triple combination therapy. Researchers reported at the 6th Conference on Retroviruses and Opportunistic Infections in February 1999 that one fusion inhibitor, T-20, significantly lowered virus amounts in a group of patients with drug-resistant viral strains.

Other therapies aimed at eradicating the virus that remains after successful combination treatment include drugs targeted at bolstering the immune system such as IL-2 (Interleukin-2) and G-CSF (Neupogen).

Though these and other potential treatments may individually or in combination help wipe out AIDS sometime in the future, what's really needed, says NIAID's Fauci, are types of drugs that don't yet exist. "These agents would ideally be potent, inexpensive, relatively nontoxic even after prolonged periods, active against viral strains resistant to currently available agents, and easy to administer."

Speeding AIDS Drug Approvals

With the emergence of AIDS, FDA put into place a program in the late 1980s that allows promising therapies for life-threatening illnesses to be approved conditionally before all necessary studies are completed. A key goal is to make treatments available to desperately ill patients who might have to wait years under the formal clinical trial and drug approval system for the same drug to be marketed.

Under the agency's accelerated approval regulations, a drug can be marketed without studies that show direct effects on clinical disease progression or death. Instead, FDA relies on surrogate markers, such as viral load, which are laboratory measurements intended to reliably predict a drug's ultimate clinical benefits.

FDA has three requirements for accelerated approval:

- The surrogate must have a reasonable certainty of predicting actual future clinical benefit.

- The drug's sponsor must complete post-marketing studies, providing the required data to verify the drug's clinical benefit.

- The sponsor must prove clinical benefit in a timely manner or FDA will revoke the accelerated approval.

Chapter 20

Pulsed Therapy and Structured Interruptions of AIDS Treatment

Research has begun on two new strategies for long-term treatment of HIV disease. Although both theories involve taking people off treatment in some way, they have different goals and expectations. These two strategies are known as pulsed therapy and structured interruptions of treatment (sometimes called drug holidays).

The first approach, best described as a form of pulsed or intermittent therapy, aims at stimulating a stronger immune response against HIV. Researchers speculate that this will empower the person's own immune system sufficiently to control HIV replication without the continual use of anti-HIV drugs.

The second approach, a type of structured interruption of treatment (or drug holiday), can take a number of different forms. On one level, it can be little more than taking people off therapy, after successfully suppressing HIV for a year or more, to simply see what happens. On another level, it assumes that measurable HIV replication will begin again sometime after treatment is stopped but tests whether this is necessarily bad. This kind of therapy interruption compares the benefits and drawbacks of constantly staying on drug therapy against those of periodically taking time off.

While each approach is getting serious attention as a research project, no one suggests that we know enough to recommend these

From Project Inform: "Pulsed Therapy and Structured Interruptions of Treatment," © 1999 Project Inform, from *PI Perspectives,* April 1999. Reprinted with permission. For more information, contact the National NIV/AIDS Treatment Hotline, 800-822-7422, or visit our website, www.projectinform.org.

strategies for anyone's personal use. They are experimental strategies whose overall harm or benefits are simply not yet known.

Pulsed Therapy

The pulsed therapy approach assumes that people should always maintain viral loads below the limit of detection to be healthy. In this approach, a person who has been treated since the earliest stage of HIV infection is taken off all therapy once viral load remains undetectable for some pre-determined length of time, perhaps six months to a year or longer.

While off therapy, the person would be carefully monitored for the return of measurable virus. If and when viral load becomes detectable again, the person would be put back on aggressive antiviral therapy. Typically, this results in the rapid disappearance of measurable viral load for the second time. After another pre-determined period on therapy, the cycle is repeated—taking the person off therapy while monitoring for return of measurable viral load.

An interesting phenomenon has been noted in a few cases of pulsed therapy, either as a structured experiment or simply as a matter of patient choice. The first time a person went off therapy, viral breakthrough (return of measurable levels of viral load) occurred after a relatively short period of time, ranging from a few days to a few weeks. After restarting therapy, viral load plummeted again, below the level of detection. Then after staying on therapy for varying periods, they stopped therapy a second time. This time, viral load remained undetectable for considerably longer than the first time, despite the lack of continued treatment.

A few people who cycled on and off therapy twice now have no return of measurable viral load, while off therapy, for periods ranging from 6-21 months. Researchers theorize that each cycle of pulsed therapy led to a progressively longer period for the body to fully control viral replication without the help of anti-HIV drugs. In a few cases, people treated with two or more cycles of pulsed therapy have been able to control viral replication with continued therapy for as long as two years (and still counting).

It is hard to draw any clear conclusions from these observations since nearly every patient involved has done something differently from others. For the most part, they were simply choosing to go on and off therapy for personal reasons. They each had varying times on and off therapy, and varied considerably in how quickly they returned to treatment when viral load reappeared. Researchers carefully studied the consequences of their actions, and were understandably surprised by the results.

What Is Going on Here?

Researchers at the Aaron Diamond AIDS Research Institute and the RIGHT group have proposed a theory: the periods in which a person is taken off therapy and viral replication is allowed to resume may be beneficial. They suspect that the returned viral load is acting somewhat like a vaccination. HIV is aggressively presented to the immune system once again, stimulating a more powerful immune response.

This makes some sense because we know when people use antiviral drugs that work for them, HIV is no longer being presented to the immune system. In theory this might allow the normal immune response against HIV to gradually decline. In turn, occasional interruptions in therapy as proposed here may reintroduce HIV into the immune system, thus stimulating a renewed immune response against the virus.

If this is indeed what is happening—and there is promising initial evidence that it is—this approach might be used to help people become less dependent on anti-HIV drugs and more reliant on their immune systems for control of HIV. Such a response might resemble the tiny percentage of HIV-infected people known as long-term nonprogressors. Such people appear able to control HIV replication without the use of anti-HIV drugs and usually have an abnormally strong immune response against HIV, very similar to that being seen in people who are treated with pulsed therapy.

Still, pulsed therapy is far more theory than reality at this point. The only thing known for sure is that a few people seem to respond in a way that resembles the theory, including the widely discussed Berlin patient reported by Dr. Franco Lori's group. Studies of many more people are necessary and already planned.

Even proponents of pulsed therapy warn that there is no evidence so far that this will work in typical, chronically infected people. The case reports noted have all come from people who began anti-HIV treatment extremely early after initial HIV infection. Such people are known to still be able to mount strong HIV-specific immune responses.

In contrast, many people with more typical chronic HIV infection (where treatment began six months or later after initial infection) frequently show no evidence of this kind of immune response. Some researchers believe that the natural capacity for this immune response is lost fairly early in the course of HIV infection. Thus, for now, the only realistic target for pulsed therapy research is in people treated from the earliest or acute stage of HIV infection, also known as primary infection.

Structured Interruptions of Treatment

The second strategy, structured interruptions of treatment, responds to a different set of goals and concerns. It assumes that people taken off therapy are likely to see a rebound of measurable viral load. What's not clear is how high the rebound will go and whether it will initially shoot up and then fall back to some lower set point level (a viral load level lower than that seen before the person began therapy).

In this approach, people are not automatically put back on antiviral therapy the minute viral load becomes detectable again. Instead, a person stays off drugs for awhile despite the presence of detectable viral load. So then a question begs to be asked: Is the harm caused by a return of measurable viral load a greater or lesser danger than constant therapy, and all the attendant side effects and development of resistance to treatment?

What is the harm of constant therapy? Even if viral load remains undetectable for long periods, there are many possible long-term consequences to constant therapy. The risks of cumulative side effects and tissue damage are perhaps the greatest concerns. This encompasses problems such as fat redistribution (lipodystrophy), high cholesterol and triglycerides, diabetes, heart disease and liver problems. These come in addition to the side effects of the older generation of drugs, such as pain in the feet, legs, and/or hands (peripheral neuropathy), red and white blood cell suppression (anemia), pancreatitis, rash, etc.

Suppression of viral load through anti-HIV drug therapy can produce improvements in overall health and prolonged survival. The challenge is to find the best possible balance—to get the most from therapy without experiencing its down sides which includes the emergence of possible long-term negative effects. For some, this might mean periodically structuring time away from the drugs, for the body to recover from side effects. Some researchers believe that periodic interruptions of therapy may not only be possible, but necessary to help people live out a normal lifetime with HIV disease.

Since we only have about three years of experience treating people with today's potent three-and four-drug combinations, it remains highly uncertain just how long people will tolerate constant use of the drugs. Few researchers, however, have enough confidence in the drugs to believe that people could use them continually for the 20-50 years needed to live a normal life span.

In contrast, we have long known that most people can tolerate long periods of untreated HIV infection without irreparable harm. On the average, people using no treatment at all can usually go for roughly ten years without progression to AIDS. For some, this period is longer, for others it's shorter. Part of the goal of treatment interruptions is to give some of this time back to people, in effect letting them coast along with the virus for awhile. They then return to medication only when signs of disease progression become apparent. Similar strategies employing periodic interruptions of treatments are routinely used for other chronic illnesses that require long-term therapy.

Another concern caused by constant therapy is simply the weariness it causes people. The longer many people remain on constant therapy the more likely they begin to miss doses or take short unstructured drug holidays. That can do harm by encouraging development of viral resistance. If structured interruptions of treatment can be offered to people in ways that are unlikely to hasten resistance, with little or no downside, commitment to proper use of therapy may increase during those periods when people use the drugs. This approach offers a compromise, but hopefully one that will provide long-term benefits.

Since we know that short or frequently repeated drug holidays speed the development of viral resistance, the model here focuses not on casual weekend holidays but rather on carefully planned, structured interruptions. An additional benefit already demonstrated in initial studies is that the break from drugs may help a person's virus increase its sensitivity to some previously used drugs. In theory, this might restore their ability to use drugs to which they had developed resistance. This would greatly enhance their options for future therapy.

Structured Treatment Interruption Research Programs

Treatment interruption programs are just beginning and plan to start with people who have undetectable levels of HIV for six months to a year or more (though this may change after more experience is gained). After that, the approaches vary. Four are outlined following.

1. Some plan to take people off therapy and monitor them to measure the immune and viral responses when therapy is stopped. Here, a person will usually restart anti-HIV therapy

as soon as viral load again becomes measurable. The hope is that this may identify the people in whom this approach would be safest and most productive. Such a study is underway at the National Institutes of Health (NIH).

2.   Some plan to take people off therapy and monitor them, but not immediately restart therapy if viral load reappears. These seek to determine whether viral load will rise to and maintain a high level peak, perhaps even higher than before the person started therapy. Or they may find that such a peak is followed by a gradual reduction back to a lower and stable level (a set point). If viral load comes back down to a modest set point, researchers may choose to withhold therapy as long as viral load remains stable with no major decline in CD4+ cell counts. Such a study is planned at the NIH.

3.   Still another approach, perhaps targeted to people with more advanced disease or those who have developed resistance to most available drugs, will keep people off therapy, regardless of viral load, for a period of a few to several months. At some fixed point, anti-HIV therapy will be restarted. The hope of this approach— sometimes called a washout period—is to see if the time off allows the virus to return to its natural state (often called wild-type virus) and regain sensitivity to previously used drugs. Restarting therapy with a mix of old and new drugs might then kick off another long period of effective viral control.

4.   Another approach takes people off therapy for a fixed period, such as two to six months or longer. This is done to let the body heal from drug side effects and rest from the constant rigor of daily therapy. Either at a fixed point in time, or after some permissible level of CD4+ cell count decreases and/or viral load increases occur, the person may be put back on anti-HIV therapy. If successful, this could theoretically be repeated over many years or even throughout a normal lifetime. The hope is that the mix of time on and off therapy might lead to the increased tolerance of therapy and the longest possible life expectancy for HIV-infected people, short of an outright cure.

Commentary

Many important new strategies for the use of anti-HIV therapy must be tested. Until recently, most research focused only on how well individual drugs worked over a period of a few months to a few years. Many people are already coming to the end of the hope offered by such narrowly defined, product-driven strategies.

Today, new strategy research on pulsed therapy or structured interruptions of treatment may well be what's needed. Such research may extend our knowledge of how to best get HIV-infected people through a lifetime, or at least well into the new millennium and not just the next few years. These strategies should not yet be considered recommendations for medical practice, nor should the fact that they are being tested encourage people to try them on their own.

We don't have enough information to know whether these procedures will help people live longer or instead cut precious time off what a person has left. If we knew, there would be no need for the research. The right approach is in the context of well-designed studies. Self experimentation seldom leads to knowledge, since there is never a way to know whether what happens to an individual is due to the strategy or drugs used, or whether it is a mere coincidence.

The next several months will see a rash of new strategy studies asking whether and how it might be possible for people to get off therapy, at least temporarily. The more people who volunteer to participate in these studies, the sooner we will know what is and isn't possible.

Chapter 21

Alternative and Complementary Treatments for AIDS

What Are Alternative Therapies?

A health treatment that does not fit into standard western medical practice is called alternative or complementary. This includes many different therapies:

- Traditional healing practices such as ayurveda, Chinese acupuncture, and Native American healing
- Physical therapies such as chiropractic, massage, and yoga
- Homeopathy or herbs
- Energy work such as polarity therapy or Reiki
- Relaxation techniques, including meditation and visualization

Some doctors don't like alternative therapies. They think there hasn't been enough research on them. They think that patients always do better if they use western medicine. Other physicians like to use alternative therapies along with western medicine. They think alternative therapies can reduce stress, relieve some of the side effects of antiviral drugs, or have other benefits.

"Alternative and Complementary Therapies," Fact Sheet Number 700, © 2002 New Mexico AIDS InfoNet; reprinted with permission. Fact sheets are regularly updated; check the website, www.aidsinfonet.org for the most recent information.

How Many People Use Alternative Therapies?

Alternative therapies are very popular. In the United States, over 70% of people with HIV have used some kind of an alternative therapy. Many people use them regularly. Some health insurance plans pay for therapies such as chiropractic or acupuncture.

Are They Safe?

Alternative therapies can have dangerous side effects. The words "natural" or "non-drug" do not guarantee safety. The FDA (Food and Drug Administration) does not approve dietary supplements or monitor their safety or contents. Some herbs can lower blood levels of antiviral drugs. Consumers need to be careful when using alternative therapies.

Do They Really Work?

It is difficult to find good information on alternative therapies. Get as much information as you can before using them. Try to find out:

- When and how was this therapy developed?
- How does it work?
- Are there any articles or studies of this therapy?
- Are the therapists trained, certified, or licensed?
- Are there any known side effects or other risks?

Sometimes this information is truly not available. However, if it seems like people don't want to answer your questions, be extra careful. You might be dealing with a health fraud.

Why Aren't There More Studies of Alternative Therapies?

Most research tests treatments for a particular disease or condition. Every patient gets exactly the same treatment.

Specific Disease or Condition: Some alternative therapies treat the whole person, not an illness. They might restore harmony, balance, or normal energy flow. Acupuncturists, for example, use the pulse to see if your body's energy is out of balance. Acupuncture for people with

HIV is based on their individual energy pattern, not on their HIV. Therapies like this might help people with HIV, but they are not designed to treat HIV.

Standardized Treatment: Few alternative therapies are standardized. Different brands of herbs can have different amounts of the active ingredient, although more standardized products are being made. Chiropractic, acupuncture, and other therapies are not standard. They are adjusted for each patient. Research is very difficult when treatments are not standardized.

Safe Treatments: The FDA wants to know that a therapy is safe before they test how well it works. Even if a treatment has been used for many years with no reports of health problems, the FDA requires a scientific study to show that it is safe.

Paying for the Study: Scientific research is very expensive. The makers of alternative therapies often cannot afford to pay for scientific studies. The government prefers to pay for studies of western medical drugs because they appear to be more effective. Patents allow manufacturers to make large profits that help pay for research. However, most alternative therapies cannot be patented.

Despite these barriers, some alternative therapies have been carefully studied. Often, this research has been conducted outside the U.S. and might not be considered by the FDA.

Working with Your Doctor

Tell your doctor as much as possible about how you want to deal with your HIV infection. Tell your doctor about all the therapies you use. This is very important if you have any kind of bad reaction to a medicine that you are taking. There could be some alternative therapies that you should not use together with your HIV medications.

Check your doctor's attitude and knowledge on alternative therapies. Ideally, your doctor can keep an open mind and help you evaluate alternative therapies that interest you.

The Bottom Line

Most people with HIV use some kind of alternative or complementary therapy. Some alternative therapies can be dangerous. Others are safe to use. Some have been carefully studied and can improve your health.

It is difficult to study alternative therapies. Find out as much as you can before you start using an alternative therapy. Let your doctor know about the therapies you are using.

Chapter 22

Marijuana and AIDS Treatment

Smoking marijuana has become a popular treatment for weight loss associated with HIV. Claims about its effectiveness are based largely on individual experience rather than data from studies. A synthetic form of the most active ingredient in marijuana, called dronabinol (Marinol), is approved by the U.S. Food and Drug Administration. It is available by prescription for treating HIV-related weight loss (anorexia), as well as treating nausea for people undergoing chemotherapy.

This chapter describes the different forms of marijuana that are currently available. Although many report that marijuana improves their appetite and weight, it's important to consider possible health risks before using it. Also, the only studies that have been conducted to assess the impact of medical marijuana in people with HIV have been very small and very brief. Much of the following information comes from research on people who do not have HIV disease.

Buyers Clubs and the Law

Marijuana is an illegal substance, yet buyers clubs have been established in some areas to provide the drug for people using marijuana for medical purposes. These clubs provide a safe, place to buy

From Project Inform: "Medical Marijuana," © 2002 Project Inform, reprinted with permission. For more information, contact the National NIV/ AIDS Treatment Hotline, 800-822-7422, or visit our website, www.projectinform.org.

marijuana. Even though they are illegal under federal law, some cities like San Francisco have local laws permitting them to operate. Some even have programs that provide medical marijuana free or at reduced cost to people with limited incomes.

Legislation was approved on a public vote in California that allows physicians to prescribe marijuana for some medical conditions. HIV-associated wasting is one of four conditions in the legislation. While some healthcare providers have voiced concern over the safety of marijuana smoking, many providers have also been impressed with positive results in weight gain, mood and quality of life in their HIV-positive patients who use medical marijuana.

Safety Concerns

There are many possibly harmful effects from smoking marijuana, just as there would be from inhaling almost any other form of smoke. Most of the studies citing these effects were conducted many years ago, and conflicting reports can often be found among all of them. Many people question whether political motives may have influenced early studies of marijuana. For people living with HIV, the largest safety concerns when using marijuana are the affects on:

- immune function,
- lung complications (particularly with smoked marijuana),
- hormones, and
- mental state.

Immune Function

Marijuana and/or its psychoactive ingredient THC have been reported to suppress many immune functions. These include the function of cells important in controlling infections commonly seen among people living with HIV. Marijuana may also increase your risk for certain infections, including herpes and a variety of other bacterial, viral and fungal infections. Some of these infections may result in increased HIV levels. None of this, however, has been clearly documented in HIV-positive people.

Some research suggests that marijuana has no significant effect—good or bad—on the immune system of people living with HIV. Studies from the Multicenter AIDS Cohort Study evaluating outcomes in 1,662 HIV-positive users of psychoactive drugs (marijuana, cocaine,

LSD, etc.) found that none of the drugs were linked to a higher rate of HIV disease progression or loss of CD4+ cell counts. Of the men who took part in the study, 89% reported using marijuana in the preceding two years. A recent study, presented in 2000, examined the short-term impact of marijuana, dronabinol or placebo on HIV levels, CD4+ cell count and HIV levels. After twenty-one days, the use of marijuana did not appear to have harmful affects. Much longer-term studies are needed before concluding that marijuana use is either safe or unsafe for people living with HIV, however.

Lung Complications

Research comparing the effects of tobacco and marijuana smoking on the lungs shows that marijuana smoke can be harmful. Smoking marijuana increases the risks of lung complications, may worsen asthma and may increase the risk of lung cancer over and above smoking tobacco.

Another possible harmful effect of smoking marijuana is that it may cause lung infections. In particular, a fungus sometimes found in marijuana called *aspergillus* is thought to be the cause of possible infections. This infection has sometimes been seen in people with advanced HIV disease.

Some recommend putting marijuana in the microwave for ten seconds to kill any fungus that might be growing on it. The exact time needed to kill the fungus will vary depending on the oven settings, the quantity and moisture content of the marijuana, and the wattage of the microwave. There are no standards for this, but in general, smaller microwave ovens put out less power and would therefore require longer cooking times to kill a fungus.

Recent studies suggest that smoking marijuana may also decrease the ability of cells in the lung to destroy *candida* and bacteria. *Candida* is the fungus responsible for candidiasis, a common condition in people living with HIV. People living with HIV who smoke marijuana may be at higher risk for lung complications. This particular effect might be minimized or eliminated by baking and eating marijuana (as in pot brownies and cakes)—rather than smoking it.

Impact on Hormones

Many men with HIV experience low testosterone levels during the course of HIV infection. Women may also experience lowered testosterone levels and changes in other hormones, both of which may be contributing factors in many menstrual irregularities seen in women living with HIV. Studies in animals and humans show that marijuana may further lower the levels of hormones, including testosterone. This information is important to people with HIV as lowered testosterone levels are associated with AIDS-related wasting. Marijuana could cause or worsen this condition, possibly leading to the necessity of testosterone replacement therapy.

Mental Status

The question of the neurological (change in mental status) effects of marijuana has been addressed by several studies in recent years. Marijuana use has been shown to have short-term impact on a person's ability to think, learn, judge and perform tasks. Moreover, marijuana use has short-term effects on memory. It's less clear if marijuana has any long-term effects on mental status or mood. It is also less clear whether the effects noted are perceived as good or bad by those who experience them. Some people feel smoking marijuana offers relief from depression, while others say it increases their anxiety levels.

Marijuana's Impact on Appetite

Extensive research on how smoked marijuana affects appetite has been conducted, although much of it was published 20 to 50 years ago. Anecdotal accounts of increased food intake have always been reported by marijuana smokers—the so-called munchies. The quality of the food (candy bars and chips vs. vegetables, fruits and protein) and quality of the weight gain (fat vs. muscle) needs to be considered.

Overall, studies suggest that people using marijuana eat more but the food they eat is generally snack food, like cookies and junk food. They also exercise less and sleep more, all of which contributes to weight gain.

It's not at all clear that this kind of weight gain, that consists more of body fat than of lean muscle, will benefit the overall health and longevity of a person with HIV-related wasting. However, if medical marijuana is combined with a comprehensive nutritional and weight maintenance program, as well as exercise, it may prove useful. Because of these concerns, it is important that evaluating the medical effects of marijuana not be limited to measuring weight gain, as this may lead to false conclusions about its value.

When considering all the safety factors associated with marijuana use, it's important to weigh these factors against the harm being done by wasting. What may sound harmful to a healthy person may seem irrelevant to another when compared to the alternatives they face.

Oral THC Versus Marijuana

The oral drug, dronabinol (Marinol), was approved in 1992 for use in treating anorexia in people with HIV-related wasting. The active ingredient in dronabinol is THC, which is one of the main psychoactive agents in marijuana and the chemical that makes someone feel "stoned." For treating HIV-related weight loss, THC probably helps as an appetite stimulant, in the same way people who are "stoned" get the munchies.

People who use dronabinol have mixed experiences. Some report a minimal drug effect while others experience far too much euphoria or feeling "stoned." This is because of the variability in how the oral drug gets into the bloodstream, or perhaps to an individuals' point of view and how they feel about such sensations. Smoking marijuana, or using edible forms of it, may be a more efficient way to get THC throughout the body. People who have tried both forms say that they are better able to control how "stoned" they get by smoking or eating marijuana and thus prefer it over the pill formulation.

Other Possible Uses for Medical Marijuana

For people living with HIV, marijuana may have other uses besides stimulating the appetite. Some research and reports of people's personal experiences support the notion that marijuana/THC can help treat nausea and vomiting. The exact reason why it works is unknown. Dronabinol is approved to ease nausea in people undergoing chemotherapy. Marijuana, therefore, may be a realistic alternative for people who don't benefit from standard anti-nausea medication. This could be an important benefit because so many people report difficulties with nausea when using anti-HIV therapies.

Marijuana has been shown to be an effective treatment for general pain associated with illness or serious injury. As with nausea, how marijuana relieves mild pain is not known. New studies suggest that marijuana may have anti-inflammatory effects.

The Future of Medical Marijuana

A recent report from the Institute of Medicine (IOM) of the U.S. National Academy of Sciences stated that certain chemicals found in marijuana may help manage certain conditions in some people, but that marijuana smoke, like tobacco smoke, is harmful. Though there is an oral medication (dronabinol) that is supposed to mimic the desired effects of smoking marijuana, many people prefer to smoke or eat marijuana in its natural form.

In an attempt to copy the effects of inhaling marijuana while eliminating the risks involved with smoking, some researchers are looking at the use of a vaporizer (or inhaler) for smokeless inhalation. Though not included in this IOM report, other sources indicate that a vaporizer is now readily available. This device heats marijuana to a certain temperature to release active chemicals without setting the dried plant on fire. Since this has only been around for a short time, it is not known how effective it is in delivering the drug. However, early results seem promising.

Overall, medical marijuana research will likely shift from study of the crude plant material to research and eventually drug development of chemicals derived from marijuana. This has already occurred with isolating THC and the development of dronabinol.

What currently holds back more studies of marijuana (or chemicals associated with marijuana) and its effects on the body is a complex matter. Aside from the obvious political concerns, research scientists are not given much incentive to work on marijuana and its derived chemicals. Namely, funding is scarce from government and private sources, and there is concern that the fruits of research will not be made public because of the controversial nature of the drug. Additionally, many researchers feel their reputations may be affected by working with marijuana because of its status as a street drug and controlled substance.

Nevertheless, more research related to marijuana could benefit many people, especially those living with HIV. There are indications that substances present in marijuana can stimulate appetite, relieve pain and stop nausea. So, research that leads to uncovering the chemicals responsible for these effects and uncovering the best way to deliver them to the body could prove helpful. And though research may not eliminate all the safety concerns associated with medical marijuana, it may make this therapy a more realistic alternative for many people.

Buying and Access

- Dronabinol is available by prescription through hospitals and pharmacies.

- Medical marijuana buying, selling and use is illegal in most of the United States.

- There are a limited number of buyer's clubs, providing a safe environment for people to buy medical marijuana. Some have programs that offer medical marijuana free or at reduced cost for people in need. The best buyer's clubs operate with the community oversight and accountability of a well-run non-profit agency.

- Not all buyer's clubs are ethical or conduct business in the best interest of people living with HIV. Buyer beware, and be aware of your options in your local area.

The Bottom Line

Medical Marijuana

- Medical marijuana may be useful in promoting appetite for people with HIV-related anorexia.

- Marijuana may also be useful in managing nausea and may help relieve pain.

- A synthetic form of an active ingredient in marijuana, dronabinol (Marinol) is approved by the FDA for treating HIV-related weight loss and for managing nausea associated with the use of chemotherapy.

Pros

- Dronabinol is FDA-approved and legally available by prescription through hospitals and pharmacies.

- People who have tried both dronabinol and medical marijuana contend that they are better able to control drug effects with medical marijuana.

- Some limited studies suggest that marijuana doesn't have negative long-term impact on HIV disease and measures of immune health, like CD4+ cell counts.

Cons

- Dronabinol has absorption problems and individuals' claim difficulty in controlling the drug effect (feeling too "stoned").

- Medical marijuana is not legally available to many people. Third-party payers, like insurance and Federal programs, do not cover its cost.

- Marijuana and its active ingredient THC has been shown in some studies to suppress immune function.

- Smoked marijuana increases the risk of lung infections and complications.

- Marijuana may be contaminated with insecticides, pesticides, fungus and/or bacteria. Ingesting these could have mild-to-severe health consequences. (Some claim that microwaving marijuana for ten seconds on high may decrease risks associated with fungus contamination.)

- Marijuana/THC has short-term impact on mental status. Long-term effects are less clear.

- Some studies suggest that marijuana/THC may decrease testosterone levels.

- It is unknown if marijuana interacts with anti-HIV drug therapies, increases HIV replication or negatively impacts HIV disease progression.

Part Three

Complications Associated with AIDS

Chapter 23

Cryptosporidiosis (Crypto)

Crypto (full name is cryptosporidiosis) is a disease caused by a microscopic parasite (a type of germ). It causes diarrhea, stomach cramps, and fever. You get crypto by putting anything in your mouth that has been in contact with the feces (solid waste, bowel movement) of a person or animal infected with crypto. You can help keep crypto out of your mouth by:

- washing your hands

- practicing safer sex

- not swallowing water when you swim

- washing and cooking your food

- drinking only safe water

What is cryptosporidiosis?

Cryptosporidiosis (krip-toe-spo-rid-e-O-sis) is a disease caused by a microscopic parasite, or germ, called *Cryptosporidium parvum.* Both the disease and the germ are often called crypto.

"You Can Prevent Crypto (Cryptosporidiosis): A Guide for People with HIV Infection," National Center for HIV, STD and TB Prevention, Centers for Disease Control and Prevention (CDC), updated March 2001; available online at http://www.cdc.gov/hiv/pubs/brochure/oi-cryp.htm.

What are the symptoms of crypto?

Most people who get crypto have watery diarrhea, stomach cramps, an upset stomach, or a slight fever. In some people, the diarrhea can be so severe that they lose weight. Other people with crypto have no symptoms.

How does crypto affect someone with AIDS or HIV?

Crypto can cause severe illness for a long time in people infected with HIV. You can die from crypto. If your CD4 (sometimes called T-helper) cell count is below 200/mm3, crypto may give you symptoms for a long time. If your CD4 cell count is above 200, your symptoms may last only 1 to 3 weeks. But even after your symptoms go away, you may still be carrying crypto. If you are carrying crypto, even without symptoms, you can give it to someone else. Also, your own symptoms may come back if your CD4 cell count later drops below 200.

How is crypto spread?

Crypto is spread in the feces (bowel movements). Crypto is not spread by contact with blood. You can get crypto by putting anything in your mouth that has touched the feces of a person or animal infected with crypto. You can't tell by looking whether something has been in contact with feces, so you need to be aware of what these things may be.

Things likely to be contaminated with feces are:

- Skin around a person's anus (especially important with sex partners)
- Animals (skin or fur of farm animals and household pets)
- Cat litter boxes
- Children in diapers
- Clothing, bedding, toilets, or bed pans used by someone with diarrhea
- Dirt (in gardens, yards, parks, etc.)
- Uncooked or unwashed food
- Water (for bathing, swimming, or drinking)

Can crypto be treated?

Yes, but no drug cures it. Anti-retroviral medicines (HIV medicines) will decrease or get rid of crypto symptoms. However, crypto is usually not cured and may come back if the immune system gets weaker. Some drugs, such as paromomycin (par-o-mo-MI-sin) may reduce the symptoms of crypto. If you suspect you may have crypto, talk with your health care provider. If you have diarrhea, you might become dehydrated. Drink plenty of fluids to prevent dehydration. Oral rehydration drinks work well.

How can I protect myself from crypto?

Wash your hands.

- Wash your hands often with soap and water. Always wash your hands well after you touch anything that might have had contact with even the smallest amounts of human or animal feces (see previous list). Even if you wear gloves when you handle these things, you should still wash your hands well when you finish.

Practice safer sex.

- People with crypto may have it on their skin in the anal and genital areas, thighs, and buttocks. You can't tell by looking if someone has crypto, so you may want to protect yourself in these ways with any sex partner:

  Avoid rimming (kissing or licking the anus). Rimming is likely to spread crypto even if you and your partner wash well before.

  Always wash your hands well with soap and water after touching your partner's anus or rectal area.

Be careful around animals.

Farm animals. If you visit a farm, try to avoid touching the animals, especially young animals (calves and lambs). Be sure not to directly touch the feces from any animal. After the visit, wash your hands well with soap and water before you prepare food or put anything in your mouth. Have someone who does not have HIV clean your shoes. If you must clean your shoes yourself, wear disposable gloves and wash your hands well after taking off the gloves.

Household pets. Most domestic animals (dogs, cats, birds) are safe as household pets. However, avoid contact with pets that may have crypto. Pets most likely to have crypto include:

- Puppies or kittens younger than 6 months
- Dogs or cats with diarrhea
- Stray pets

Have someone who does not have HIV clean litter boxes or cages. If you must do the cleaning yourself, wear disposable gloves and wash your hands well with soap and water after taking off the gloves. Have any new puppy or kitten younger than 6 months or any pet with diarrhea tested for crypto.

Be careful when swimming or using hot tubs.

Do not swallow water when you swim or use a hot tub. Crypto may be present in fresh water, salt water, or even swimming pool water. Protect yourself and others—do not swim or use public hot tubs if you have diarrhea. Crypto is not killed by the amount of chlorine used in swimming pools, hot tubs, and at water parks.

Wash and/or cook your food.

The outsides of vegetables and fruits may have crypto on them. Washing removes crypto from the surface, and cooking kills crypto.

- Wash all vegetables or fruit you will eat raw. If you can, peel fruit before eating.
- Cook food whenever possible. Cooked food and processed or packaged foods should be safe if, after cooking or processing, the food is not handled by someone with crypto.

Drink safe water.

- Do not drink water straight from lakes, ponds, rivers, streams, or springs.
- Do not drink tap water without boiling it if the public health department announces that tap water may not be safe for drinking.
- You may choose to take extra steps to lower the risk of getting crypto from tap water. These steps may take time and may cost

money, so you may want to talk about these with your doctor. If you take these extra steps, you should do so all the time, not just at home. Also, remember that water and ice from a refrigerator ice maker and drinks made at a fountain are often made with tap water.

The following are ways to be sure your water is safe:

- Boil the water. Boiling is the best way to kill crypto. Heat the water at a rolling boil for 1 minute. After it cools, put it in a clean container, seal it with a lid, and store it in the refrigerator. Use this water for drinking, cooking, or making ice. Clean containers and ice trays with soap and water before use. Do not touch the inside of them after cleaning.

- Distill the water. You can also remove crypto from your water by using a home distiller. These devices use heat to remove crypto. Store distilled water the same way you would store boiled water.

- Filter the water. Filters trap crypto from the water flowing through them. You must replace filter cartridges regularly and properly or the filter will fail. Have someone who does not have HIV change the filter cartridges for you. If you change the cartridge yourself, wear gloves and wash your hands well with soap and water when done. Filters may not remove crypto as well as boiling does because even good filters may let some crypto through. Not all home water filters remove crypto.

The following filters are most effective for removing crypto:

- Filters that work by reverse osmosis

- Filters that have absolute 1-micron pores

- Filters that meet National Sanitation Foundation (NSF) Standard #53. Contact NSF for a list of Standard 53 Cyst Filters.

- Drink bottled water. Bottled water from a protected well or protected spring is less likely to contain crypto than bottled water from a river, stream, or lake; but you cannot be sure it is safe. Any bottled water that has been distilled or treated by one or more of the methods listed under filter the water should be safe.

- Take extra care when traveling. Poor water treatment and food sanitation in developing countries may increase your risk for getting crypto. Take the same precautions you would at home. Avoid especially food and drink from street vendors, uncooked foods, tap water, and unpasteurized drinks. Talk with your health care provider about other advice on travel abroad.

Chapter 24

Cytomegalovirus (CMV)

CMV infection is very common; between 50 and 85 percent of all Americans have CMV by age 40. In people with HIV, CMV can cause retinitis (ret-in-I-tis), which can cause blindness. You can take steps to reduce your chance of infection with CMV and to protect yourself from CMV-related diseases.

What is CMV?

CMV, or cytomegalovirus (si-to-MEG-a-lo-vi-rus), is a virus that is found in all parts of the world. For someone with HIV or AIDS, CMV can cause retinitis (blurred vision and blindness), painful swallowing, diarrhea, and pain, weakness, and numbness in the legs.

How is CMV spread?

CMV spreads from one person to another in saliva (spit), semen, vaginal secretions, blood, urine, and breast milk. You can get CMV when you touch these fluids with your hands, then touch your nose or mouth. People can also get CMV through sexual contact, breast-feeding, blood transfusions, and organ transplants.

"You Can Prevent CMV (Cytomegalovirus): A Guide for People with HIV Infection," National Center for HIV, STD and TB Prevention, Centers for Disease Control and Prevention (CDC), updated September 1999; available online at http://www.cdc.gov/hiv/pubs/brochure/oi_cmv.htm.

How can I protect myself from CMV?

You may already have CMV. However, you can take steps to avoid CMV, such as:

- washing your hands frequently and thoroughly
- using condoms
- talking to your doctor if you expect to receive a blood transfusion. Most blood banks don't screen blood for CMV.

If you work in a day care center, you should take these special precautions:

- wash your hands thoroughly after contact with urine or saliva
- avoid oral contact with saliva or objects covered with saliva (such as cups, pacifiers, toys, etc.)
- talk with your doctor about whether you should continue to work in a day care center.

How do I know if I have CMV?

A blood test can tell you if you have CMV, but this test is not commonly performed. CMV doesn't always cause symptoms. Some people have fatigue, swollen glands, fever, and sore throat when they first get CMV. But these are also symptoms of other illnesses, so most people don't know it when they get CMV.

How is CMV different for someone with HIV?

Once CMV enters a person's body, it stays there. Most people with CMV never get CMV-related diseases. However, in people with HIV or AIDS, the virus can cause severe disease.

How can I prevent CMV disease?

The most important thing you can do is to get the best care you can for your HIV infection. Take your antiretroviral medicine just the way your doctor tells you to. If you get sick from your medicine, call your doctor for advice. CMV disease mostly affects HIV-infected people whose CD4 cell counts are below 100. Oral (taken by mouth) ganciclovir (gan-CY-clo-veer) may be used to prevent CMV disease, but it is expensive, has side effects, and may not work for all people. Normally, ganciclovir is not recommended, but you may want to talk with your doctor about it.

Chapter 25

Co-Infection with HIV and Hepatitis C Virus

About one quarter of HIV-infected persons in the United States are also infected with hepatitis C virus (HCV). HCV is one of the most important causes of chronic liver disease in the United States and HCV infection progresses more rapidly to liver damage in HIV-infected persons. HCV infection may also impact the course and management of HIV infection.

The latest U.S. Public Health Service/Infectious Diseases Society of America (USPHS/IDSA) guidelines recommend that all HIV-infected persons should be screened for HCV infection. Prevention of HCV infection for those not already infected and reducing chronic liver disease in those who are infected are important concerns for HIV-infected individuals and their health care providers.

Who is likely to have HIV-HCV co-infection?

The hepatitis C virus (HCV) is transmitted primarily by large or repeated direct percutaneous (i.e., passage through the skin by puncture) exposures to contaminated blood. Therefore, co-infection with HIV and HCV is common (50%-90%) among HIV-infected injection drug users (IDUs). Co-infection is also common among persons with hemophilia who received clotting factor concentrates before concentrates

---

"Frequently Asked Questions and Answers about Co-infection with HIV and Hepatitis C Virus," National Center for HIV, STD and TB Prevention, Centers for Disease Control and Prevention (CDC), updated August 2001; available online at http://www.cdc.gov/hiv/pubs/facts/HIV-HCV_Coinfection.htm.

179

were effectively treated to inactivate both viruses (i.e., products made before 1987). The risk for acquiring infection through perinatal or sexual exposures is much lower for HCV than for HIV. For persons infected with HIV through sexual exposure (e.g., male-to-male sexual activity), co-infection with HCV is no more common than among similarly aged adults in the general population (3%-5%).

What are the effects of co-infection on disease progression of HCV and HIV?

Chronic HCV infection develops in 75%-85% of infected persons and leads to chronic liver disease in 70% of these chronically infected persons. HIV-HCV co-infection has been associated with higher titers of HCV, more rapid progression to HCV-related liver disease, and an increased risk for HCV-related cirrhosis (scarring) of the liver. Because of this, HCV infection has been viewed as an opportunistic infection in HIV-infected persons and was included in the 1999 *USPHS/IDSA Guidelines for the Prevention of Opportunistic Infections in Persons Infected with Human Immunodeficiency Virus*. It is not, however, considered an AIDS-defining illness. As highly active antiretroviral therapy (HAART) and prophylaxis of opportunistic infections increase the life span of persons living with HIV, HCV-related liver disease has become a major cause of hospital admissions and deaths among HIV-infected persons.

The effects of HCV co-infection on HIV disease progression are less certain. Some studies have suggested that infection with certain HCV genotypes is associated with more rapid progression to AIDS or death. However, the subject remains controversial. Since co-infected patients are living longer on HAART, more data are needed to determine if HCV infection influences the long-term natural history of HIV infection.

How can co-infection with HCV be prevented?

Persons living with HIV who are not already co-infected with HCV can adopt measures to prevent acquiring HCV. Such measures will also reduce the chance of transmitting their HIV infection to others.

Not injecting or stopping injection drug use would eliminate the chief route of HCV transmission; substance-abuse treatment and relapse-prevention programs should be recommended. If patients continue to inject, they should be counseled about safer injection practices; that is, to use new, sterile syringes every time they inject drugs and never reuse or share syringes, needles, water, or drug preparation equipment.

Toothbrushes, razors, and other personal care items that might be contaminated with blood should not be shared. Although there are no data from the United States indicating that tattooing and body piercing place persons at increased risk for HCV infection, these procedures may be a source for infection with any bloodborne pathogen if proper infection control practices are not followed.

Although consistent data are lacking regarding the extent to which sexual activity contributes to HCV transmission, persons having multiple sex partners are at risk for other sexually transmitted diseases (STDs) as well as for transmitting HIV to others. They should be counseled accordingly.

How should patients co-infected with HIV and HCV be managed?

General Guidelines

Patients co-infected with HIV and HCV should be encouraged to adopt safe behaviors (as described in the previously) to prevent transmission of HIV and HCV to others.

Individuals with evidence of HCV infection should be given information about prevention of liver damage, undergo evaluation for chronic liver disease and, if indicated, be considered for treatment. Persons co-infected with HIV and HCV should be advised not to drink excessive amounts of alcohol. Avoiding alcohol altogether might be wise because the effects of even moderate or low amounts of alcohol (e.g., 12 oz. of beer, 5 oz. of wine or 1.5 oz. hard liquor per day) on disease progression are unknown. When appropriate, referral should be made to alcohol treatment and relapse-prevention programs. Because of possible effects on the liver, HCV-infected patients should consult with their health care professional before taking any new medicines, including over-the-counter, alternative or herbal medicines.

Susceptible co-infected patients should receive hepatitis A vaccine because the risk for fulminant hepatitis associated with hepatitis A is increased in persons with chronic liver disease. Susceptible patients should receive hepatitis B vaccine because most HIV-infected persons are at risk for HBV infection. The vaccines appear safe for these patients and more than two-thirds of those vaccinated develop antibody responses. Prevaccination screening for antibodies against hepatitis A and hepatitis B in this high-prevalence population is generally cost-effective.

Postvaccination testing for hepatitis A is not recommended, but testing for antibody to hepatitis B surface antigen (anti-HBs) should be performed 1-2 months after completion of the primary series of hepatitis B vaccine. Persons who fail to respond should be revaccinated with up to three additional doses.

HAART has no significant effect on HCV. However, co-infected persons may be at increased risk for HAART-associated liver toxicity and should be closely monitored during antiretroviral therapy. Data suggest that the majority of these persons do not appear to develop significant and/or symptomatic hepatitis after initiation of antiretroviral therapy.

Treatment for HCV Infection

A Consensus Development Conference Panel convened by The National Institutes of Health in 1997 recommended antiviral therapy for patients with chronic hepatitis C who are at the greatest risk for progression to cirrhosis. These persons include anti-HCV positive patients with persistently elevated liver enzymes, detectable HCV RNA, and a liver biopsy that indicates either portal or bridging fibrosis or at least moderate degrees of inflammation and necrosis. Patients with less severe histological disease should be managed on an individual basis.

In the United States, two different regimens have been approved as therapy for chronic hepatitis C: monotherapy with alpha interferon and combination therapy with alpha interferon and ribavirin. Among HIV-negative persons with chronic hepatitis C, combination therapy consistently yields higher rates (30%-40%) of sustained response than monotherapy (10%-20%). Combination therapy is more effective against viral genotypes 2 and 3, and requires a shorter course of treatment; however, viral genotype 1 is the most common among U.S. patients. Combination therapy is associated with more side effects than monotherapy, but, in most situations, it is preferable. At present, interferon monotherapy is reserved for patients who have contraindications to the use of ribavirin.

Studies thus far, although not extensive, have indicated that response rates in HIV-infected patients to alpha interferon monotherapy for HCV were lower than in non-HIV-infected patients, but the differences were not statistically significant. Monotherapy appears to be reasonably well tolerated in co-infected patients. There are no published articles on the long-term effect of combination therapy in co-infected patients, but studies currently underway suggest it is superior to monotherapy. However, the side effects of combination therapy are greater in co-infected patients. Thus, combination therapy should be used with caution until more data are available.

The decision to treat people co-infected with HIV and HCV must also take into consideration their concurrent medications and medical conditions. If CD4 counts are normal or minimally abnormal (>400/ ul), there is little difference in treatment success rates between those who are co-infected and those who are infected with HCV alone.

Other Treatment Considerations

Persons with chronic hepatitis C who continue to abuse alcohol are at risk for ongoing liver injury, and antiviral therapy may be ineffective. Therefore, strict abstinence from alcohol is recommended during antiviral therapy, and interferon should be given with caution to a patient who has only recently stopped alcohol abuse. Typically, a 6-month abstinence is recommended for alcohol abusers before starting therapy; such patients should be treated with the support and collaboration of alcohol abuse treatment programs.

Although there is limited experience with antiviral treatment for chronic hepatitis C of persons who are recovering from long-term injection drug use, there are concerns that interferon therapy could be associated with relapse into drug use, both because of its side effects and because it is administered by injection. There is even less experience with treatment of persons who are active injection drug users, and an additional concern for this group is the risk for reinfection with HCV. Although a 6-month abstinence before starting therapy also has been recommended for injection drug users, additional research is needed on the benefits and drawbacks of treating these patients. Regardless, when patients with past or continuing problems of substance abuse are being considered for treatment, such patients should be treated only in collaboration with substance abuse specialists or counselors. Patients can be successfully treated while on methadone maintenance treatment of addiction.

Because many co-infected patients have conditions or factors (such as major depression or active illicit drug or alcohol use) that may prevent or complicate antiviral therapy, treatment for chronic hepatitis C in HIV-infected patients should be coordinated by health care providers with experience in treating co-infected patients or in clinical trials. It is not known if maintenance therapy is needed after successful therapy, but patients should be counseled to avoid injection drug use and other behaviors that could lead to reinfection with HCV and should continue to abstain from alcohol.

Infections in Infants and Children

The average rate of HCV infection among infants born to women co-infected with HCV and HIV is 14% to 17%, higher than among infants born to women infected with HCV alone. Data are limited on the natural history of HCV infection in children, and antiviral drugs for chronic hepatitis C are not FDA-approved for use in children under aged 18 years. Therefore, children should be referred to a pediatric hepatologist or similar specialist for management and for determination for eligibility in clinical trials.

What research is needed on HIV-HCV co-infection?

Many important questions remain about HIV-HCV co-infection:

- By what mechanism does HIV infection affect the natural history of hepatitis C?

- Does HAART affect the impact of HIV on the natural history of HCV infection?

- Does HCV affect the natural history of HIV and, if so, by what mechanism?

- How can we effectively and safely treat chronic hepatitis C in HIV-infected patients?

- How can we distinguish between liver toxicity caused by antiretrovirals and that caused by HCV infection?

- What is the best protocol for treating both HIV and chronic hepatitis C in the co-infected patient?

Chapter 26

Lipodystrophy

One of the most common and distressing side effects associated with combination therapy today concerns visible changes in body composition and appearance. Although some aspects of this phenomenon were reported in earlier years of the epidemic, the frequency of reports has greatly increased since the beginning of the protease inhibitor era in 1996.

These changes in appearance are brought about by several different forms of redistribution of body fat—fat moving away from the face, arms, butt and legs, and then collecting around the gut (central obesity), at the base of the neck (buffalo hump) and/or in the breasts (breast enlargement). Less frequently seen are accumulations of lumpy fat tissue, similar in appearance to cellulite, on the back below the shoulder blades. Associated with these changes, and possibly causally related, are striking increases in a number of blood test markers, such as triglycerides and cholesterol level, and insulin resistance. These blood changes have sometimes been linked to increased risk of heart disease and to the development of diabetes.

The cause of these changes is unknown or at least uncertain. Is it a consequence of HIV disease progression? Is the virus itself interfering with the way the body processes fat and protein? If so, why is it more common today than before? Are these changes a result of protease

From Project Inform: "Lipodystrophy," © 1999 Project Inform, from *PI Perspectives,* April 1999. Reprinted with permission. For more information, contact the National NIV/AIDS Treatment Hotline, 800-822-7422, or visit our website, www.projectinform.org.

inhibitor therapy, as is commonly thought? If so, why have they occurred in some people who haven't used protease inhibitors, or any anti-HIV therapy at all? Are some of the drugs used today more or less likely than others to contribute to these problems? Are there any treatments that can prevent or treat these changes? What is the long-term consequence of these changes, and what percentage of HIV infected people are experiencing them?

Sadly, all these questions currently remain unanswered. Changes in body composition and all laboratory (e.g. blood work results) abnormalities associated with these changes have not been clearly defined, but are currently grouped together and referred to as lipodystrophy (pronounced, lip-oh-dis-troh-fee).

What Is Lipodystrophy?

Currently there is not an official definition for lipodystrophy, which makes it difficult to study in any systematic way. The following working definition lumps together the thinking of a number of groups. Much of this information may prove useful for doctors and their patients in monitoring for possible early signs of lipodystrophy.

Noted changes in body composition (self-reported by a patient, diagnosed or confirmed by a physician with the aid of tests such as magnetic resonance imaging (MRI), comparative photographs and measurements, or made apparent review of medical records). These changes include at least one of the following:

- Peripheral fat wasting (a significant decrease in fat from the face, arms, butt and legs), resulting in a thin or drawn look;

- Central obesity (truncal obesity or protease paunch). This build-up of fat behind the stomach muscle is generally not mushy but rather fairly firm/hard; this fat is different than the normal increases in fat associated with aging;

- Development of a dorsal fat pad (buffalo hump), a build-up of fat at the base of the back of the neck between the shoulders;

- Breast enlargement. This is a build up of fat in the breasts and has been observed in both women and men.

The changes in body composition are commonly accompanied by abnormal lab results including at least two of the following:

- Elevated triglyceride levels, >2mmol/l

- Elevated cholesterol, >5.5mmol/l
- Elevated C-peptide, >2.5mmol/l
- Glucose intolerance
- Impaired fasting glucose, 6.0-7.0mmol/l
- Impaired glucose intolerance, 7.8-11.1mmol/l
- Diabetes mellitus, >7.0mmol/l fasting or >11.1mmol/l non-fasting

Because other HIV-related conditions might effect body composition, if an individual has had a serious HIV-related condition (e.g. an AIDS-defining condition) within the past three months, it can't be certain that changes in body composition are a result of lipodystrophy, but might be due to other infections.

We know that certain therapies (anabolic steroids) also affect body composition. If changes in body composition occur while someone is taking these therapies, it is unclear if the changes are HIV-related, related to anti-HIV therapies and/or related to the anabolic steroids.

Can Lipodystrophy Be Treated?

While lipodystrophy clearly affects an increasing number of people, there have been no controlled studies investigating how to treat the condition. Reports of individual successes cannot be considered predictive of whether the treatments will work for others.

Three separate reports claim some success in treating lipodystrophy associated with the use of protease inhibitor-containing regimens. Those reports occurred as a result of switching people off protease inhibitors and substituting a non-nucleoside reverse transcriptase inhibitor (NNRTI). Physicians reported some reductions in central obesity (fat around the gut); however, not everyone had a return of peripheral fat (fat in the arms and legs). Reductions were also reported in lipid levels (cholesterol and triglycerides) and a reversal of insulin resistance (which is associated with diabetes).

One potential area of concern from a study showed that 10% of the group who switched to a NNRTI-class drug had increases in HIV levels. This could be just coincidence. It is possible these people would have had an increase in HIV levels if they stayed on their protease inhibitors. Nevertheless, this observation does cause some concern. Despite these seemingly positive findings, the number of people involved was very small and some individual physicians have reported contradictory results in their own medical practices.

A physician in New York has observed that growth hormone (Serostim) had some effect in reducing central obesity and buffalo hump in a few patients. But Serostim had no effect on facial and limb wasting or on decreasing lipid levels. One person had to stop growth hormone therapy because of side effects and had a rapid return of central obesity. It was again reduced when the growth hormone was restarted. Considering the extremely high cost of Serostim and the apparent need for continuous therapy, it is hard to consider this approach particularly hopeful.

A number of people have reported success with using liposuction technology to remove disfiguring buffalo humps; however, there is every reason to fear that such humps will slowly grow back over time, since the underlying cause has not changed. Liposuction is not recommended for treatment of central obesity, since the fat is stored deeply behind the abdominal muscles and cannot be easily removed. Some women have resorted to breast reduction surgery when excessive growth lead to pain and difficulty walking. Surgical solutions such as these should only be considered in the most extreme cases, especially since their long-term success is unknown.

Several small studies looked at the use of specific drugs to treat some of the laboratory abnormalities associated mainly with the use of protease inhibitor therapy. One study showed that the combination of gemfibrozil (Lopid) and atorvastatin (Lipitor) lowered lipid levels to the normal range in about 50% of people. Another study showed that metformin (Glucophage) reduced central obesity and insulin resistance but also led to an average 2kg weight loss. Finally, one other study showed that troglitazone (Rezulin) reduced glucose levels but had no effect on lipid levels.

Many of these therapies have potential drug interactions with protease inhibitors. Doctors and patients who consider experimenting with these approaches to manage lab abnormalities should talk to a pharmacist about possible drug interactions and any necessary dose adjustments to therapies.

Commentary

It is difficult to conduct studies to treat lipodystrophy because of the need for an agreed upon case definition. An Australian group is likely to have some new results that may give us a better definition for lipodystrophy. A large U.S. study will start shortly to look at the prevalence of lipodystrophy. That study may also provide us a better working definition to use in other studies as well as in clinics.

To date, much of the effort to study lipodystrophy has been driven by pressure from AIDS activists. Even though the problem has been evident for nearly three years, it has taken a very long time for pharmaceutical companies and the research community in general to take positive steps toward further understanding it. It appears that community pressure has once again been helpful since several new studies will soon be underway, by both government and industry.

Many groups are studying the cause of lipodystrophy. Glaxo Wellcome scientists have recently reported that they have conducted laboratory studies which seem to have identified two possible causes of fat redistribution. Both mechanisms are similar to, but not exactly the same as, that posed by the Australian group previously. The Glaxo theory suggests that the problem might be caused by one mechanism by ritonavir, saquinavir, and nelfinavir, and/or a somewhat different mechanism related to indinavir. For the moment, they believe that their own protease inhibitor, amprenavir, poses neither problem, but only time will tell if this is accurate or merely self-reporting.

Unfortunately, in the meantime, there is very little information available for people on how to diagnose and treat this syndrome. For most people, fat redistribution does not become physically dangerous. However, triglyceride and cholesterol levels can become so severely elevated that many physicians worry about increased risks of heart disease and other serious conditions. Careful and frequent monitoring of lab tests, along with regular physical examinations, should become part of the medical routine for people on combination therapies. When lab marker changes reach what appear to be life threatening levels, physicians should act appropriately, just as they would any other time these tests show alarming results.

It is unclear just how widespread these problems are, with various groups reporting incidence levels ranging from roughly 15% to as high as 75%. This widespread difference probably reflects variations in the underlying definition used for lipodystrophy. There is as yet no reason to suspect that these problems will affect everyone, but there is certainly enough evidence to suggest that a serious problem exists which demands greater attention than it has been given.

Lipodystrophy Studies in Women

Several studies on body composition changes and abnormal changes in laboratory values (i.e. blood work results) associated with the use of anti-HIV therapy were presented at the recent conference in Chicago. The first examined the relationship between body composition (fat distribution) and two laboratory measures being associated with lipodystrophy, insulin levels and cholesterol levels, in 33 women treated with protease inhibitor-containing anti-HIV regimens. It found that women treated with protease inhibitors were more likely to have elevated waist-to-hip ratios (WHR) compared to HIV negative women and that this increase was independent of any overall change in weight (i.e. weight gain). This means that women with HIV receiving protease inhibitors were more likely to have larger waste sizes, relative to their hip size compared to HIV-negative women.

Whether women living with HIV not receiving protease inhibitors also have higher WHR compared to HIV-negative women will be important in understanding the contribution of protease inhibitor therapy to this observation. Another interesting finding was that the elevated WHR was significantly correlated with higher levels of triglycerides, glucose levels. While this study was relatively small, it suggests important clues about the relationship between physical and chemical changes some women on protease inhibitors appear to be experiencing.

A second study compared changes in body shape between women receiving protease inhibitors (PI) and women not using protease inhibitor-containing anti-HIV regimens. Ninety-five women on protease inhibitors and 35 women not receiving protease inhibitor regimens were examined. While increases in breast and waist size were reported among both groups, women on protease inhibitors tended to have a more dramatic size increase in both measurements (three or more size increase for bras and four or more size increase for pants). The difference among the two groups, however, was not dramatic enough to be able to equate increases in breast or waist size, overall, strictly to the use of protease inhibitor-containing regimen. Despite the increase in breast and waist size, changes in overall body weight for both groups was minimal (a median gain of 7.8 pounds for women on PI versus 3.8 pounds). Finally, 7% of women participating in the study discontinued PI therapy because of changes in body shape.

Further confirming these findings was a study showing similar patterns of body shape changes in women taking anti-HIV regimens that did not include protease inhibitors. Among 306 women participating in the study, enlargement of the breasts and waist (abdomen), and wasting of the butt, thighs and calves were reported in 32 women (10.5%). All of the women reporting fat redistribution were receiving a regimen containing 3TC (lamivudine, Epivir), a nucleoside analog reverse transcriptase inhibitors (NARTI). Twelve of the 32 women reporting body shape changes were taking double combination therapy (including 3TC) that did not include a protease inhibitor. Additionally, among women taking 3TC, the risk of developing changes in body shape was significantly lower in those also taking AZT (zidovudine, Retrovir) and higher in women taking D4T (stavudine, Zerit). Thus, the study suggests a strong association between body shapes changes and the use of 3TC, including women who had never taken a protease inhibitor. While far from confirmed, these data suggest that the mechanism causing changes in body shape in women on anti-HIV therapy may not necessarily be related to protease inhibitors.

Chapter 27

Disseminated Mycobacterium Avium Complex Disease (MAC)

Mycobacterium avium [MY-co-bak-TEER-ee-um A-vee-um] complex, also known as MAC, is the name of a group of germs. These germs can infect people who are living with HIV. Adults with HIV usually don't get MAC disease until their T-cell count drops below 50. Because MAC disease occurs later in the course of HIV infection, it usually is not the first sickness a person with HIV gets. Most people with HIV have already been diagnosed with AIDS before they get MAC.

- About 20 to 30 percent of people with AIDS get MAC disease.

- Adults usually don't get MAC disease until their T-cell count drops below 50, but children can get it earlier.

- You can get MAC disease more than once.

- There are several drugs you can take to prevent MAC disease.

Can children get MAC disease?

Yes. The risk of MAC for children with HIV goes up as their T-cell count goes down, just as it does for adults. However, children who get MAC disease usually get it before their T-cell count falls to 50. Children with HIV usually have higher T-cell counts than adults with HIV.

"You Can Prevent MAC (Mycobacterium Avium Complex Disease)," National Center for HIV, STD and TB Prevention, Centers for Disease Control and Prevention (CDC), May 1999; available online at http://www.cdc.gov/hiv/pubs/brochure/oi_mac.htm.

What are the symptoms of MAC disease?

Although MAC usually infects persons through their lungs or intestines, it spreads quickly through the bloodstream, causing widespread or disseminated disease. People with disseminated MAC disease can have fever, night sweats, weight loss, abdominal pain, tiredness, and diarrhea.

How is MAC disease diagnosed?

MAC disease is diagnosed by laboratory tests that can identify the MAC germ in samples of blood, bone marrow, or tissue.

How do people get MAC disease?

People with AIDS probably get MAC disease through normal contact with air, food, and water. MAC disease has been found in many types of animals, including birds, chickens, pigs, cows, rabbits, and dogs. MAC germs can be found in most sources of drinking water, including treated water systems, and in dirt and household dust. MAC disease does not seem to be spread from one person to another.

How can I avoid MAC disease?

Because MAC germs are found in food, water, and soil, there is no easy way to avoid them. However, there are drugs that can prevent MAC germs from causing disease.

When should I get treatment to prevent MAC disease?

Because MAC disease occurs in people with very low T-cell counts, you should not get treatment to prevent MAC disease until your T-cell count is below 50. Your doctor will tell you when you or your child need to begin treatment for preventing MAC disease.

What drugs are used to prevent MAC?

Drugs which can reduce your chances of getting MAC disease are:

- clarithromycin [kla-REE-thro-MY-sin]
- azithromycin [a-ZEE-thro-MY-sin]
- rifabutin [rif-a-BU-tin]

Ask your doctor whether you should take one of these drugs.

Can the drugs used to prevent MAC disease cause side effects?

Yes. Rifabutin can cause eye irritation. If you are taking rifabutin or other drugs to prevent MAC, see your doctor regularly and report any side effects.

If I have already had MAC disease, can I get it again?

Yes. If you have had MAC disease, continue to take drugs to treat and prevent further MAC disease. MAC disease is most commonly treated with a combination of clarithromycin and ethambutol [eth-AM-bu-tol], with or without rifabutin.

Chapter 28

Pneumocystis Carinii
Pneumonia (PCP)

Pneumocystis carinii (NEW-mo-SIS-tis CA-RIN-nee-eye) pneumonia, or PCP, is a severe illness found in people with HIV. It is caused by a germ called *Pneumocystis carinii*. Most people infected with this germ don't get pneumonia because their immune systems are normal. People whose immune systems are badly damaged by HIV can get PCP. People with HIV are less likely to get PCP today than in earlier years. However, PCP is still the most common serious infection among people with AIDS in the United States.

How do I know if I have PCP?

If you have PCP, you probably will have fever, cough, or trouble breathing. People with PCP may die if the infection is not treated quickly. See your doctor immediately if you have these symptoms. PCP can be diagnosed only by laboratory tests of fluid or tissue from the lungs.

How do you catch PCP?

Most scientists believe PCP is spread in the air, but they don't know if it lives in the soil or someplace else. The PCP germ is very common. Since it is difficult to prevent exposure to PCP, you should get medical care to prevent PCP.

"You Can Prevent PCP: A Guide for People with HIV Infection," National Center for HIV, STD, and TB Prevention, Centers for Disease Control and Prevention (CDC), updated March 1999; available online at http://www.cdc.gov/hiv/pubs/brochure/pcpb.htm.

How can I protect myself from PCP?

PCP can be prevented. The best drug for preventing PCP is trimethoprim-sulfamethoxazole (try-METH-o-prim - sul-fa-meth-OX-uh-sole), or TMP-SMX. TMP-SMX is a combination of two medicines. It has many different brand names, such as Bactrim, Septra, and Cotrim. Adults and older children can take TMP-SMX as a tablet. You can also get TMP-SMX as a liquid.

I was vaccinated for pneumonia. Won't that protect me against PCP?

No. The pneumonia vaccine protects you against another kind of pneumonia, but not against PCP. There is no vaccine for PCP.

When should I start treatment to prevent PCP?

You should have your blood tested regularly to check the strength of your immune system. Your doctor should prescribe TMP-SMX to prevent PCP if your CD4 cell count falls below 200. Your doctor may also put you on TMP-SMX if you show certain symptoms, such as having a temperature above 100°F that lasts for 2 weeks or longer, or if you get a fungal infection in the mouth or throat (commonly called thrush). Having thrush is believed to raise your risk for getting PCP.

What are the side effects of TMP-SMX?

TMP-SMX can make some people have a rash or feel sick. If the drug reaction is not severe, TMP-SMX should be continued because it works so much better than any other medicine to prevent PCP.

Are there other medicines to prevent PCP?

Yes. Check with your doctor about the possibility of other treatments. Take all of your medicines as prescribed by your doctor. Don't change how many pills you are taking without speaking with your doctor.

Can I get PCP more than once?

Yes. If you have already had PCP you can get it again. TMP-SMX can prevent second infections with PCP. Therefore, you should take TMP-SMX even after you have had PCP to prevent getting it again.

Can children get PCP?

Yes. Children with HIV or AIDS can also get PCP. To learn more about children and PCP, call the AIDS Treatment Information Service at 1-800-448-0440.

Is PCP sexually transmitted?

No. PCP is not sexually transmitted.

Chapter 29

Tuberculosis and HIV

Tuberculosis (TB) is a disease caused by a germ called Mycobacterium (my-ko-bak-TEER-I-um) tuberculosis. TB most often affects the lungs, but TB germs can infect any part of the body. TB may be latent or active TB. Latent means that the germs are in the person's body but are not causing illness. If you have latent TB you will not have symptoms and cannot spread TB. However, if HIV has made your immune system too weak to stop the TB germs from growing, they can multiply and cause active TB (also called TB disease).

In people with HIV, TB in the lungs or anywhere else in the body is called an AIDS-defining condition. In other words, a person with both HIV and active TB has AIDS.

How is TB spread?

TB is spread from one person to another through the air. When a person who has TB disease of the lung or throat coughs, sneezes, or sings, tiny, moist drops that contain TB germs are sent into the air. A person who breathes air that contains these drops may get TB. People with TB disease are most likely to spread it to people they spend time with every day, such as family members, friends, or co-workers.

You can't get TB from shaking hands, sitting on a toilet seat, or sharing dishes or utensils.

"Tuberculosis: A Guide for Adults and Adolescents with HIV," National Center for HIV, STD, and TB Prevention, Centers for Disease Control and Prevention (CDC), updated April 1999; available online at http://www.cdc.gov/hiv/pubs/brochure/oi_tb.htm.

How can I avoid TB?

Some activities and jobs may increase your chances of spending time with people who have TB and getting TB. These include working in a health care setting (a hospital, a clinic, a doctor's office), in jails and prisons, and in shelters for homeless people. You and your doctor should decide whether you should working such a place. If you do things that may increase your chances of getting TB, you and your doctor may decide that you need to be tested for TB more often than once a year.

If you can, avoid spending time with someone who has active TB but is not taking medicine or has just started taking medicine. A person who has been taking medicine for a few weeks can normally no longer spread TB to you. That person's doctor will say when it's safe for other people to spend time with him or her.

If you are exposed to a person with active TB, you should ask your doctor about getting treatment, even if your skin test was negative for TB.

How do I know if I might have active TB?

Your symptoms depend on where in your body the TB germs are growing. TB germs usually grow in the lungs. TB in the lungs may cause:

- a bad cough that lasts longer than 3 weeks
- pain in the chest
- coughing up blood or phlegm from deep inside the lungs

Other symptoms are:

- weakness or fatigue
- weight loss
- no appetite
- chills
- fever
- sweating at night

Does TB affect only the lungs?

No. Active TB most often affects the lungs. But it can also affect almost any other body organ, such as the kidneys or the spine. A person whose TB is not in the lungs or throat usually cannot give TB to other people.

Am I at greater risk of getting TB because I have HIV?

Yes. Latent TB is much more likely to become active TB in someone with HIV. This is because HIV weakens the immune system, which makes it harder for the body to fight off diseases like TB.

Since I have HIV, should I be tested for TB?

Yes. If you have not already had TB or if you had a positive result from a skin test for TB in the past, get a tuberculin skin test, or TST at the health department or your doctor's office. When you have the test, a health care worker will inject a small amount of testing fluid (called tuberculin) just under the skin on the lower part of your arm. After 2 or 3 days, the health care worker will check your arm to see whether you had a positive reaction to the test.

If you have a positive test result (which usually means you have latent TB), you may need other tests to see whether you have TB disease (active TB). These tests usually include a chest x-ray and a test of the phlegm you cough up. Because TB can grow somewhere else in your body, other tests may be done.

If you have a negative test result you should be tested again at least once a year, depending on your chances of getting TB. Discuss your chances of getting TB with your doctor.

If you are an HIV-infected mother whose baby was born after you got HIV, have your baby tested for TB when the baby is 9 to 12 months old.

If I have latent TB, can drugs help prevent it from becoming active TB?

Yes. The drug isoniazid can help prevent latent TB from becoming active TB. People with HIV infection who need to take isoniazid are also given a vitamin called pyridoxine to prevent peripheral neuropathy (a disorder of the nervous system).

Get tested for latent TB, with a TST, as soon as possible after you learn you have HIV. If your skin test result is positive (but you do not have active TB), you will most likely be given 12 months of treatment with isoniazid to prevent active TB. You need to take your medicine for the full 12 months because TB germs die very slowly. Take your medicine exactly as your doctor or nurse tells you.

If you are a woman who is pregnant, you may still take isoniazid to fight TB. However, your doctor may tell you not to take the medicine until after the first 3 months of your pregnancy. The germs that caused your latent TB might not be killed by isoniazid. In that case, you will be given another drug (probably rifampin) that is used to prevent TB.

If I have active TB, can it be cured?

Yes. The drugs that fight TB work as well as in people with HIV as they do in people who do not have HIV.

Several drugs are used to treat active TB. You will need to take more than one drug for several weeks. Your symptoms may go away within a few weeks after you start taking the medicine. TB germs die very slowly, so you need to keep taking your medicine exactly as your doctor or nurse tells you (the right amount at the right time for the right length of time).

Can I give TB to other people?

Yes. If you have TB disease of the lungs or throat, you can probably spread TB to other people. You may need to stay home from work or school or other activities for a few weeks. After you've taken your medicine for a few weeks, you will probably no longer be able to spread TB to others, but you need to continue taking your medicine for 6 to 9 months to be totally cured. Your doctor or nurse will tell you when you can return to work or school or other activities. The medicine should not affect your strength, your sexual function, or your ability to work. Taking the medicine as prescribed will keep you from again becoming sick with TB disease.

I am taking protease inhibitors to fight HIV infection. Can I also take medicine to cure TB?

Yes. But you should know that medicines for TB and the protease inhibitors affect each other. Your doctor will decide which combination of medicines will work best for you.

What is drug-resistant TB?

When TB germs are not killed by a certain drug, that TB is called drug-resistant. TB germs may become resistant when patients do not take their medicine long enough or in the right amount at the right times. Follow your doctor's advice when taking medicines.

People who have drug-resistant TB can transmit it to others. Drug-resistant TB is found often in people who come from areas where TB is common (for example, Africa, Southeast Asia, Latin America) but it also occurs in parts of the United States.

When several different drugs can't kill TB germs, the TB is called multidrug-resistant TB (MDR TB). A patient with MDR TB may need to see a doctor who is an expert on drug-resistant TB and who can recommend the best combination of drugs to fight the germs.

Chapter 30

AIDS-Related Kaposi's Sarcoma (KS)

Kaposi's sarcoma (KS) is a disease in which cancer (malignant) cells are found in the tissues under the skin or mucous membranes that line the mouth, nose, and anus. KS causes red or purple patches (lesions) on the skin and/or mucous membranes and spreads to other organs in the body, such as the lungs, liver, or intestinal tract.

Until the early 1980's, Kaposi's sarcoma was a very rare disease that was found mainly in older men, patients who had organ transplants, or African men. With the acquired immunodeficiency syndrome (AIDS) epidemic in the early 1980's, doctors began to notice more cases of Kaposi's sarcoma in Africa and in gay men with AIDS. Kaposi's sarcoma usually spreads more quickly in these patients.

If there are signs of KS, a doctor will examine the skin and lymph nodes carefully (lymph nodes are small bean-shaped structures that are found throughout the body; they produce and store infection-fighting cells). The doctor also may order other tests to see if the patient has other diseases.

The chance of recovery (prognosis) depends on what type of Kaposi's sarcoma the patient has, the patient's age and general health, and whether or not the patient has AIDS.

"Kaposi's Sarcoma (PDQ®): Treatment," National Cancer Institute (NCI), updated September 2002. Additional information about cancer-related topics is available from the National Cancer Institute's website online at http://www.cancer.gov.

Stage Information

There is no accepted staging system for Kaposi's sarcoma. Patients are grouped depending on which type of Kaposi's sarcoma they have. There are three types of Kaposi's sarcoma.

Classic

Classic Kaposi's sarcoma usually occurs in older men of Jewish, Italian, or Mediterranean heritage. This type of Kaposi's sarcoma progresses slowly, sometimes over 10 to 15 years. As the disease gets worse, the lower legs may swell and the blood may not be able to flow properly. After some time, the disease may spread to other organs. Many patients with classic Kaposi's sarcoma may develop another type of cancer later on in their lives.

Immunosuppressive Treatment Related

Kaposi's sarcoma may occur in people who are taking drugs to make their immune systems weaker (immunosuppressants). The immune system helps the body fight off infection. People who have had an organ transplant (such as a liver or kidney transplant) have to take drugs to prevent their immune system from attacking the new organ.

Epidemic

Kaposi's sarcoma in patients who have Acquired Immunodeficiency Syndrome (AIDS) is called epidemic Kaposi's sarcoma. AIDS is caused by a virus called the Human Immunodeficiency Virus (HIV), which attacks and weakens the immune system. Infections and other diseases can then invade the body, and the immune system cannot fight against them. Kaposi's sarcoma in people with AIDS usually spreads more quickly than other kinds of Kaposi's sarcoma and often is found in many parts of the body.

Recurrent

Recurrent disease means that the KS has come back (recurred) after it has been treated. It may come back in the area where it first started or in another part of the body.

Treatment Option Overview

There are treatments for all patients with Kaposi's sarcoma. Four kinds of treatment are used:

- surgery (taking out the cancer)
- chemotherapy (using drugs to kill cancer cells)
- radiation therapy (using high-dose x-rays to kill cancer cells)
- biological therapy (using the body's immune system to fight cancer)

Radiation therapy is a common treatment of Kaposi's sarcoma. Radiation therapy uses high-dose x-rays or other high-energy rays to kill cancer cells and shrink tumors. Radiation for Kaposi's sarcoma comes from a machine outside the body (external beam radiation therapy).

Surgery means taking out the cancer. A doctor may remove the cancer using one of the following:

- Local excision cuts out the lesion and some of the tissue around it.
- Electrodesiccation and curettage burns the lesion and removes it with a sharp instrument.
- Cryotherapy freezes the tumor and kills it.

Chemotherapy uses drugs to kill cancer cells. Chemotherapy may be taken by pill, or it may be put into the body by a needle in a vein or muscle. Chemotherapy is called a systemic treatment because the drug enters the bloodstream, travels through the body, and can kill cancer cells outside the original site. Chemotherapy for Kaposi's sarcoma also may be injected into the lesion (intralesional chemotherapy).

Biological therapy tries to get the body to fight the cancer. It uses materials made by the body or made in a laboratory to boost, direct, or restore the body's natural defenses against disease. Biological therapy is sometimes called biological response modifier (BRM) therapy or immunotherapy.

Treatment by Stage

Treatment of Kaposi's sarcoma depends on the type of Kaposi's sarcoma the patient has, and the patient's age and general health.

Standard treatment may be considered because of its effectiveness in patients in past studies, or participation in a clinical trial may be considered. Not all patients are cured with standard therapy and some standard treatments may have more side effects than are desired. For these reasons, clinical trials are designed to find better ways to treat cancer patients and are based on the most up-to-date information. Clinical trials are ongoing in most parts of the country for most stages of Kaposi's sarcoma.

Classic Kaposi's Sarcoma

Treatment may be one of the following:

- Radiation therapy.
- Local excision.
- Systemic or intralesional chemotherapy.
- Chemotherapy plus radiation therapy.

Immunosuppressive Treatment Related Kaposi's Sarcoma

Depending on the patient's condition, the cancer may be controlled if immunosuppressive drugs are stopped. If the patient cannot stop taking these drugs or if this does not work, treatment may be one of the following:

- Radiation therapy.
- A clinical trial of chemotherapy.

Epidemic Kaposi's Sarcoma

Treatment may be one of the following:

- Surgery (local excision, electrodesiccation and curettage, or cryotherapy) with or without radiation therapy.
- Systemic chemotherapy. Clinical trials are testing new drugs and drug combinations.
- Biological therapy.
- A clinical trial evaluating new treatments.

Recurrent Kaposi's Sarcoma

Treatment of recurrent Kaposi's sarcoma depends on the type of Kaposi's sarcoma, and the patient's general health and response to earlier treatments. The patient may want to take part in a clinical trial.

Chapter 31

AIDS Dementia Complex (ADC)

AIDS dementia complex (ADC) is one of the most frequent and serious neurologic complications of HIV. It is characterized by cognitive dysfunction (trouble with concentration, memory and attention), declining motor performance (strength, dexterity, coordination) and behavioral changes. It occurs primarily in more advanced HIV infection when the CD4 cell counts are relatively low. While the progression of dysfunction is variable, it is regarded as a serious complication historically predicting death in less than one year. Diagnosis is made by neurologists who carefully rule out alternative diagnoses. This routinely requires a careful neurological examination, brain scan (MRI or CT) and a lumbar puncture to evaluate the cerebrospinal fluid. No single test is available to confirm the diagnosis, but the constellation of history, laboratory findings, and examination reliably establish the diagnosis when performed by experienced clinicians.

The cause of ADC is not fully known at present. Presence of the HIV virus is required, and there is good evidence that successful antiretroviral therapy, if started early enough, can induce a degree of improvement in neurologic performance. Evidence that antiviral therapy prevents ADC is incomplete and in some cases contradictory. However, most investigators recommend at a minimum that aggressive antiretroviral therapy with maximally central nervous system

---

(CNS) penetrating drugs be used when this diagnosis is likely. Since the amount of virus in the brain does not correlate well with the degree of dementia, most investigators believe that secondary mechanisms are also important in the manifestation of ADC. Current hypotheses with variable levels of scientific support include contributions by cytokines such as tumor necrosis factor, toxic portions of the viral molecule (such as gp120 from the viral envelope and tat), excitatory amino acid mediated mechanisms, and calcium mediated neurotoxicity as playing some role in this disorder.

Recently completed experimental studies include:

- ACTG 301 has completed enrollment, but subjects continue in followup on this study. It tests a neuroprotective substance, memantine, in a controlled trial adding this potentially neuroprotective drug to best anti-retroviral therapy. This important trial seeks to test the role of neurotoxic mechanisms while patients continue to get maximal antiretroviral therapy. This drug may also play a beneficial role for peripheral neuropathy in HIV, and patients with both cognitive-motor deficits and neuropathy may participate. All patients will have access to memantine at the conclusion of the controlled portion of the trial.

- NARC 003 has also concluded enrollment and will be analyzed in the third quarter of 2000. This trial tests CPI-1189, an agent that has an effective tumor necrosis alpha antagonist property and in vitro properties suggesting potential efficacy for neurologic toxicity. Participating sites: Washington University (St. Louis), Columbia University (New York), Johns Hopkins University (Baltimore), University of Rochester (NY), Northwestern University (Chicago) and University of San Diego (CA).

- A5090 is a trial for treatment of HIV related motor cognitive disorder. This study is jointly sponsored by NARC and the ACTG system, and will test the safety and efficacy of selegiline (deprenyl) patches for this disorder. It follows up an earlier small study that suggested efficacy for this agent in the setting of AIDS dementia. The study will be placebo controlled for the first 24 weeks, then open label for an additional 24 weeks.

In all cases, it remains important to seek a maximally effective HIV treatment regimen when dementia develops. Efforts to bring viral load to the lowest possible level in serum (and probably in cerebral spinal fluid (CSF)) should be primary goal for all treating physicians. Antivirals with good CNS penetration including zidovudine, D4T, nevirapine, and abacavir may be used preferentially if they have not already failed.

These trials are important because they extend the range of therapies available, and also because they are serious efforts to correlate the clinical manifestations of ADC with prospectively collected samples of serum and CSF in patients with dementia to further study the pathophysiology of this disorder. With more certain understanding of the pathophysiology, more appropriate and specific therapies can be designed for the future. Additional studies to evaluate brain metabolism in this disorder by such means as positron emission tomography or magnetic resonance spectroscopy are available at selected centers. Other centers are actively attempting to evaluate the role of viral loads in the cerebrospinal fluid as it relates to the development of dementia, and to follow this parameter over the course of treatment.

Chapter 32

Peripheral Neuropathy

Peripheral neuropathy is a very common and disabling problem encountered in HIV infection. It develops primarily in relatively advanced patients with low CD4 counts, and may be exacerbated by the neurotoxicity of several of the drugs commonly used to treat HIV including ddC, ddI, and D4T. However, it is clear that the viral infection itself results in a typical symmetric, painful, distal sensory neuropathy. This entity almost always presents with variable loss of sensation in the feet and a variety of uncomfortable sensations of swelling, prickling, throbbing or other painful sensations in the feet. This may extend up the legs as it worsens and may eventually start to effect the hands. It occurs in around 20% of AIDS patients, and similar symptoms occur in an even greater number when the drug induced neuropathy is included. In general, when neuropathy is caused by one of the drugs, eliminating or reducing the dose of the drug may relieve the symptoms after 4-8 weeks.

Treatment of neuropathic pain such as is encountered in neuropathy is notoriously difficult. Minimizing neurotoxic drugs, optimizing diet, assuring that there are no contributing vitamin deficiencies (especially B12 and thiamine) are important first steps. Alcohol is often a neurotoxin, and continued heavy alcohol use may worsen symptoms. Routine analgesics such as aspirin and ibuprofen generally provide little relief. Even narcotics may not fully relieve this kind of pain. The most commonly helpful therapy is use of low doses of tricycle antidepressant drugs such as amitriptyline or imipramine, not because they can relieve depression, but because they change the pain processing in the brain, thus providing symptomatic relief for the patient. Newer antidepressants (Prozac and similar drugs) are generally less helpful than the older tricyclic compounds for this indication.

Treatment of painful neuropathy is a major current focus for the Neurologic AIDS Research Consortium and of the AIDS Clinical Trial Group. The recently completed trial of nerve growth factor (NGF) (ACTG 291) has been reported in *Neurology 2000*; 54:1080-1088. NGF did provide significant relief to pain in patients with neuropathy based on Gracely Pain Scale scores. However, during the 18 week trial, quantitative sensory testing did not document return of function in the peripheral nerves. At present, subjects that participated in ACTG 291 continue to have access to NGF.

A recently completed trial of lamotrigine for peripheral neuropathy is being analyzed in early 2001. Results are pending at this time.

NARC is developing a study probing the pathophysiology of painful neuropathy resulting from dideoxynucleoside toxicity in HIV patients. This study, being developed in the ACTG system, is A5117, led by Dr. Anthony Geraci and Dr. David Simpson at Mt. Sinai Medical Center in New York. The study will provide critical information about the measures reflecting damage in the peripheral nerves when pain develops, and will be the basis for a future treatment trial seeking to prevent this serious complication.

Chapter 33

Other Major Neurologic Complications in AIDS

Toxoplasma Encephalitis

Toxoplasma encephalitis is a frequently encountered neurologic complication in AIDS probably occurring in around 10% of cases. Incidence depends on the prevalence of prior infection, and on the pattern of prophylactic antibiotic usage. Current sulfa prophylaxis used especially for Pneumocystis pneumonia prevention, also reduces reactivation of toxoplasma. When toxoplasma encephalitis occurs, it presents with a subacute encephalopathy which may be generalized (increasing confusion, lethargy, signs of increased intracranial pressure) due to multifocal involvement, or may present with any focal neurologic deficit or seizures. Imaging studies generally show a multifocal encephalitis with variable mass effect and contrast enhancement. Since this encephalitis often responds promptly to therapy, diagnosis is most often suggested by successful therapeutic trial. The optimal therapy combines sulfadiazine with pyrimethamine. However, in sulfa allergic patients, clindamycin is generally substituted for sulfadiazine. If a patient continues to deteriorate on this therapy, or fails to improve in 7-14 days, consideration of a brain biopsy to seek alternate diagnoses is appropriate. Such cases should probably be referred to neurologic referral centers with greater experience with these complications.

217

Cryptococcal Meningitis

Cryptococcal meningitis is a very frequent complication of advancing HIV infection, occurring in about 10% of subjects. It may present with subtle neurologic changes, unaccustomed headaches, new fever, or systemic symptoms. Marked meningismus is uncommon in HIV, making it important to maintain a high level of alertness for this diagnosis, and study the spinal fluid when symptoms referable to the brain occur. Imaging studies are generally unrewarding. In symptomatic cases, most clinicians believe optimal response is achieved by a consolidation therapy with amphotericin B administered intravenously, followed by permanent suppression with fluconazole. Clinical follow-up including repeat cerebral spinal fluid (CDF) examinations, and monitoring serum cryptococcal antigen response is critical. In severe cases with marked elevations of pressure, direct therapy to reduce elevated CFS pressure, and use of steroids may be required. Successful therapy of this complication is rewarding, with excellent recovery and long term control a reasonable expectation.

Syphilis

Syphilis is a concurrent venereal disease which much be considered when neurologic complications are encountered in HIV. Therapy for syphilis that is effective when the immune system is intact likely is insufficient in the setting of immunodeficiency. Eradication of neurosyphilis is particularly problematic, and even extended courses of intravenous penicillin or ceftriaxone cannot be assured of eradicating this opportunistic infection. Careful monitoring for neurosyphilis and aggressive treatment with close follow-up is required.

Central Nervous System (CNS) Lymphoma

CNS lymphoma is a particularly serious and common neurologic complication of advanced immunodeficiency. The primary CNS lymphoma is not associated with systemic lymphoma, and presents as single or multiple brain tumors, generally with significant mass effect and contrast enhancement on imaging studies. These tumors in AIDS are almost always associated with Epstein-Barr Virus which is found in the tissue of the tumor. CSF analysis for the DNA of EBV is generally positive in the setting of CNS lymphoma in AIDS, and may help to suggest the diagnosis. However, a brain biopsy is generally required to confirm the diagnosis in most cases. Unfortunately, the prognosis for this tumor is particularly poor in the setting of HIV. Radiation therapy may be palliative, but almost always the tumor is associated with death within six months. Supplementing radiation with chemotherapy is under consideration, but because of advancing immunodeficiency, this is difficult, and has not in general led to clinically meaningful prolongation of quality survival.

Chapter 34

HIV Wasting Syndrome

Wasting syndrome is involuntary weight loss greater than 10%, accompanied by more than 30 days of diarrhea, weakness, or fever. It was one of the first noted HIV-related systemic conditions and, before antiretrovirals, one of the most common HIV-related conditions.

Individuals with wasting are more likely to develop an HIV-related infection or cancer, and they are more likely to die from AIDS. In particular, a weight loss of 3% in one month, 5% in 6 months, or 10% in 12 months predicts the development of HIV related illnesses.

What Causes Wasting?

HIV infection affects the body in many ways that result in an increased demand for calories and compounded by a poor intake of calories, results in weight loss and poor nutrition:

Altered metabolism. Baseline metabolism is the rate at which the body burns calories. HIV infection (without illness) increases the baseline metabolism by 10%, meaning that a person with HIV needs more calories to maintain their body weight. In an HIV-infected person who has an infection or cancer, the baseline metabolism increases by about 30%, requiring even more calories to maintain a normal body weight.

Low food intake. Many people with HIV, especially those with an HIV-related infection or cancer, do not eat enough food to maintain their body weight. They may have a low appetite or may not eat when they are hungry because so many AIDS drugs must be taken on an empty stomach; opportunistic infections in the mouth may make it difficult to eat; infections in the intestines may make eating unpleasant; or they may not have the energy to prepare food.

Poor nutrient absorption. In healthy people, nutrients are absorbed from food by the small intestine. In people with HIV, nutrients are not absorbed very well because of intestinal infections, diarrhea, and perhaps the virus itself.

Hormonal and biochemical changes. The majority of weight lost in HIV wasting is lean body mass, the working tissue of the body. Normally, a person with poor nutrition and a high metabolism burns off fat first and then muscle. People with HIV tend to burn off muscle first, then fat because of hormonal and biochemical changes. For example, people with HIV have reduced levels of testosterone, a hormone that helps maintain lean body mass.

Treatment

Antiretroviral therapy and treatment for HIV-related infections or cancers decreases the metabolism. A decreased metabolic rate means calories are not used up as quickly and weight loss is slowed.

Good nutrition is essential. People who are experiencing wasting may benefit from a nutritionist.

Several medications are used to treat wasting by increasing appetite, lean body mass, or body fat, either singly, or in combination. They include the following:

- Megestrol acetate was the first medication approved by the FDA to treat wasting. It is a powerful appetite stimulant. It results in a reduced testosterone level in men and women and the weight gained is primarily fat.

- Dronabinol, an active ingredient in marijuana, is an appetite stimulant and does not have a direct effect on fat or muscle.

- Human growth hormone increases appetite and lean body mass.

- Thalidomide increases appetite, lean body mass, and fat.

- Oxandrolone, nandrolone, and testosterone are steroids that increase appetite and a sense of well-being. The weight gained is predominantly lean body mass.

Chapter 35

Drug Interactions in HIV Treatment

Drug Interactions

With the number of drugs available to treat HIV and prevent or treat opportunistic infections (OIs), the potential for drug interactions becomes an increasing concern. Developing a health management plan and deciding which therapies to include in that plan seems a daunting task. Not only does each particular therapy have potential side effects, but each therapy might augment or diminish the benefit of other drugs. Many people are taking a variety of therapies simultaneously, ranging from experimental and approved antivirals to complimentary approaches and over-the-counter medications. Drug interactions are not always considered when developing a treatment strategy, but may play a major role in the success of any plan for managing HIV disease. The following are some guidelines to help prevent drug interactions.

The first section in this chapter is from Project Inform: Excerpted from "Drug Interactions," © 2002 Project Inform, reprinted with permission. An extensive chart listing drug interactions is available on the Project Inform website at http://www.projectinform.org/fs/drugin.html. For more information, contact the National HIV/AIDS Treatment Hotline, 800-822-7422, or visit our website, www.projectinform.org. The second section is reprinted with permission from "Cocktails and Party Favors" by Meredith A. Potochnic, Pharm.D., STEP *Perspective,* Volume 2, Number 1, Spring 2002, © 2002 Seattle Treatment Education Project. For additional information contact the Seattle Treatment Education Project at PMB 998 1122 East Pike Street, Seattle, WA 98122-3934, (206) 329-4857, info@stepproject.org, or visit http://www.thebody.com/step/steppage.html.

- Brown Bag Medicine Checkup: Each time you see your health care provider, put all your medications, including over-the-counter and complimentary products, in a bag and have your physician conduct a personalized review of your medicine for safety, appropriateness, compatibility and instructions for use.

- Each time you are prescribed a new medication, ask your physician if it can be combined safely with your other therapies.

- Talk to your health care provider about making a "medicine checkup" part of your regular visits, and discuss how best to monitor for potential drug interactions. Bring the medicine with you to your appointment.

Drug interactions can take various forms, occurring immediately or over several weeks. Some drugs simply should not be used together, while others can be combined only if accompanied by careful monitoring to detect emergency problems. Interactions can occur when one therapy affects how another is absorbed, broken down (metabolized), distributed or excreted. Interactions can also occur when one therapy alters the effect of another. A common interaction can occur when two drugs have similar toxicity profiles. For example, both ddI and ddC can cause peripheral neuropathy, a tingling or pain in the legs, hands or feet. It is not recommended that they be used together because the similar side effects of the two drugs may increase the potential for neuropathy. Similarly, AZT and ganciclovir, a treatment for CMV (cytomegalovirus), may both cause bone marrow suppression, resulting in anemia. However, the addition of a third drug, G-CSF (Neupogen), can help manage this interaction. In addition, higher blood levels of a drug increase the chance of potential toxicity.

As it has become standard medical practice to prevent multiple OIs (opportunistic infections) with a number of different drugs, drug interactions are of increasing concern. In some prevention regimens, drug interactions may even cause more harm than good. For example, one drug might reduce blood levels of another drug, leading to the development of drug resistance. In other words, drug interactions could result in the development of a disease unresponsive to standard treatment. The added toxicity of numerous combined therapies may also outweigh their potential benefit for preventing disease. Therefore, health care providers and people with HIV should make informed decisions about combination therapies and OI prevention regimens and should monitor carefully for drug interactions and other side effects.

Unfortunately, most drug interaction studies have compared only two drugs, although most people with HIV often take many more than two drugs. As a result, very little is known about how all the commonly used drugs interact with each other.

In the mean time, it is important to discuss potential drug interactions with a health care provider and a pharmacist. Before starting a new therapy—be it approved, experimental or complimentary—factor in potential drug interactions and side effects. Not everyone experiences side effects of drugs and many drug interactions can be managed by monitoring carefully, adjusting the doses, or discontinuing the therapy as needed.

An extensive chart listing drug interactions is available on the Project Inform website at http://www.projectinform.org/fs/drugin.html. This chart should only be used as a guide for drug interactions. Some of these interactions have been reported in medical literature while others are purely anecdotal. Remember that these drug interactions might occur in some people, but not in others. The chart was put together through information from package inserts, anecdotal reports, discussions with pharmacologists and physicians who treat HIV disease, and discussions with pharmaceutical companies.

Cocktails and Party Favors

The club drug epidemic is spreading. According to a *Drug Abuse Trend* report published by the National Institute on Drug Abuse (a division of the National Institutes of Health), there appears to be an alarming increase in the use of ecstasy, GHB, and ketamine in almost all cities surveyed. Methamphetamine use appears to remain concentrated on the West Coast and has been associated with an increased number of emergency room visits in Seattle. Other drugs of abuse identified by this report include cocaine, heroin, marijuana, benzodiazepines (clonazepam [Klonopin], alprazolam [Xanax], diazepam [Valium]), sildenafil (Viagra), and various prescription narcotics. With the increasing popularity of such drugs, there is concern that their use can potentially lead to serious health problems. For example, what happens when club drugs are mixed with HIV medications?

There has been a lot of interest regarding how recreational drug use may affect HIV infection and antiretroviral therapy. The most obvious concerns are as follows:

- There is concern that some recreational drugs may weaken the immune system, possibly speeding up the progression of HIV disease.

- There is concern that recreational drug use could interfere with one's ability to adhere to antiretroviral therapy, possibly leading to viral resistance.

- There is concern that combining HIV medications with recreational drugs might result in a drug interaction, which could either decrease the effectiveness of one's antiretroviral therapy, or cause a serious side effect.

The intention of this section is to focus on the area of drug interactions between HIV medications and recreational drugs. It will help to first understand the definition of a drug interaction.

A drug interaction happens when a person takes two drugs and one or both of the drugs behave differently when taken together than they would if taken alone. In other words, one of the medications changes the effects of the other. In some situations, drug interactions are not a problem. In other situations, drug interactions can affect one's therapy or even cause serious harm. The most common type of drug interaction that is seen with HIV medications is related to how a drug is metabolized (broken down) by the body.

The liver is the major organ that is involved in the metabolism of most HIV medications (particularly protease inhibitors and non-nucleosides). The liver is also used to break down some recreational drugs. To confuse things, some drugs, especially protease inhibitors, can also slow down (inhibit) how the liver clears other medications from the body. When two medications in the body are waiting in line to be broken down by the liver, they often have to compete. Protease inhibitors, such as ritonavir, are stronger and often win the competition. In this situation, the second medication is not cleared as quickly, often resulting in increased levels in the bloodstream. If drugs such as recreational drugs are present in the bloodstream in larger than usual concentrations, they can be dangerous.

On the flip side, some medications can speed up (induce) how the liver clears other medications from the body. When this happens, the second medication is cleared faster from the body and there is not enough medication around to do its work. Inducers can cause some HIV medications to be removed from the bloodstream and this can lead to viral resistance.

Quite a bit is known about drug interactions with protease inhibitors and other HIV medications. Unfortunately, there is minimal information available regarding drug interactions with recreational drugs. Little research is being done on this topic because there is a lack of financial incentive for drug companies to fund research due to ethical concerns and the fear of being recognized as supporters of illicit drug use. Based on what we already know about how certain drugs are cleared from the body, we can guess that mixing certain combinations together could lead to danger.

The best way to avoid potentially serious interactions is to not mix recreational drugs with antiretroviral therapy. However, if you choose to mix them, you should at least be aware of the risks involved. Following is a description of suspected drug interactions that may occur between HIV medications and recreational drugs.

Alcohol

Antiretrovirals (ARVs)

There is not a direct interaction between alcohol and ARVs. However, it is possible that chronic alcohol use can increase the risk of drug toxicities such as liver damage (with protease Inhibitors, nevirapine, d4T), pancreatitis (with ddI, ddC), and neuropathy (with ddI, d4T, ddC).

There is an established association between excessive alcohol use and poor adherence to ARVs. It would be ideal to achieve sobriety prior to starting HAART. If sobriety is not a possibility and there is a need to start HAART, avoid a ddI-containing regimen as it may increase the risk of pancreatitis.

GHB

GHB and alcohol are both central nervous system (CNS) depressants. When mixed together, alcohol can increase the potential for seizures, difficulty breathing, and GHB coma. Avoid mixing with GHB.

Sedatives

Sedatives such as diazepam (Valium), triazolam (Halcion), temazepam (Restoril), and many others, are, like alcohol, CNS depressants. When mixed together, they can lead to prolonged sleep and possibly decreased breathing. Avoid mixing with sedatives.

Amyl Nitrate (Poppers)

Viagra

May result in extremely low blood pressure which can potentially be fatal. Do not mix.

Cocaine (Coke, Blow)

Antiretrovirals (ARVs)

There are no known interactions between cocaine and ARVs. There is one test-tube study to suggest that cocaine may cause HIV to reproduce 20 times faster than normal. However, a definite correlation between cocaine use and viral load has not been established.

Long-term cocaine use can lead to problems with attention and concentration, memory loss, and decreased speed in processing information. Cocaine usage promotes a disorganized behavior, which can lead to missing ARV doses and ultimately to drug resistance.

Crystal Methamphetamine (Crystal Meth, Crystal, Speed, Ice)

Protease Inhibitors (PIs)

There is a theoretical concern that PIs, particularly ritonavir, can decrease the clearance of crystal. This interaction could result in a 2- to 3-fold buildup of crystal in the blood, possibly leading to an overdose.

Start with lower doses of crystal (1/3 to 1/2 of normal dose) to account for possible enhanced activity by protease inhibitors. If injecting, use clean and safe technique. As with cocaine and other binge drugs, there is a concern that the use of crystal can lead to a lapse in taking HIV medications.

Long Term Crystal Use

Long-term use of crystal can lead to weight loss, poor nutrition, lack of sleep, and fatigue which might lead to further immunosuppression.

Ecstasy (E, X, MDMA)

Antiretrovirals (ARVs)

Antiretrovirals (ARVs), particularly PIs (ritonavir) and delavirdine, may cause a 3- to 10-fold increase in ecstasy levels in the bloodstream, leading to an overdose.

To date, there has been at least one death caused by an ecstasy overdose that may be the result of an interaction between ecstasy and the PI ritonavir.

Mixing "X" with PIs is likely to increase levels of "X" as well as prolong the "high." If mixing the two, it is advisable to start with 1/4 to 1/2 tablet and wait for effect. "X" can increase your body temperature and cause you to sweat, especially if you are dancing in a hot environment. Take frequent breaks to cool off. It is important to drink plenty of fluids, especially if taking indinavir (Crixivan) or if combining ecstasy with alcohol. Alcohol will increase the risk of dehydration.

If you have high blood pressure, diabetes, a heart condition, or asthma, "X" could be a dangerous drug for you.

Antidepressants

MAO inhibitors (Nardil) should not be used in combination with "X" as mixing them might cause an increased blood pressure which could be life threatening. Do not mix.

Selective serotonin reuptake inhibitors (SSRIs) such as fluoxetine (Prozac), sertraline (Zoloft), paroxetine (Paxil), and many others may have a reduced effect when mixed with "X." There is information to suggest that even short-term use of "X" may cause permanent changes in brain chemistry, which could increase the risk of depression.

If you are suffering from depression, it may be best to avoid ecstasy as it may either aggravate or complicate the treatment of depression.

GHB (G, Liquid Ecstasy)

Protease Inhibitors (PIs)

Protease inhibitors (PIs) may potentially increase levels of GHB in the bloodstream. This interaction is not well documented. However, there is a case report of a life-threatening reaction to GHB when given in combination with the PIs (ritonavir and saquinavir).

GHB is difficult to measure since it is only available as a liquid. It is best to start with no more than one teaspoonful and wait about 30 minutes for effects to begin before taking more. In some people, effects can last for about 4 hours, depending on the dose and/or the possibility of drug interactions.

GHB overdoses can occur pretty quickly and may present with drowsiness, nausea, vomiting, headache, decreased breathing, loss of reflexes, and loss of consciousness. It is best to be on the buddy system when taking GHB.

Alcohol

Alcohol and GHB are both central nervous system (CNS) depressants. When mixed together, alcohol can increase the potential for seizures, difficulty breathing, and GHB coma.

Avoid mixing with alcohol and sedatives.

Sedatives

Sedatives (Valium, Halcion, Restoril, and many others) and GHB are both CNS depressants. When mixed together, they can increase your risk of GHB coma and breathing failure.

Heroin (Smack, Junk, China White)

Protease Inhibitors (PIs)

Protease inhibitors such as ritonavir may decrease heroin levels by 50%, thus decreasing the possibility of an overdose.

Don't try to compensate for this possible interaction. Start with your normal dose and only increase if you experience a lesser effect. Use clean and safe injection technique.

Heroin generally doesn't mix well with other party drugs so avoid mixing.

Ketamine (Special K, K, Vitamin K, Kitty Valium)

Antiretrovirals

Antiretrovirals such as protease inhibitors and delavirdine may increase the levels of "K" in the bloodstream, possibly leading to increased heart rate, increased blood pressure, or difficulty breathing.

A New York HIV doctor has reported two cases of chemical hepatitis that may be the result of mixing ritonavir with "K."

If mixing "K" with ARVs, less drug will go further. Start with 1/3 to 1/2 of your usual dose and wait for effect. Don't take another bump unless you feel OK. Otherwise, you may end up in a semi-conscious K-hole.

Avoid mixing with alcohol, GHB, or sedatives as all four can cause CNS depression.

Like GHB, it is best to be on the buddy system when taking "K."

Marijuana (THC)

Protease Inhibitors (PIs)

Protease inhibitors may increase levels of THC in the bloodstream. However, there are no known cases of marijuana overdose, so this interaction should not be dangerous. Smoking marijuana may increase one's risk for pneumonia.

THC may be helpful to control nausea and to increase appetite. As an alternative to smoking, there is an oral form available (Marinol).

Marinol may cause more tiredness and fatigue as compared to inhaled marijuana. If given with a protease inhibitor, Marinol can be introduced at a lower dose and increased for effect.

Sedatives (Benzodiazepines)

Protease Inhibitors (PIs)

Protease inhibitors may block the breakdown of certain sedatives, leading to increased blood levels of these drugs. Sedatives to avoid with P's include triazolam (Halcion), midazolam (Versed), flurazepam (Dalmane), and diazepam (Valium).

Alternative sedatives that appear to be safer when combined with protease inhibitors include lorazepam (Ativan), temazepam (Restoril), oxazepam (Serax).

Alcohol

Alcohol, GHB, and Ketamine are all CNS depressants and if mixed will increase the risk of decreased breathing or coma. Avoid mixing with alcohol, GHB, or "K."

Viagra

Protease Inhibitors (PIs)

Protease inhibitors may decrease the clearance of Viagra, leading to high blood levels of Viagra. Side effects of interaction may include abnormal changes in blood pressure and chest pain.

Recommended starting dose of Viagra is 25 mg. Dose may be increased if needed and/or tolerated.

Amyl Nitrate ("Poppers")

May result in extremely low blood pressure which can potentially be fatal. Do not mix.

Conclusion

The best way to avoid potentially serious interactions is to not mix recreational drugs with antiretroviral therapy. However, if you choose to mix them, you should at least be aware of the risks involved.

Please note that this is not a complete list of all drug interactions that occur with antiretrovirals or other HIV-related medications. The intention is to focus on drug interactions that occur primarily with recreational drugs. If you have questions regarding drug interactions with other prescription and non-prescription medications or with recreational drugs not mentioned in this chapter, please consult your physician or pharmacist to ensure the safety of that combination. It is important that you feel comfortable talking to your healthcare provider without the fear of being judged.

Additionally, recommendations made to reduce the harm of certain combinations cannot be validated by studies, as there are none. There is no guarantee that a serious adverse reaction won't occur when combining certain drugs not listed in this chapter. It is important to accept the reality that people are mixing cocktails and party favors on a regular basis. It is simply the hope that after weighing the risks, you make an informed decision to choose what is best for you.

To further reduce the harm of mixing cocktails, here are some general guidelines:

- If you are trying a recreational drug for the first time, try it alone, before mixing it with other substances.

- Avoid mixing psychedelics with alcohol.

- Be conservative and not greedy. Product batches are not always consistent. Just because you tolerated a dose this time, doesn't mean you won't overdose next time.

- Realize that every person reacts differently. Just because your friend can tolerate a combination, doesn't mean that you can.

- Party with friends who know what you are taking in case of an overdose.

- Stay hydrated.

- Get plenty of rest and let your immune system recover.

- Antiretroviral therapy should not be interrupted, as interruption of therapy could lead to viral resistance. Talk to your doctor if you are thinking about stopping your medications.

Part Four

Living with AIDS

Chapter 36

Living with HIV/AIDS: An Overview

Although HIV is a serious infection, people with HIV and AIDS are living longer, healthier lives today, thanks to new and effective treatments. This chapter will help you understand how you can live with HIV and how you can keep yourself healthy.

You probably have many questions about HIV, such as: What is HIV and how did I get it? What is the difference between HIV and AIDS? How can I stay healthy longer? How do I protect other people from my HIV? Where can I find help in fighting HIV? This chapter will give you answers to many of your questions. You should feel free to ask your doctor any question about HIV.

What is HIV and how did I get it?

The first cases of AIDS were identified in the United States in 1981, but it most likely existed here and in other parts of the world for many years before that. In 1984 scientists proved that HIV causes AIDS.

You might have caught HIV by having unprotected sex—sex without a condom—with someone who has HIV. Or you might have shared a needle to inject drugs or shared drug works with someone who has HIV. Babies born to women with HIV also can become infected. Although in the past you could get HIV from a blood transfusion, today

---

National Center for HIV, STD and TB Prevention, Centers for Disease Control and Prevention (CDC), updated September 1998; available online at http://www.cdc.gov/hiv/pubs/brochure/livingwithhiv.htm. Despite the older date of this document, the overview provided is still helpful.

it is unlikely you got infected that way because all blood in the United States has been tested for HIV since 1985. You could not have gotten HIV just from working with or being around someone who has HIV— and no one can get it from you that way. Also, HIV is not spread by insect bites or stings, on toilet seats, or through everyday things like sharing a meal.

What is the difference between HIV and AIDS?

When HIV enters your body, it infects your CD4 cells and kills them. CD4 cells sometimes called T-helper cells) help your body fight off infection and disease. Usually, CD4 cell counts in someone with a healthy immune system range from 500 to 1800.

When you lose CD4 cells, your immune system breaks down and you can't fight infections and diseases as well. When your CD4 cell count goes under 200, doctors say you have AIDS. Doctors also say you have AIDS if you have HIV and certain diseases, such as tuberculosis or *Pneumocystis carinii* [NEW-mo-SIS-tis CA-RIN-nee-eye] pneumonia (PCP), even if your CD4 cell count is over 200.

How can I stay healthy longer?

There are many things you can do for yourself to stay healthy. Here are a few:

- Make sure you have a doctor who knows how to treat HIV.

- Follow your doctor's instructions. Keep your appointments. Your doctor may prescribe medicine for you. Take the medicine just the way he or she tells you to because taking only some of your medicine gives your HIV infection more chance to fight back. If you get sick from your medicine, call your doctor for advice— don't change how you take your medicine on your own or because of advice from friends.

- Get immunizations (shots) to prevent infections such as pneumonia and flu. Your doctor will tell you when to get these shots. If you smoke or if you use drugs not prescribed by your doctor, quit.

- Eat healthy foods. This will help keep you strong, keep your energy and weight up, and help your body protect itself.

- Exercise regularly to stay strong and fit.

- Get enough sleep and rest.

- Take time to relax. Many people find prayer or meditation, along with exercise and rest, helps them cope with the stress of having HIV infection or AIDS.

There also are many things you can do to protect your health when you prepare food or eat, when you travel, and when you're around pets and other animals. You can read more about these things in the brochures in the CDC Opportunistic Infections Series. You can get these brochures and other information on HIV from the CDC National AIDS Hotline at (800)342-2437 or at the CDC web site at http://www.cdc.gov.

What can I expect when I go to the doctor?

At your first appointment your doctor will ask you questions, do a checkup, draw blood, and do a tuberculosis skin test and other tests. Your doctor also may give you some immunizations (shots). Tell your doctor about any health problems you are having so that you can get treatment. You also should ask your doctor any questions you have about HIV or AIDS, such as what to do if your medicine makes you sick, where to get help in quitting smoking or drug use, or how to eat healthy foods.

When your doctor draws blood, it is used for many tests, including the CD4 cell count and viral load testing. Viral load testing measures the amount of HIV in your blood. Viral load tests help predict what will happen next with your HIV infection if you don't get treatment. They are used with CD4 cell counts to decide when to start and when to change your drug therapies.

Keep your follow-up appointments with your doctor. At follow-up appointments you and your doctor will talk about your test results, and he or she may prescribe medicine for you.

What is the treatment for HIV or AIDS?

HIV and HIV-related illnesses vary from person to person. People can live with HIV for many years. Your doctor will design a medical care plan for you. Your doctor will tell you about the risks and benefits of the drugs for HIV and when you need to start taking them. Many drugs are used together to treat HIV. These drugs often include antiretroviral medicines. These medicines are powerful drugs, but they are not cures for HIV. If your doctor prescribes any of these drugs for you, take them exactly as prescribed.

If your HIV infection gets worse and your CD4 cell count falls be-low 200, you are more likely to get other infections. Your doctor will prescribe TMP-SMX (trimethoprim-sulfamethoxazole [try-METH-o-prim—sul-fa-meth-OX-uh-zole])—also known as Bactrim®, Septra®, or Cotrim®—or other drugs, to prevent PCP.

Your doctor also may prescribe other drugs for you, depending on your CD4 count. Most people have no problem with these medicines. But if you get a rash or have other problems, call your doctor right away to discuss other treatments. Don't change the way you are tak-ing any of your medicines without first talking with your doctor. If you don't take your medicines the right way, you might give your HIV infection a better chance to fight back.

What are some of the other diseases I could get?

In addition to PCP, you also have a higher chance of getting other diseases, depending on your CD4 count. These are called opportunis-tic infections because a person with HIV can get the infection if his or her weakened immune system gives it the opportunity to develop. More than 100 germs can cause opportunistic infections. Some of these infections include:

- MAC (mycobacterium avium [my-ko-bak-TEER-i-um a-VEE-i-um] complex)

- CMV (cytomegalovirus [si-to-MEG-eh-lo-vi-res])

- TB (tuberculosis [too-burr-qu-LO-sis])

- toxo (toxoplasmosis [tok-so-plaz-MO-sis])

- crypto (cryptosporidiosis [krip-to-spo-rid-e-O-sis])

You can learn more about how to prevent the most serious oppor-tunistic infections from the brochures in the CDC Opportunistic In-fections Series, which you can get by calling the CDC National AIDS Hotline at (800) 342-2437.

Watch out for certain symptoms:

- breathing problems

- mouth problems, such as thrush (white spots), sores, change in taste, dryness, trouble swallowing, or loose teeth

- fever for more than two days

- weight loss

- poor vision or floaters (moving lines or spots in your vision)

- diarrhea

- skin rashes or itching

Tell your doctor right away if you have any of these problems. Your doctor can treat most of your HIV-related problems, but sometimes he or she may need to send you to a specialist. Visit a dentist at least twice a year, or more often if you have mouth problems.

How do I protect other people from my HIV?

- Don't have unprotected sex—sex without a condom. Abstinence—not having sex—is the best way to protect other people. If you have sex, use a new latex condom (rubber) each and every time.

- If you use a lubricant, use a water-based lubricant. You should not use new petroleum-based jelly, cold cream, baby oil, or other oils because they can weaken a condom and it may break.

- If you are allergic to latex, you can use polyurethane (a type of plastic) condoms.

- If male condoms are not available, use female condoms.

- If you choose to use a spermicide (a cream, foam, or gel used to kill sperm) use it as the instructions say. You can use condoms with or without spermicide.

- For oral sex, use protection such as a condom, dental dam (a square piece of latex used by dentists), or plastic food wrap. Do not reuse these items.

- Keep sex toys for your own use only and don't use someone else's sex toys.

- Don't share drug needles or drug works. In many places there are needle exchange programs. Use them. Better yet, seek help if you inject drugs. You can fight HIV much better if you don't have a drug habit.

- Tell people you've had sex with that you have HIV. This will not be easy, but it will help them get the help they need. Your local public health department may help you find these people and tell them they have been exposed to HIV. If they have HIV, this may help them get care and avoid spreading HIV to others.

- If a woman you had sex with is pregnant, even if you are not the father, it is very important that you tell her you have HIV. If she has HIV, she needs to get early medical care for her own health and to protect her baby.

- Don't donate blood, plasma, or organs.

- Keep razors or toothbrushes for your own use only and don't use someone else's razor or toothbrush. HIV can be spread through fresh blood on such items.

Family Planning and Pregnancy

Is there any special advice for women with HIV?

Yes. If you are a woman with HIV, your doctor should check you for sexually transmitted diseases (STDs) and perform a Pap test at least once a year.

Women with HIV are more likely to have abnormal Pap tests. If your Pap test is abnormal, your doctor may need to repeat it or do other tests. If you have had an abnormal Pap test in the past, tell your doctor.

If you are thinking about either avoiding pregnancy or becoming pregnant, talk with your doctor about important issues such as:

- What birth control methods are best for me?

- Will HIV cause problems for me during pregnancy or delivery?

- Will my baby have HIV?

- Will treatment for my HIV infection cause problems for my baby?

- If I am pregnant and want an abortion, where can I go for it? What if they won't help me because I have HIV?

- If I choose to get pregnant, what medical and community programs and support groups can help me and my baby?

- What if I become pregnant?

If you become pregnant, talk to your doctor right away about medical care for you and your baby. You also need to plan for your child's future in case you get sick. Your HIV treatment will not change very much from what it was before you became pregnant. You should have a Pap test and tests for STDs during your pregnancy. Your doctor will order tests and suggest medicines for you to take. Talk with him or her about all the pros and cons of taking medicine while you are pregnant.

If you decide to have your baby, talk with your doctor about how you can prevent giving HIV to your baby. It is very important that you get good care early in your pregnancy. The chances of passing HIV to your baby before or during birth are about 1 in 4, or 25%, but treatment with zidovudine [zy-DAH-vue-deen], sometimes called ZDV, AZT, or Retrovir®, has been shown to greatly lower this risk. Your doctor will want to have you on a drug treatment that includes ZDV.

Although you are pregnant, you should still use condoms each time you have sex, to avoid catching other diseases and to avoid spreading HIV. Even if your partner already has HIV, he should still use condoms.

After birth, your baby will need to be tested for HIV, even if you took ZDV and/or other drugs while you were pregnant. Your baby will need to take medicine to prevent HIV infection and PCP. Talk with your doctor about your baby's special medical needs. Because HIV infection can be passed through breast milk, you should not breast-feed your baby.

Where can I find help in fighting HIV?

If you are living with HIV or AIDS, you need many kinds of support—medical, emotional, psychological, and, yes, financial. Your doctor, your local health and social services departments, your local AIDS service organization, and your local library can aid you in finding all kinds of help:

- answers to your questions about HIV and AIDS
- doctors, insurance, and help in making health care decisions
- food, housing, and transportation
- planning to meet financial and daily needs
- support groups for you and your loved ones
- home nursing care
- help in legal matters, including Americans with Disabilities Act (ADA) claims
- confidential help in applying for Social Security disability benefits

You also can get information on these things from the CDC National AIDS Hotline at (800) 342-2437. Many people living with HIV feel better if they can talk with other people who also have HIV. Here are some ways to find others with HIV:

- Contact your local AIDS service organization. Look under AIDS or Social Service Organizations in the yellow pages of your telephone book.

- Contact a local hospital, church, or American Red Cross chapter for referrals.

- Read HIV newsletters or magazines.

- Join support groups or Internet forums.

- Volunteer to help others with HIV.

- Be an HIV educator or public speaker, or work on a newsletter.

- Attend social events to meet other people who have HIV.

Thousands of people are living with HIV, and AIDS, today. Many are leading full, happy, and productive lives. You can too if you work with your doctor and others and take the steps outlined in this chapter to stay healthy.

Chapter 37

Depression and HIV/AIDS

Research has enabled many men and women, and young people living with human immunodeficiency virus (HIV), the virus that causes acquired immunodeficiency syndrome (AIDS), to lead fuller, more productive lives. As with other serious illnesses such as cancer, heart disease or stroke, however, HIV often can be accompanied by depression, an illness that can affect mind, mood, body and behavior. Treatment for depression helps people manage both diseases, thus enhancing survival and quality of life.

Despite the enormous advances in brain research in the past 20 years, depression often goes undiagnosed and untreated. Although as many as one in three persons with HIV may suffer from depression,[1] the warning signs of depression are often misinterpreted. People with HIV, their families and friends, and even their physicians may assume that depressive symptoms are an inevitable reaction to being diagnosed with HIV. But depression is a separate illness that can and should be treated, even when a person is undergoing treatment for HIV or AIDS. Some of the symptoms of depression could be related to HIV, specific HIV-related disorders, or medication side effects. However, a skilled health professional will recognize the symptoms of depression and inquire about their duration and severity, diagnose the disorder, and suggest appropriate treatment.

Excerpted from "Depression and HIV/AIDS," National Institute of Mental Health (NIMH), NIH Publication Number 02-5005, 2002.

Depression Facts

Depression is a serious medical condition that affects thoughts, feelings, and the ability to function in everyday life. Depression can occur at any age. NIMH-sponsored studies estimate that 6 percent of 9- to 17-year-olds in the U.S. and almost 10 percent of American adults, or about 19 million people age 18 and older, experience some form of depression every year.[2,3] Although available therapies alleviate symptoms in over 80 percent of those treated, less than half of people with depression get the help they need.[3,4]

Depression results from abnormal functioning of the brain. The causes of depression are currently a matter of intense research. An interaction between genetic predisposition and life history appear to determine a person's level of risk. Episodes of depression may then be triggered by stress, difficult life events, side effects of medications, or the effects of HIV on the brain. Whatever its origins, depression can limit the energy needed to keep focused on staying healthy, and research shows that it may accelerate HIV's progression to AIDS.[5,6]

Get Treatment for Depression

While there are many different treatments for depression, they must be carefully chosen by a trained professional based on the circumstances of the person and family. Prescription antidepressant medications are generally well-tolerated and safe for people with HIV. There are, however, possible interactions among some of the medications and side effects that require careful monitoring. Specific types of psychotherapy, or talk therapy, also can relieve depression.

Some individuals with HIV attempt to treat their depression with herbal remedies. However, use of herbal supplements of any kind should be discussed with a physician before they are tried. Scientists recently discovered that St. John's wort, an herbal remedy sold over-the-counter and promoted as a treatment for mild depression, can have harmful interactions with other medications, including those prescribed for HIV. In particular, St. John's wort reduces blood levels of the protease inhibitor indinavir (Crixivan®) and probably the other protease inhibitor drugs as well. If taken together, the combination could allow the AIDS virus to rebound, perhaps in a drug-resistant form. (See the alert on the NIMH Web site: http://www.nimh.nih.gov/events/stjohnwort.cfm.)

Treatment for depression in the context of HIV or AIDS should be managed by a mental health professional—for example, a psychiatrist, psychologist, or clinical social worker—who is in close communication with the physician providing the HIV/AIDS treatment. This is especially important when antidepressant medication is prescribed, so that potentially harmful drug interactions can be avoided. In some cases, a mental health professional that specializes in treating individuals with depression and co-occurring physical illnesses such as HIV/AIDS may be available. People with HIV/AIDS who develop depression, as well as people in treatment for depression who subsequently contract HIV, should make sure to tell any physician they visit about the full range of medications they are taking.

Recovery from depression takes time. Medications for depression can take several weeks to work and may need to be combined with ongoing psychotherapy. Not everyone responds to treatment in the same way. Prescriptions and dosing may need to be adjusted. No matter how advanced the HIV, however, the person does not have to suffer from depression. Treatment can be effective.

It takes more than access to good medical care for persons living with HIV to stay healthy. A positive outlook, determination and discipline are also required to deal with the stresses of avoiding high-risk behaviors, keeping up with the latest scientific advances, adhering to complicated medication regimens, reshuffling schedules for doctor visits, and grieving over the death of loved ones.

Other mental disorders, such as bipolar disorder (manic-depressive illness) and anxiety disorders, may occur in people with HIV or AIDS, and they too can be effectively treated. For more information about these and other mental illnesses, contact NIMH.

Remember, depression is a treatable disorder of the brain. Depression can be treated in addition to whatever other illnesses a person might have, including HIV. If you think you may be depressed or know someone who is, don't lose hope. Seek help for depression.

For more information about depression and NIMH activities and programs in HIV and AIDS research, contact:

National Institute of Mental Health (NIMH)
Office of Communications and Public Liaison
Information Resources and Inquiries Branch
6001 Executive Blvd., Rm. 8184, MSC 9663
Bethesda, MD 20892-9663
Tel: 301-443-4513
TTY: 301-443-8431
Fax: 301-443-4279
Mental Health FAX 4U: 301-443-5158

National Institute of Mental Health (NIMH) (continued)
Internet: http://www.nimh.nih.gov
E-Mail: nimhinfo@nih.gov

NIMH Depression Publications
Toll-Free: 800-421-4211

National Institute of Allergy and Infectious Diseases (NIAID)
Office of Communications and Public Liaison
31 Center Drive
Room 7A50, MSC 2520
Bethesda, MD 20892-2520
Tel: 301-496-5717
HIV/AIDS Treatment Information Service: 800-HIV-0440
AIDS Clinical Trials Information Service: 800-TRIALS-A
Internet: http://www.niaid.nih.gov

References

1. Bing EG, Burnam MA, Longshore D, et al. The estimated prevalence of psychiatric disorders, drug use and drug dependence among people with HIV disease in the United States: results from the HIV Cost and Services Utilization Study. *Archives of General Psychiatry*, in press.

2. Shaffer D, Fisher P, Dulcan MK, et al. The NIMH Diagnostic Interview Schedule for Children Version 2.3 (DISC-2.3): description, acceptability, prevalence rates, and performance in the MECA Study. Methods for the Epidemiology of Child and Adolescent Mental Disorders Study. *Journal of the American Academy of Child and Adolescent Psychiatry*, 1996; 35(7): 865-77.

3. Regier DA, Narrow WE, Rae DS, et al. The de facto mental and addictive disorders service system. Epidemiologic Catchment Area prospective 1-year prevalence rates of disorders and services. *Archives of General Psychiatry*, 1993; 50(2): 85-94.

4. National Advisory Mental Health Council. Health care reform for Americans with severe mental illnesses. *American Journal of Psychiatry*, 1993; 150(10): 1447-65.

5. Leserman J, Petitto JM, Perkins DO, et al. Severe stress, depressive symptoms, and changes in lymphocyte subsets in human immunodeficiency virus-infected men. *Archives of General Psychiatry*, 1997; 54(3): 279-85.

6. Page-Shafer K, Delorenze GN, Satariano W, et al. Comorbidity and survival in HIV-infected men in the San Francisco Men's Health Survey. *Annals of Epidemiology*, 1996; 6(5): 420-30.

Chapter 38

Nutrition Strategies for AIDS

Introduction

Proper nutrition is a powerful tool for the successful management of HIV disease. Medical research confirms that weight loss—especially muscle tissue wasting—often leads to malnutrition and is a fatal manifestation of AIDS. Malnutrition has also been identified as a distinct cofactor contributing to HIV disease progression. Nourishing food, medications, and nutritional supplements all work synergistically to fight the immune suppression initiated by HIV. Appropriate dietary changes can significantly mitigate the side effects of AIDS medications and the symptoms associated with opportunistic infections.

The availability of protease inhibitors can improve the action of nucleoside and non-nucleoside analog drugs to more effectively manage HIV disease. The medical advances of combination therapies—for those who can afford and adhere to them—only increase the important role of nutrition. However, even the most promising treatments have side effects, and there have been many associated with combination therapy including lipodystrophy (a type of fat redistribution syndrome), and an increased risk of developing chronic conditions such as diabetes and heart disease. In cases where new treatments prolong the lives

"Introduction," "General Nutrition Recommendations (Fact Sheet 3)" and "Food and Medication Interactions Can Be Very Harmful (Fact Sheet 32)," © 2001 AIDS Nutrition Services Alliances, reprinted with permission; available online at http://www.aidsnutrition.org.

251

of people living with HIV/AIDS, long-term survivors will benefit substantially from proper nutrition.

There are many people living with HIV/AIDS for whom combination therapy has failed. Moreover, the majority of HIV-positive people live in developing countries, where 90% of the AIDS cases occur, and they will not have access to combination therapy in the near future. Consequently, life-sustaining food and safe clean fluids may be the most realistic and cost-effective approaches to manage HIV disease.

General Nutrition Recommendations

Calories

To maintain your weight use the following equation:

Example: 145 pounds x 17 = 2464 calories

To gain weight add 500 calories each day:

145 x 17 = 2464 + 500 = 2965 calories

Protein

You need to eat between 100-120 grams each day. You get protein in a lot of foods not just meat. Eat a high protein food with at least 20 grams of protein at least 3 times a day.

Fat

30-35% of your calories can be from fat. Eat less saturated fat such as butter, lard and tropical oils. Eat better fats such as olive oil and canola oil.

Fluids

Drink at least 10 cups of water or juice a day.

General Vitamin and Mineral Recommendations

- 2 multivitamins each day (use multi with less than 10 mg iron).

- 400 I.U. of Vitamin E if you are taking AZT or have high cholesterol or triglycerides.

- 500-1000 mg Vitamin C if you are a smoker, have an infection or have high triglycerides or cholesterol.

- B complex each day.

Talk to your dietitian or doctor to see what other vitamins or minerals may be helpful to you.

Sample Menu

Breakfast
  1 slice of lean ham
  toast with butter
  herb tea or juice

Snack
  2 ounces cheese and crackers
  1 cup juice
  apple

Lunch
  2 cups juice
  peanut butter and jelly sandwich
  4 fig bars

Snack
  granola bar
  2 cups juice

Dinner
  turkey sandwich (with 5 ounces turkey)
  1 cup soup
  salad
  pudding
  2 cups juice

Total: 2,800 calories, 104 grams protein, 31% fat calories.

Five easy things you can do to boost your nutrition:

1. Drink 10 cups of water, juice, herb tea, or decaffeinated beverages.

2. Eat a serving of fruit and a serving of vegetable each day.

3. Eat 3 times a day or more.

4. Take your multivitamin.

5. Go for a walk or do some exercise each day.

Food and Medication Interactions Can Be Very Harmful

Following is a list of common medications that should not be taken with certain foods.

- Blood pressure medication called calcium channel blockers such as Procardia

    Warning: Do not drink grapefruit juice less than 2 hours before or 5 hours after taking medication. Can be fatal.

- Antihistamines such as Claritin, Allegra or Benadryl

    Warning: Do not drink grapefruit juice as can cause serious heart problems.

- Crixivan (Indinavir), a protease inhibitor

    Warning: Do not drink grapefruit juice as it can lower the levels of meds in the blood and increase change of resistance.

- Cyclosporin, medication which fights organ rejection in transplant recipients

    Warning: Do not drink grapefruit juice less than 2 hours before or 5 hours after taking medication. Can cause trembling or confusion.

- Blood thinner medication called coumadin

    Warning: Do not take Vitamin E supplements with medication as it can cause serious bleeding. Do not eat foods high in Vitamin K such as broccoli, spinach and turnip greens as it can reduce effectiveness of medication.

- Antidepressants called MAO inhibitors

    Warning: Do not take with St. John's Wart. Do not take with tyramine containing foods such as cheese, red wine and sausage as it can cause a potentially fatal rise in blood pressure.

- Certain antibiotics such as Cipro

- Certain ulcer medications such as Tagamet, Zantac or Pepcid

- Bronchodilator called theophylline

  Warning: Do not drink more than 1 cup of coffee or other caffeinated colas total in 1 day. These medication increase level of caffeine in blood causing jitters, stomach irritation, nausea, palpitation or seizure (theophylline).

- Heart medication called ACE inhibitors such as Capoten and Vasotec

  Warning: Do not eat more than 1 banana a day or take potassium supplements since it can cause harmful buildup of potassium which can cause heart problems.

Chapter 39

HIV and Preventing Infection from Unsafe Food and Water

Food and water can carry germs that cause illness. Germs in food or water may cause serious infections in people with HIV. You can protect yourself from many infections by preparing food and drinks properly.

What illnesses caused by germs in food and water do people with HIV commonly get?

Germs in food and water that can make someone with HIV ill include Salmonella, Campylobacter, Listeria and Cryptosporidium. They can cause diarrhea, upset stomach, vomiting, stomach cramps, fever, headache, muscle pain, bloodstream infection, meningitis, or encephalitis.

Do only people with HIV get these illnesses?

No, they can occur in anyone. However, these illnesses are much more common in people with HIV.

Are these illnesses the same in people with HIV as in other people?

No. The diarrhea and nausea are often much worse and more difficult to treat in people with HIV. These illnesses are also more likely

"Safe Food and Water: A Guide for People Living with HIV Infection," National Center for HIV, STD and TB Prevention, Centers for Disease Control and Prevention (CDC), updated February 1999; available online at http://www.cdc.gov/hiv/pubs/brochure/food.htm.

to cause serious problems in people with HIV, such as bloodstream infections and meningitis. People with HIV also have a harder time recovering fully from these illnesses.

If I have HIV, can I eat meat, poultry, and fish?

Yes. Meat, poultry (such as chicken or turkey), and fish can make you sick only if they are raw, undercooked, or spoiled. To avoid illness:

- Cook all meat and poultry until they are no longer pink in the middle. If you use a meat thermometer, the temperature inside the meat or poultry should be over 165° F. Fish should be cooked until it is flaky, not rubbery.

- After handling raw meat, poultry, and fish, wash your hands well with soap and water before you touch any other food.

- Thoroughly wash cutting boards, cooking utensils, and countertops with soap and hot water after they have had contact with raw meat, poultry, or fish.

- Do not let uncooked meat, poultry, or fish or their juices touch other food or each other.

- Do not let meat, poultry, or fish sit at room temperature for more than a few minutes. Keep them in the refrigerator until you are ready to cook them.

- Eat or drink only pasteurized milk or dairy products.

Can I eat eggs if I have HIV?

Yes. Eggs are safe to eat if they are well cooked. Cook eggs until the yolk and white are solid, not runny. Do not eat foods that may contain raw eggs, such as hollandaise sauce, cookie dough, homemade mayonnaise, and Caesar salad dressing. If you prepare these foods at home, use pasteurized eggs instead of eggs in the shell. You can find pasteurized eggs in the dairy case at your supermarket.

Can I eat raw fruits and vegetables?

Yes. Raw fruits and vegetables are safe to eat if you wash them carefully first. Wash, then peel fruit that you will eat raw. Eating raw alfalfa sprouts and tomatoes can cause illness, but washing them well can reduce your risk of illness.

How can I make my water safe?

Don't drink water straight from lakes, rivers, streams, or springs.

Because you cannot be sure if your tap water is safe, you may wish to avoid tap water, including water or ice from a refrigerator ice-maker, which is made with tap water. Always check with the local health department and water utility to see if they have issued any special notices for people with HIV about tap water.

You may also wish to boil or filter your water, or to drink bottled water. Processed carbonated (bubbly) drinks in cans or bottles should be safe, but drinks made at a fountain might not be because they are made with tap water. If you choose to boil or filter your water or to drink only bottled water, do this all the time, not just at home.

Boiling is the best way to kill germs in your water. Heat your water at a rolling boil for 1 minute. After the boiled water cools, put it in a clean bottle or pitcher with a lid and store it in the refrigerator. Use the water for drinking, cooking, or making ice. Water bottles and ice trays should be cleaned with soap and water before use. Don't touch the inside of them after cleaning. If you can, clean your water bottles and ice trays yourself.

What should I do when shopping for food?

- Read food labels carefully. Be sure that all dairy products that you purchase have been pasteurized. Do not buy any food that contains raw or undercooked meat or eggs if it is meant to be eaten raw. Be sure that the "sell by" date has not passed.

- Put packaged meat, poultry, or fish in separate plastic bags to prevent their juices from dripping onto other groceries or each other.

- Check the package that the food comes in to make sure that it isn't damaged.

- Do not buy food that has been displayed in unsafe or unclean conditions. Examples include meat that is allowed to sit without refrigeration or cooked shrimp that is displayed with raw shrimp.

- After shopping, put all cold and frozen foods into your refrigerator or freezer as soon as you can. Do not leave food sitting in the car. Keeping cold or frozen food out of refrigeration for even a couple of hours can give germs a chance to grow.

Is it safe for me to eat in restaurants?

Yes. Like grocery stores, restaurants follow guidelines for cleanliness and good hygiene set by the health department. However, you should follow these general rules in restaurants:

- Order all food well done. If meat is served pink or bloody, send it back to the kitchen for more cooking. Fish should be flaky, not rubbery, when you cut it.

- Order fried eggs cooked on both sides. Avoid eggs that are sunny-side up. Scrambled eggs should be cooked until they are not runny. Do not order foods that may contain raw eggs, such as Caesar salad or hollandaise sauce. If you aren't sure about the ingredients in a dish, ask your waiter before you order.

- Do not order any raw or lightly steamed fish or shellfish, such as oysters, clams, mussels, sushi, or sashimi. All fish should be cooked until done.

Should I take special measures with food and water in other countries?

Yes. Not all countries have high standards of food hygiene. You need to take special care abroad, particularly in developing countries. Follow these rules when in other countries:

- Do not eat uncooked fruits and vegetables unless you can peel them. Avoid salads.

- Eat cooked foods while they are still hot.

- Boil all water before drinking it. Use only ice made from boiled water. Drink only canned or bottled drinks or beverages made with boiled water.

- Steaming-hot foods, fruits you peel yourself, bottled and canned processed drinks, and hot coffee or tea should be safe.

- Talk with your health care provider about other advice on travel abroad.

Chapter 40

Traveling with AIDS: Protect Yourself from Opportunistic Infections

In the United States or abroad? For business or pleasure? When you travel, you risk coming into contact with germs you might not find at home. Many of these germs can make you very sick.

For people with special health needs, travel can be risky to their health. If you have human immunodeficiency virus (HIV)—the virus that causes AIDS—you should have all the facts. Travel, especially to developing countries, can increase your risk of getting opportunistic infections. (They are called opportunistic because a person may get the infection when their weakened immune system gives it the opportunity to develop.) The best thing you can do when you travel is to know the medical risks and to take steps to protect yourself.

Before You Travel

Talk to your doctor or an expert in travel medicine about health risks in the area you plan to visit. They can tell you how to keep yourself healthy when you travel to places where certain illnesses are a problem. They also can tell you about places that might not be safe

"Preventing Infections during Travel: A Guide for People with HIV Infection," National Center for HIV, STD and TB Prevention, Centers for Disease Control and Prevention (CDC), updated November 1998; available online at http://www.cdc.gov/hiv/pubs/brochure/travel.htm. Despite the older date of this article, it provides general information about preventing infection while traveling with AIDS. For current information about travel precautions, visit CDC's Travelers' Health website at www.cdc.gov/travel.

for you to visit. Ask them if they know of doctors who treat people with HIV in the region you plan to visit. Plan in advance for problems that might come up.

Traveler's diarrhea is a common problem. Carry a 3- to 7-day supply of medicine (antibiotics) to treat it. A common drug for traveler's diarrhea is ciprofloxacin (SIP-ro-flocks-uh-sin). If you are pregnant, your doctor may suggest you take TMP- SMX (trimethoprim-sulfamethoxazole [try- METH-o-prim - sul-fa-meth-OX-uh-sole]) instead.

Insect-borne diseases are also a major problem in many areas. Take a good supply of an insect repellent that contains 30 percent or less DEET with you. Plan to sleep under a mosquito net, preferably one treated with permethrin, in places where there is malaria or dengue [DEN-gay] fever. Unless you need to go there, avoid areas where yellow fever is found.

Ask your doctor if you need to take medicine or get special vaccinations before you travel. He or she will know which vaccines are safe for you. Your doctor will also know the best ways to protect you from such things as malaria, typhoid fever, and hepatitis. Make sure all your routine vaccinations are up to date. This is very important for HIV-infected children who are traveling.

If you are leaving the United States, make sure you know if the countries you plan to visit have special health rules for visitors. These rules can include vaccinations that may not be safe for HIV-infected people to take. Your doctor or local health department can help you with this.

If you have medical insurance, check to see what it covers when you are away from home. Many insurance plans have limited benefits outside the United States. Very few plans cover the cost of flying you back to the United States if you become very sick. Make sure your paperwork is in order, and take along proof of insurance when you travel.

When You Travel

Food and water in developing countries may not be as clean as they are at home. These items might contain bacteria, viruses, or parasites that could make you sick.

Do not eat raw fruit and vegetables that you do not peel yourself, raw or undercooked seafood or meat, unpasteurized dairy products, or anything from a street vendor. Also, do not drink tap water, drinks made with tap water, or with ice made from tap water, or unpasteurized milk.

Food and drinks that are generally safe include steaming-hot foods, fruits that you peel yourself, bottled (especially carbonated) drinks, hot coffee or tea, beer, wine, and water that you bring to a rolling boil for1 full minute. If you can't boil your water, you can filter and treat it with iodine or chlorine, but this will not work as well as boiling.

Tuberculosis, or TB, is very common worldwide, and can be severe in people with HIV. Avoid hospitals and clinics where coughing TB patients are treated. When back in the United States, have your doctor test you for TB.

In many places, animals may roam more freely than they do in the area where you live. If you think animals have left droppings on beaches or other areas, always wear shoes and protective clothing and sit on a towel to avoid direct contact with the sand or soil.

Swimming can make you sick if you swallow water. You should never swim in water that might contain even very small amounts of sewage or animal waste. To make sure that you get the most fun from your trip, protect your health (and the health of others) just as you do at home.

Take all medications as prescribed by your doctor.

If your doctor has you on a special diet, stick with it.

Take the same precautions that you take at home to prevent giving HIV to others.

Chapter 41

Household Pets: Special Precautions for People with AIDS

You do not have to give up your pet. Although the risks are low, you can get an infection from pets or other animals. Several simple precautions are all you need to take with pets or other animals. HIV can not be spread by, or to, cats, dogs, birds, or other pets.

Should I keep my pets?

Yes. Most people with human immunodeficiency virus (HIV) can and should keep their pets. Owning a pet can be rewarding. Pets can help you feel psychologically and even physically better. For many people, pets are more than just animals—they are like members of the family. However, you should know the health risks of owning a pet or caring for animals. Animals may carry infections that can be harmful to you. Your decision to own or care for pets should be based on knowing what you need to do to protect yourself from these infections.

What kinds of infections could I get from an animal?

Animals can have cryptosporidiosis (crypto), toxoplasmosis (toxo), Mycobacterium avium complex (MAC), and other diseases. These diseases can give you problems like severe diarrhea, brain infections, and skin lesions.

"Preventing Infections from Pets," National Center for HIV, STD and TB Prevention, Centers for Disease Control and Prevention (CDC), June 1999; available online at http://www.cdc.gov/hiv/pubs/brochure/oi_pets.htm.

What can I do to protect myself from infections spread by animals?

- Always wash your hands well with soap and water after playing with or caring for animals. This is especially important before eating or handling food.

- Be careful about what your pet eats and drinks. Feed your pet only pet food or cook all meat thoroughly before giving it to your pet. Don't give your pet raw or undercooked meat. Don't let your pets drink from toilet bowls or get into garbage. Don't let your pets hunt or eat another animal's stool (droppings).

- Don't handle animals that have diarrhea. If the pet's diarrhea lasts for more than 1or 2 days, have a friend or relative who does not have HIV take your pet to your veterinarian. Ask the veterinarian to check the pet for infections that may be the cause of diarrhea.

- Don't bring home an unhealthy pet. Don't get a pet that is younger than 6 months old—especially if it has diarrhea. If you are getting a pet from a pet store, animal breeder, or animal shelter (pound), check the sanitary conditions and license of these sources. If you are not sure about the animal's health, have it checked out by your veterinarian.

- Don't touch stray animals because you could get scratched or bitten. Stray animals can carry many infections.

- Don't ever touch the stool of any animal.

- Ask someone who is not infected with HIV and is not pregnant to change your cat's litter box daily. If you must clean the box yourself, wear vinyl or household cleaning gloves and immediately wash your hands well with soap and water right after changing the litter.

- Have your cat's nails clipped so it can't scratch you. Discuss other ways to prevent scratching with your veterinarian. If you do get scratched or bitten, immediately wash the wounds well with soap and water.

- Don't let your pet lick your mouth or any open cuts or wounds you may have.

- Don't kiss your pet.

- Keep fleas off your pet.

- Avoid reptiles such as snakes, lizards, and turtles. If you touch any reptile, immediately wash your hands well with soap and water.

- Wear vinyl or household cleaning gloves when you clean aquariums or animal cages and wash your hands well right after you finish.

- Avoid exotic pets such as monkeys, and ferrets, or wild animals such as raccoons, lions, bats, and skunks.

- If you are bitten, you may need to seek medical advice.

I have a job that involves working with animals. Should I quit?

Jobs working with animals (such as jobs in pet stores, animal clinics, farms, and slaughterhouses) carry a risk for infections. Talk with your doctor about whether you should work with animals. People who work with animals should take these extra precautions:

- Follow your worksite's rules to stay safe and reduce any risk of infection. Use or wear personal protective gear, such as coveralls, boots, and gloves.

- Don't clean chicken coops or dig in areas where birds roost if histoplasmosis [his-to-plaz-MO-sis] is found in the area.

- Don't touch young farm animals, especially if they have diarrhea.

Can someone with HIV give it to their pets?

No. HIV can not be spread to, from, or by cats, dogs, birds, or other pets. Many viruses cause diseases that are like AIDS, such as feline leukemia virus, or FeLV, in cats. These viruses cause illness only in a certain animal and cannot infect other animals or humans. For example, FeLV infects only cats. It does not infect humans or dogs.

Are there any tests a pet should have before I bring it home?

A pet should be in overall good health. You don't need special tests unless the animal has diarrhea or looks sick. If your pet looks sick, your veterinarian can help you choose the tests it needs.

What should I do when I visit friends or relatives who have animals?

When you visit anyone with pets, take the same precautions you would in your own home. Don't touch animals that may not be healthy. You may want to tell your friends and family about the need for these precautions before you plan any visits.

Should children with HIV handle pets?

The same precautions apply for children as for adults. However, children may want to snuggle more with their pets. Some pets, like cats, may bite or scratch to get away from children. Adults should be extra watchful and supervise an HIV-infected child's hand washing to prevent infections.

Chapter 42

Caring for Someone with AIDS at Home

One of the best places for people with AIDS to be cared for is at home, surrounded by the people who love them. Many people living with AIDS can lead an active life for long periods of time. Most of the time, people with AIDS do not need to be in a hospital. Being at home is often cheaper, more comfortable, more familiar, and gives them more control of their life. In fact, people with AIDS-related illnesses often get better faster and with less discomfort at home with the help of their friends and loved ones.

If you are caring for someone with AIDS at home, remember that each person with AIDS is different and is affected by HIV, the virus that causes AIDS, in different ways. You should get regular updates from the person's doctor or nurse on what kind of care is needed. Many times what is needed is not medical care, but help with the normal chores of life: shopping, getting the mail, paying bills, cleaning the house, and so on.

Also remember that AIDS causes stress on both the person who is sick and on you as you care for them. Caring for someone with AIDS is a serious responsibility. You will have to work with the person with AIDS to decide what needs to be done, how much you can do, and when additional help is needed. But, by rising to the challenges of caring for someone with HIV infection and AIDS, you can share emotionally satisfying experiences, even joy, with those you love. You can also find

"Caring for Someone with AIDS at Home: A Guide," Centers for Disease Control and Prevention (CDC), revised June 2001; available online at http://www.cdc.gov/hiv/pubs/brochure/careathome.htm.

new strengths within yourself. But you need to take care of yourself as well as the person with AIDS.

How to Get Ready to Take Care of Someone at Home

Every situation is different, but here are some tips to get you started.

Read this information. Have the person living with HIV or AIDS read it. Have other people living in the same house as the person with AIDS read it. The information in this chapter is for both people with diagnosed AIDS and people with HIV infection who are sick and need care.

Take a home care course, if possible. Learn the skills you need to take care of someone at home and how to manage special situations. Your local Red Cross chapter, Visiting Nurses Association, State health department, or HIV/AIDS service organization can help you find a home care course.

Talk with the person you will be caring for. Ask them what they need. If you are nervous about caring for them, say so. Ask if it is OK for you to talk to their doctor, nurse, social worker, case manager, other health care professional, or lawyer when you need to. Together you can work out what is best for both of you.

Talk with the doctor, nurse, social worker, case manager, and other health care workers who are also providing care. They may need the patient's permission, sometimes in writing, to talk to you, but you need to talk to these people to find out how you can help. Work with them and the person you are caring for to develop a plan for who does what.

Get clear, written information about medicines and other care you'll give. Ask what each drug does and what side effects to look out for.

Ask the doctor or nurse what changes in the person's health or behavior to watch for. For example, a cough, fever, diarrhea, or confusion may mean an infection or problem that needs a new medicine or even putting the person in the hospital.

You also need to know whom to call for help or information and when to call them. Make a list of doctors, nurses, and other people you might need to talk to quickly, their phone numbers, and when they are available. Keep this list by the phone.

Talk to a lawyer or AIDS support organization. For some medical care or life support decisions, you may need to be legally named as the care coordinator. If you are going to help file insurance claims, apply for government aid, pay bills, or handle other business for the person with AIDS, you may also need a power of attorney. There are many sources of help for people with AIDS, and you can help the person with AIDS get what they are entitled to.

Think about joining a support group or talking to a counselor. Taking care of someone who is sick can be hard emotionally as well as physically. Talking about it with people with the same kind of worries helps sometimes. You can learn how other people cope and realize that you are not alone.

Take care of yourself. You can't take care of someone else if you are sick or upset. Get the rest and exercise you need to keep going. You also need to do some things you enjoy, such as visit your friends and relatives. Many AIDS service organizations can help with respite care and send someone to be with the person you're caring for while you get out of the house for awhile.

Giving Care

People living with AIDS should take care of themselves as much as they can for as long as they can. They need to be and feel as independent as possible. They need to control their own schedules, make their own decisions, and do what they want to do as much as they are able. They should develop their own exercise program and eating plan. In addition to regular visits to the doctor, many people with AIDS work at staying healthy by eating properly, sleeping regularly, doing physical exercises, praying or meditating, or other things. If the person you care caring for finds something that helps them, encourage them to keep it up. An exercise program can help maintain weight and muscle tone and can make a person feel better if it is tailored to what the person can do. Well-balanced, good-tasting meals help people feel good, give them energy, and help their body fight illness. People with HIV infection are better off if they don't drink alcoholic drinks, smoke, or use illegal drugs. Keeping up-to-date on new treatments and understanding what to expect from treatments the person is taking are also important.

There are some simple things you can do to help someone with AIDS feel comfortable at home.

- Respect their independence and privacy.

- Give them control as much as possible. Ask to enter their room, ask permission to sit with them, etc., saying "Can I help you with that?" lets them keep control.

- Ask them what you can do to make them comfortable. Many people feel shy about asking for help, especially help with things like using the toilet, bathing, shaving, eating, and dressing.

- Keep the home clean and looking bright and cheerful.

- Let the person with AIDS stay in a room that is near a bathroom.

- Leave tissues, towels, a trash basket, extra blankets, and other things the person might need close by so these things can be reached from the bed or chair.

If the person you care caring for has to spend most of their time in bed, be sure to help them change position often. If possible, a person with AIDS should get out of bed as often as they can. A nurse can show you how to help someone move from a bed to a chair without hurting yourself or them. This helps prevent stiff joints, bedsores, and some kinds of pneumonia. They may also need your help to turn over or to adjust the pillows or blankets. A medical trapeze over the bed can help the person shift position by themselves if they are strong enough. If they are so weak they can't turn over, have a nurse show you how to use a sheet to help roll the person in bed from side to side. Usually a person in bed needs to change position at least every 4 hours.

Bedsores

Bedsores or other broken skin can be serious problems for someone with AIDS. In addition to changing position in bed often, to help keep skin healthy, put extra-soft material (sheepskin, egg crate foam, or water mattresses) under the person, keep the sheets dry and free from wrinkles, and massage the back and other parts of the body (like hips, elbows, and ankles) that press down on the bed. Report any red or broken areas on the skin to the doctor or nurse right away.

Exercises

Even in bed, a person can do simple arm, hard, leg, and foot exercises. These are usually called range of motion exercises. These exercises help prevent stiff, sore points and help keep the blood moving. A doctor, nurse, or physical therapist can show you how to help.

Breathing

If someone is having trouble breathing, sitting them up may help. Raise the head of a hospital-type bed or use extra pillows or some other soft back support. If they have severe trouble breathing, they need to see a doctor.

Comfort

A good back rub can help a person relax as well as help their circulation. A nurse, physical therapist, or book on massage can give you some tips on how to give a good back rub. Put books, remote controls, water, tissues, and a bell to call for help within easy reach. If the person can't get up, put a urinal or bedpan within easy reach.

Providing Emotional Support

You are caring for a person, not just a body; their feelings are important too. Since every person is different, there are no rules about what to do or say, but following are some ideas that may help.

- Keep them involved in their care. Don't do everything for them or make all their decisions. Nobody likes feeling helpless.

- Have them help out around the house if they can. Everybody likes to feel useful. They want to be part of the group, contributing what they can.

- Include them in the household. Make them part of normal talk about books, TV shows, music, what is going on in the world, and so on. Many people will want to feel involved in the things that are happening around them. But you don't always have to talk, just being there is sometimes enough. Just watching TV together or sitting and reading in the same room is often comforting.

- Talk about things. Sometime they may need to talk about AIDS or talk through their own situation as a way to think out loud. Having AIDS can make a person angry, frustrated, depressed, scared, and lonely, just like any other serious illness. Listening, trying to understand, showing you care, and helping them work through their emotions is a big part of home care. A support group of other people with AIDS can also be a good place for them to talk things out. Contact the National Association of People with AIDS for information about support groups in your area. If they want professional counseling, help them get it.

- Invite their friends over to visit. A little socializing can be good for everyone.

- Touch them. Hug them, kiss them, pat them, hold their hands to show that you care. Some people may not want physical closeness, but if they do, touch is a powerful way of saying you care.

- Get out together. If they are able, go to social events, shopping, riding around, walking around the block, or just into the park, yard, or porch to sit in the sun and breath fresh air.

Guarding against Infections

People living with AIDS can get very sick from common germs and infections. Hugging, holding hands, giving massages, and many other types of touching are safe for you, and needed by the person with AIDS. But you have to be careful not to spread germs that can hurt the person you are caring for.

Wash Your Hands

Washing your hands is the single best way to kill germs. Do it often. Wash your hands after you go to the bathroom and before you fix food. Wash your hands again before and after feeding them, bathing them, helping them go to the bathroom, or giving other care. Wash your hands if you sneeze or cough; touch your nose, mouth, or genitals; handle garbage or animal litter; or clean the house. If you touch anybody's blood, semen, urine, vaginal fluid, or feces, wash your hands immediately. If you are caring for more than one person, wash your hands after helping one person and before helping the next person. Wash your hands with warm, soapy water for at least 15 seconds. Clean under your finger nails and between your fingers. If your hands get dry or sore, put on hand cream or lotion, but keep washing your hands frequently.

Cover Your Sores

If you have any cuts or sores, especially on your hands, you must take extra care not to infect the person with AIDS or yourself. If you have cold sores, fever blisters, or any other skin infection, don't touch the person or their things. You could pass your infection to them. If you have to give care, cover your sores with bandages, and wash your hands before touching the person. If the rash or sores are on your hands, wear disposable gloves. Do not use gloves more than one time; throw them away and get a new pair. If you have boils, impetigo, or shingles, if at all possible, stay away from the person with AIDS until you are well.

Keep Sick People Away

If you or anybody else is sick, stay away from the person with AIDS until you're well. A person with AIDS often can't fight off colds, flu, or other common illnesses. If you are sick and nobody else can do what needs to be done for the person with AIDS, wear a well-fitting, surgical-type mask that covers your mouth and nose and wash your hands before coming near the person with AIDS.

Watch Out for Chickenpox

Chickenpox can kill a person with AIDS. If the person you are caring for has already had the chickenpox, they probably won't get it again. But, just to be on the safe side:

- Never let anybody with chickenpox in the same room as a person with AIDS, at least not until all the chickenpox sores have completely crusted over.

- Don't let anybody who recently has been near somebody with chickenpox in the same room as a person who has AIDS. After 3 weeks, the person who was exposed to the chickenpox can visit, if they aren't sick. Most adults have had chickenpox, but you have be very careful about children visiting or living in the house if they have not yet had chickenpox. If you are the person who was near somebody with chickenpox and you have to help the person with AIDS, wear a well-fitting, surgical-type mask, wash your hands before doing what you have to do for the person with AIDS, and stay in the room as short a time as you can. Tell the person with AIDS why you are staying away from them.

- Don't let anybody with shingles (*herpes zoster*) near a person with AIDS until all the shingles have healed over. The germ that causes shingles can also cause chickenpox. If you have shingles and have to help the person with AIDS, cover all the sores completely and wash your hands carefully before helping the person with AIDS.

- Call the doctor as soon as possible if the person with AIDS does get near somebody with chickenpox or shingles. There is a medicine that can make the chickenpox less dangerous, but it must be given very soon after the person has been around someone with the germ.

Get Your Shots

Everybody living with or helping take care of a person with AIDS should make sure they took all their childhood shots (immunizations). This is not only to keep you from getting sick, but also to keep you from getting sick and accidentally spreading the illness to the person with AIDS. Just to be sure, ask your doctor if you need any shots or boosters for measles, mumps, or rubella since these shots may not have been available when you were a child. Discuss any vaccinations with your doctor and the doctor of the person with AIDS before you get the shot. If the person with AIDS is near a person with measles, call the doctor that day. There is a medicine that can make the measles less dangerous, but it has to be given very soon after the person is around the germ.

Children or adults who live with someone with AIDS and who need to get vaccinated against polio should get an injection with inactivated virus vaccine. The regular oral polio vaccine has weakened polio virus that can spread from the person who got the vaccine to the person with AIDS and give them polio.

Everyone living with a person with AIDS should get a flu shot every year to reduce the chances of spreading the flu to the person with AIDS. Everyone living with a person with AIDS should be checked for tuberculosis (TB) every year.

Be Careful with Pets and Gardening

Pets can give love and companionship. Having a pet around can make a person with AIDS feel better and enjoy life more. However, people with HIV or AIDS should not touch pet litter boxes, feces, bird droppings, or water in fish tanks. Many pet animals carry germs that don't make healthy people sick, but can make the person with AIDS very sick. A person with AIDS can have pets, but must wash their hands with soap and water after handling the pet. Someone who does not have HIV infection must clean the litter boxes, cages, fish tanks, pet beds, and other things. Wear rubber gloves when you clean up after pets and wash your hands before and after cleaning. Empty litter boxes every day, don't just sift. Just like the people living with AIDS, pets need yearly checkups and current vaccinations. If the pet gets sick, take it to the veterinarian right away. Someone with AIDS should not touch a sick animal.

Gardening can also be a problem. Germs live in garden or potting soil. A person with AIDS can garden, but they must wear work gloves while handling dirt and must wash their hands before and after handling dirt. You should do the same.

Personal Items

A person with HIV infection should not share razors, toothbrushes, tweezers, nail or cuticle scissors, pierced earrings or other pierced jewelry, or any other item that might have their blood on it.

Laundry

Clothes and bed sheets used by someone with AIDS can be washed the same way as other laundry. If you use a washing machine, either hot or cold water can be used, with regular laundry detergent. If clothes or sheets have blood, vomit, semen, vaginal fluids, urine, or feces on them, use disposable gloves and handle the clothes or sheets as little as possible. Put them in plastic bags until you can wash them. You can but you don't need to add bleach to kill HIV; a normal wash cycle will kill the virus. Clothes may also be dry cleaned or hand-washed. If stains from blood, semen, or vaginal fluids are on the clothes, soaking them in cold water before washing will help remove the stains. Fabrics and furniture can be cleaned with soap and water or cleansers you can buy in a store; just follow the directions on the box. Wear gloves while cleaning.

Cleaning House

Cleaning kills germs that may be dangerous to the person with AIDS. You may want to clean and dust the house every week. Clean tubs, showers, and sinks often; use household cleaners, then rinse with fresh water. You may want to mop floors at least once a week. Clean the toilet often; use bleach mixed with water or a commercial toilet bowl cleaner. You may clean urinals and bedpans with bleach after each use. Replace plastic urinals and bedpans every month or so. About 1/4 cup of bleach mixed with 1 gallon of water makes a good disinfectant for floors, showers, tubs, sinks, mops, sponges, etc. (Or 1 tablespoon for bleach in 1 quart of water for small jobs). Make a new batch each time because it stops working after about 24 hours. Be sure to keep the bleach and the bleach and water mix, like other dangerous chemicals, away from children.

Food

Someone with AIDS can eat almost anything they want; in fact, the more the better. A well-balanced diet with plenty of nutrients, fiber, and liquids is healthy for everybody. Fixing food for a person with AIDS takes a little care, although you should follow these same rules for fixing food for anybody.

- Don't use raw (unpasteurized) milk.

- Don't use raw eggs. Be careful: raw eggs may be in homemade mayonnaise, hollandaise sauce, ice cream, fruit drinks (smoothies), or other homemade foods.

- All beef, pork, chicken, fish, and other meats should be cooked well done, with no pink in the middle.

- Don't use raw fish or shellfish (like oysters).

- Wash your hands before handling food and wash them again between handling different foods.

- Wash all utensils (knives, spatulas, mixing spoons, etc.) before reusing them with other foods. If you taste food while cooking, use a clean spoon every time you taste; do not stir with the spoon you taste with.

- Don't let blood from uncooked beef, pork, or chicken or water from shrimp, fish, or other seafood touch other food.

- Use a cutting board to cut things on and wash it with soap and hot water between each food you cut.

- Wash fresh fruits and vegetables thoroughly. Cook or peel organic fruits and vegetables because they may have germs on the skins. Don't use organic lettuce or other organic vegetables that cannot be peeled or cooked.

A person living with AIDS does not need separate dishes, knives, forks, or spoons. Their dishes don't need special cleaning either. Just wash all the dishes together with soap or detergent in hot water.

A person with AIDS can fix food for other people. Just like everybody else who fixes food, people with AIDS should wash their hands first and not lick their fingers or the utensils while they are cooking. However, no one who has diarrhea should fix food.

To keep food from spoiling, serve hot foods hot and cold foods cold. Cover leftover food and store it in the refrigerator as soon as possible.

Protect Yourself

A person who has AIDS may sometimes have infections that can make you sick. You can protect yourself, however. Talk to the doctor or nurse to find out what germs can infect you and other people in the house. This is very important if you have HIV infection yourself.

For example, diarrhea can be caused by several different germs. Wear disposable gloves if you have to clean up after or help a person with diarrhea and wash your hands carefully after you take the gloves off. Do not use disposable gloves more than one time.

Another cause of diarrhea is the cryptosporidiosis parasite. It is spread from the feces of one person or animal to another person or animal, often by contaminated water, raw food, or food that isn't cooked well enough. Again, wash your hands after using the bathroom and before fixing food. You can check with your local health department to see if cryptosporidiosis is in the water. If you hear that the water in your community may have cryptosporidiosis parasites, boil your drinking water for at least 1 minute to kill the parasite, then let the water cool before drinking. You may want to buy bottled (distilled) water for cooking and drinking if the cryptosporidiosis parasite or other organisms that might make a person with HIV infection sick could be in the tap water.

If the person with AIDS has a cough that lasts longer than a week, the doctor should check them for TB. If they do have TB, then you and everybody else living in the house should be checked for TB infection, even if you aren't coughing. If you are infected with TB germs, you can take medicine that will prevent you from developing TB.

If the person with AIDS gets yellow jaundice (a sign of acute hepatitis) or has chronic hepatitis B infection, you and everybody else living in the house and any people the person with AIDS has had sex with should talk to their doctor to see if anyone needs to take medicine to prevent hepatitis. All children should get hepatitis B vaccine whether or not they are around a person with AIDS.

If the person with AIDS has fever blisters or cold sores (herpes simplex) around the mouth or nose, don't kiss or touch the sores. If you have to touch the sores to help the person, wear gloves and wash your hands carefully as soon as you take the gloves off. This is especially important if you have eczema (allergic skin) since the herpes simplex virus can cause severe skin disease in people with eczema. Throw the used gloves away; never use disposable gloves more than once.

Many persons with or without AIDS are infected with a virus called cytomegalovirus (CMV), which can be spread in urine or saliva. Wash your hands after touching urine or saliva from a person with AIDS. This is especially important for someone who may be pregnant because a pregnant woman infected with CMV can also infect her unborn child. CMV causes birth defects such as deafness.

Remember, to protect yourself and the person with AIDS from these diseases and others, be sure to wash your hands with soap and water before and after giving care, when handling food, after taking gloves of, and after going to the bathroom.

Gloves

Because the virus that causes AIDS is in the blood of infected persons, blood or other body fluids (such as bloody feces) that have blood in them could infect you. You can protect yourself by following some simple steps. Wear gloves if you have to touch semen, vaginal fluid, cuts or sores on the person with AIDS, or blood or body fluids that may have blood in them. Wear gloves to give care to the mouth, rectum, or genitals of the person with AIDS. Wear gloves to change diapers or sanitary pads or to empty bedpans or urinals. If you have any cuts, sores, rashes, or breaks in your skin, cover them with a bandage. If the cuts or sores are on your hands, use bandages and gloves. Wear gloves to clean up urine, feces, or vomit to avoid all the germs, HIV and other kinds, that might be there.

There are two types of gloves you can use. Use disposable, hospital-type latex or vinyl gloves to take care of the person with AIDS if there is any blood you might touch. Use these gloves one time, then throw them away. Do not use latex gloves more than one time even if they are marked reusable. You can buy hospital-type gloves by the box at most drug stores, along with urinals, bedpans, and many other medical supplies. Many insurance companies and Medicaid will pay for these gloves if the doctor writes a prescription for them. For cleaning blood or bloody fluids from floors, bed, etc., you can use household rubber gloves, which are sold at any drug or grocery store. These gloves can be cleaned and reused. Clean them with hot, soapy water and with a mixture of bleach and water (about 1/4 cup bleach to 1 gallon of water). Be sure not to use gloves that are peeling, cracked, or have holes in them. Don't use the rubber gloves to take care of a person with AIDS; they are too thick and bulky.

To take gloves off, peel them down by turning them inside out. This will keep the wet side on the inside, away from your skin and other people. When you take the gloves off, wash your hands with soap and water right away. If there is a lot of blood, you can wear an apron or smock to keep your clothes from getting bloody. (If the person with AIDS is bleeding a lot or very often, call the doctor or nurse.) Clean up spilled blood as soon as you can. Put on gloves, wipe up the blood with paper towels or rags, put the used paper towels or rags in plastic bags to get rid of later, then wash the area where the blood was with a mix of bleach and water.

Since HIV can be in semen, vaginal fluid, or breast milk just as it can be in blood, you should be as careful with these fluids as you are with blood.

If you get blood, semen, vaginal fluid, breast milk, or other body fluid that might have blood in it in your eyes, nose, or mouth, immediately pour as much water as possible over where you got splashed, then call the doctor, explain what happened, and ask what else you should do.

Needles and Syringes

A person with AIDS may need needles and syringes to take medicine for diseases caused by AIDS or for diabetes, hemophilia, or other illnesses. If you have to handle these needles and syringes, you must be careful not to stick yourself. That is one way you could get infected with HIV.

Use a needle and syringe only one time. Do not put caps back on needles. Do not take needles off syringes. Do not break or bend needles. If a needle falls off a syringe, use something like tweezers or pliers to pick it up; do not use your fingers. Touch needles and syringes only by the barrel of the syringe. Hold the sharp end away from yourself.

Put the used needle and syringe in a puncture-proof container. The doctor, nurse, or an AIDS service organization can give you a special container. If you don't have one, use a puncture-proof container with a plastic top, such as a coffee can. Keep a container in any room where needles and syringes are used. Put it well out of the reach of children or visitors, but in a place you can easily and quickly put the needle and syringe after they are used. When the container gets nearly full, seal it and get a new container. Ask the doctor or nurse how to get rid of the container with the used needles and syringes.

If you get stuck with a needle used on the person with AIDS, don't panic. The chances are very good (better than 99%) that you will not be infected. However, you need to act quickly to get medical care. Put the needle in the used needle container, then wash where you stuck yourself as soon as you can, using warm, soapy water. Right after washing, call the doctor or the emergency room of a hospital, no matter what time it is, explain what happened, and ask what else you should do. Your doctor may want you to take medicine, such as AZT. If you are going to take AZT, you should begin taking it as soon as possible, certainly within a few hours of the needlestick.

Wastes

Flush all liquid waste (urine, vomit, etc.) that has blood in it down the toilet. Be careful not to splash anything when you are pouring liquids into the toilet. Toilet paper and tissues with blood, semen, vaginal fluid, or breast milk may also be flushed down the toilet.

Paper towels, sanitary pads and tampons, wound dressings and bandages, diapers, and other items with blood, semen, or vaginal fluid on them cannot be flushed should be put in plastic bags. Put the items in the bag, then close and seal the bag. Ask the doctor, nurse, or local health department about how to get rid of things with blood, urine, vomit, semen, vaginal fluid, or breast milk on them. If you can't have plastic bags handy, wrap the materials in enough newspaper to stop any leaks. Wear gloves when handling anything with blood, semen, vaginal fluids, or breast milk on it.

Sex

If you used to or still do have sex with a person with HIV infection, and you didn't use latex condoms the right way every time you had sex, you could have HIV infection, too. You can talk to your doctor or a counselor about taking an HIV antibody test. Call the CDC National AIDS Hotline at 1-800-342-AIDS for information about HIV antibody testing and referrals to places in your area that you can get confidential or anonymous HIV testing. The idea of being tested for HIV may be scary. But, if you are infected, the sooner you find out and start getting medical care, the better off you will be. Talk to your sex partner about what will need to change. It is very important that you protect yourself and your partner from transmitting HIV infection and other sexually transmitted diseases. Talk about types of sex that don't risk HIV infection. If you decide to have sexual intercourse (vaginal, anal, or oral), use condoms. Latex condoms can protect you from HIV infection if they are used the right way every time you have sex. Ask your doctor, counselor, or call the CDC National AIDS Hotline at 1-800-342-AIDS for more information about safer sex.

Other Help You Can Give

Dealing with hospitals or insurance companies, filling out forms, and looking up records can be difficult even if you are well. Many people with AIDS need help with these tasks.

- Getting a ride to the doctor's office, clinic, drug store, or other places can be a problem. Don't wait to be asked, offer to help.

- Keeping a diary of medical events and other information for the person you are taking care of can help them and any other people who are helping. Be sure the person you are caring for knows what you are writing and helps keep the diary if they can.

- Keeping a record of medicine and other care for the doctor or the other people providing care can help a lot. Make sure you know what drugs the person is taking, how often they should take them, and what side effects to watch out for. The doctor, nurse, or pharmacist can tell you what to do. People who are sick sometimes forget to take medicine or take too much or too little. Divided pill boxes or a chart showing what medicines to take, when to take them, and how much of each to take can help.

- If the person you are caring for has to go into the hospital, you can still help. Take a special picture or other favorite things to the hospital. Tell the hospital staff of any special needs or habits the person has or if you see any problems. Most of all, visit often.

Children with AIDS

Infants and children with HIV infection or AIDS need the same things as other children—lots of love and affection. Small children need to be held, played with, kissed, hugged, fed, and rocked to sleep. As they grow, they need to play, have friends, and go to school, just like other kids. Kids with HIV are still kids, and need to be treated like any other kids in the family.

Kids with AIDS need much of the same care that grown-ups with AIDS need, but there are a few extra things to look out for.

- Watch for any changes in health or the way the child acts. If you notice anything unusual for that child, let the doctor know. For a child with AIDS, little problems can become big problems very quickly. Watch for breathing problems, fever, unusual sleepiness, diarrhea, or changes in how much they eat. Talk to the child's doctor about what else to look for and when to report it.

- Talk to the doctor before the child gets any immunizations (including oral polio vaccine) or booster shots. Some vaccines could make the child sick. No child with HIV or anyone in the household should ever take oral polio vaccine.

- Stuffed and furry toys can hold dirt and might hide germs that can make the child sick. Plastic and washable toys are better. If the child has any stuffed toys, wash them in a washing machine often and keep them as clean as possible.

- Keep the child away from litter boxes and sandboxes that a pet or other animal might have been in.

- Ask the child's doctor what to do about pets that might be in the house.

- Try to keep the child from getting infectious diseases, especially chickenpox. If the child with HIV infection gets near somebody with chickenpox, tell the child's doctor right away. Chickenpox can kill a child with AIDS.

- Bandage any cuts or scrapes quickly and completely after washing with soap and warm water. Use gloves if the child is bleeding.

Taking care of a child who is sick is very hard for people who love that child. You will need help and emotional support. You are not alone. There are people who can help you get through this.

Changing Symptoms

People with AIDS seem to get very sick, then get better, then get very sick, then better, and so on. Sometimes they get sicker and sicker. You can't always tell if they are going to live through a particular illness or not. These times are very rough on everyone involved. If you know what to expect, you can deal with these rough times better.

Dementia

Dementia (having trouble thinking) can be a problem for a person with AIDS. AIDS can affect the brain and cause poor memory; short attention span; trouble moving, speaking, or thinking; less alertness;

loss of interest in things; and wide mood swings. These problems can upset the person with AIDS as well as the people around them. Mental problems can make it hard to follow the planned routines for care and make it difficult to protect the person with AIDS from infections. Be prepared to recognize these problems, understand what is happening, and talk to the doctor, nurse, social worker, or mental health worker about what to do.

If the person you are caring for does develop mental problems, you can help:

- Keep important things in the same place all the time, a place that is easy to reach and easy to see.

- If you need to, remind the person you are caring for where they are and who you are.

- Put a clock and a calendar where the person you are caring for can see them. Mark off the days on the calendar. Write in what will happen each day.

- Put up pictures of people who might be in the house with their names on the pictures where the person with AIDS can see them.

- Speak in short, simple sentences.

- Don't be afraid to be firm. Remove things like dangerous objects from reach.

- Keep the sound from TVs, radios, and other noises down so the person doesn't get confused by unexpected sounds.

- Talk to a health care worker who deals with people with dementia about how to handle problems.

As AIDS Progresses

Here are some of the things to expect as AIDS enters its final stages and ways to try to cope. Like other people nearing death, a person with AIDS who is near death:

- Sleeps more and more and is hard to wake up. Try to talk to them and do things during those times when they do seem alert.

- Becomes confused about where they are, the time or date, or who people are. Tell them where they are, what time and day it is, and who people are. Don't scold them for forgetting, just tell them.

- Begins to wet their pants or lose bowel control. Clean them, using gloves, and use powder or lotion to prevent rashes. A catheter for passing urine may become necessary.

- Has skin that feels cool to the touch and may turn darker on the side of their body touching the bed as the circulation slows down. Keep them covered with warm blankets, but don't use electric blankets because they can burn a person with poor circulation.

- May have trouble seeing or hearing. Even so, never talk to other people as if the person with AIDS can't hear you. Always talk to the person with AIDS or anyone else in the room as if the person with AIDS hears you.

- May seem restless, pulling at the sheets on the bed or acting as if they see things that you don't. Stay calm, speak slowly, and reassure the person. Comfort them with gentle reminders about who you are and where they are.

- May stop eating and drinking. Wipe their mouth often with a wet cloth. Keep their lips wet with lip moisturizer.

- May almost stop urinating. If there is a catheter, it may need to be rinsed or flushed to keep it from getting blocked. A nurse can show you how to do this.

- Has noisy breathing because they can't cough up the fluids that collect in the back of their throat. Talk to their doctor; the doctor may suggest raising the head of the bed or putting extra pillows under their head. Turning them on their side may also help. If they can swallow, feed them some ice chips. If they have trouble swallowing, a cool, wet washcloth on the lips can keep their mouth and lips moist and may satisfy their thirst. If they begin to have irregular breathing or seem to stop breathing for a minute, call the doctor.

Hospice Care

Many people have found hospice care (programs for people who are dying and their caregivers) for adults and children a big help. Others feel that hospice care isn't right for them. Hospice services can help caregivers, family, and other loved ones, as well as help the dying person

deal with the concerns and fears that may come near the e͞͞
life. You should be able to find hospice organizations list͞͞
local phone book.

Final Arrangements

A person with AIDS, like every other adult, should have a will. This can be a difficult subject to discuss, but a will may need to be written before there is any question of the mental competence of the person with AIDS. You may want to be sure the person you are caring for has a will and that you know where it is.

Living wills, which specify what medical care the person with AIDS wants or does not want, also have to be written before their mental competence could be questioned. You, as the caregiver, may be the person asked to see that the doctors follow the wishes of the person with AIDS. This can be a very hard experience to deal with, but is another way of showing respect for a dying person. You may want to be sure the person you are caring for knows that they can control their medical care through living wills.

Often, people who know that they will die soon choose to make their own funeral or memorial arrangements. This helps make sure that the funeral will be done the way they want it done. It also makes things easier for those left behind. They no longer have to guess what their friend or loved one would have wanted. You may be asked to help the person with AIDS plan the funeral, make arrangements with the funeral home, and select a cemetery plot or mausoleum. You may be able to help the person with AIDS decide how they wish to be buried or if they want to be cremated.

After the death, there will still be things to do. Programs that have been providing help, such as Supplemental Security Income, will have to be officially informed of the death. Some money already sent or received may have to be returned. The will may name you, a relative, or another person as the one to handle these tasks.

Dying at Home

Whether or not to die at home is a big decision, but it may not have to be made right away. As the health of the person with AIDS changes, you and they may change your minds several times. However, it is something you should talk about with the person with AIDS ahead of time. Plans should be made; legal papers may need to be signed. What the dying person wants and needs, the needs and abilities of caregivers and other loved ones, the advice of the doctors and other medical professionals, the advice of clergy or other spiritual leaders, may all need to be considered in deciding what is best. Consideration must be given to everyone living in the home. Small children and others may not be ready to cope with death in their home. Others in the home may prefer to face the final moments of the person with AIDS in familiar surroundings. Just be sure the person with AIDS knows that they will not die alone, that the people they love will try to be with them, wherever they choose to die. You also should get help to deal with your own grief after the death.

Help for You

Taking care of someone who is very sick is hard. It wears you down physically and emotionally and creates stress. You can get very angry watching a person you love get sicker and sicker no matter how hard you work or how much you care. You have to do something with this anger. Many people can talk out their anger with other people who have the same problems or with counselors, ministers, rabbis, friends, family, or health workers. Many AIDS service organizations can help you find people to talk to.

You should not try to be the only person taking care of someone with AIDS. You need some time for yourself. The sicker the person you are taking care of becomes, the more important this is. If you try to do everything yourself, you will wear yourself out and not be able to go on. You are not alone. Other people have done this before. Learn from them.

Places to Call for Help

Call the CDC National AIDS Hotline for answers to questions about HIV infection or AIDS, materials on sex and AIDS, or referrals to local organizations in your community. One of the referrals you should ask for is the telephone number of your local Red Cross chapter. The telephone number of the Hotline is 1-800-342-AIDS (1-800-342-2437). If you want to speak in Spanish, call 1-800-344-7432. If you have hearing problems and have a TTY machine, call 1-800-243-7889.

The CDC National AIDS Clearinghouse can provide other materials about HIV and AIDS. The Clearinghouse can also check computer records for organizations in your area dealing with AIDS or materials about HIV or AIDS from health departments, the American Red Cross, or other community-based organizations. The telephone number is 1-800-458-5231. The international number is 00-301-217-0023. The fax number is 1-301-738-6616.

The HIV/AIDS Treatment Information Service can answer questions about treatments for AIDS and diseases linked to AIDS. The telephone number in the United States and Canada is 1-800-448-0440. The international number is 00-301-217-0023. To send a fax, dial 1-301-738-6616. If you have a hearing problem and have a TTY machine, call 1-800-243-7012.

The AIDS Clinical Trials Information Service can provide information about current trials of new drugs for AIDS or diseases linked to AIDS. The telephone number is 1-800-TRIALS-A (1-800-874-2572).

The National Association of People With AIDS (NAPWA) is an association of people who have HIV infection or AIDS. To contact them, call 1-202-898-0414.

Your local phone book should have listings for the local American Red Cross chapter, nursing homes, hospice organizations, the state and local health departments, local HIV or AIDS service organizations, and local medical organizations or referral agencies.

Your local American Red Cross chapter may have special programs on HIV infection and AIDS for African-Americans, Hispanics, and managers and workers on the job. Some Red Cross chapters may offer other training or help with transportation. Both the CDC National AIDS Clearinghouse and the American Red Cross can provide brochures and other materials about HIV and AIDS intended for women, young people, parents, teachers, and those at high risk for or infected with HIV.

Chapter 43

Social Security Benefits for People Living with AIDS

Social Security can provide a lifeline of support to people with HIV infection. That lifeline comes in the form of monthly Social Security disability benefits and Supplemental Security Income (SSI) payments, Medicare and Medicaid coverage and a variety of other services available to people who receive disability benefits from Social Security.

If you are disabled because of HIV infection, this chapter will help you understand the kinds of disability benefits you might be eligible for from the Social Security or SSI programs.

Background Information

Acquired immunodeficiency syndrome (AIDS) is characterized by the inability of the body's natural immunity to fight infection. It is caused by a retrovirus known as human immunodeficiency virus, or HIV. Generally speaking, people with HIV infection fall into two broad categories:

1. those with symptomatic HIV infection, including AIDS; and

2. those with HIV infection but no symptoms.

Although thousands of people with HIV infection are receiving Social Security or SSI disability benefits, we believe there may be

"A Guide to Social Security and SSI Disability Benefits for People with HIV Infection," U.S. Social Security Administration (SSA), Publication Number 05-10020, October 2000.

others who might be eligible for these benefits. Social Security is committed to helping all men, women and children with HIV infection learn more about the disability programs we administer. And if you qualify for benefits, we are just as committed to ensuring that you receive them as soon as possible.

You should also be aware that the Social Security Administration's criteria for evaluating HIV infection are not linked to the Center for Disease Control's (CDC) definition of AIDS. This is because the goals of the two agencies are different. The CDC defines AIDS primarily for surveillance purposes, not for the evaluation of disability.

What Benefits Are You Eligible for?

We pay disability benefits under two programs: Social Security disability insurance, sometimes referred to as SSDI, and Supplemental Security Income, often called SSI. The medical requirements are the same for most people under both programs, and your disability is determined by the same process. However, there are major differences in the nonmedical factors, which are explained in the next two sections.

Social Security Disability Insurance Benefits: The Nonmedical Rules of Eligibility

Here are examples of how people qualify for SSDI:

- Most people qualify for Social Security disability by working, paying Social Security taxes, and in turn, earning credits toward eventual benefits. The maximum number of credits you can earn each year is four. The number of credits you need to qualify for disability depends on your age when you became disabled. Nobody needs more than 40 credits and younger people can qualify with as few as six credits.

- Disabled widows and widowers age 50 or older could be eligible for a disability benefit on the Social Security record of a deceased spouse.

- Disabled children age 18 or older could be eligible for dependent's benefits on the Social Security record of a parent who is getting retirement or disability benefits or on the record of a parent who has died. (The disability must have started before age 22.)

- Children under the age of 18 qualify for dependents benefits on the record of a parent who is getting retirement or disability benefits or on the record of a parent who has died, merely because they are under age 18.

How Much Will My Benefits Be?

How much your Social Security benefit will be depends on your earnings history. Generally, higher earnings translate into higher Social Security benefits. You can find out how much you will get by contacting Social Security and asking for an estimate of your benefits. We'll give you a form you can use to send for a free statement that contains a record of your earnings and an estimate of your benefits.

In addition to checking your benefit estimate, we encourage you to use this statement to verify that your earnings have been properly recorded in our files. It's important that you do this because any missing or unreported wages could lower your Social Security benefit or even prevent you from qualifying for disability benefits. If you find a problem, contact your local Social Security office right away, show them proof of your actual wages, and the record will be corrected. This can be particularly important for people who have tested positive for HIV but have not developed symptoms, so that any potential benefits will not be delayed by wage correction efforts.

Disabled widows, widowers and children eligible for benefits as a dependent on a spouse's or parent's Social Security record receive an amount that is a percentage of the worker's Social Security benefit.

Supplemental Security Income: The Nonmedical Rules of Eligibility

SSI is a program that pays monthly benefits to people with low incomes and limited assets who are 65 or older, or blind or disabled.

Supplemental Security Income supplements a person's income up to a certain level that can go up every year based on increases in the cost-of-living. The level varies from one state to another, so check with your local Social Security office to find out more about SSI benefit levels in your state. We don't count all the income you have when we figure out if you qualify for SSI. And if you work, there are special rules we use for counting your wages. Again, check with Social Security to find out if you can get SSI.

In addition to rules about income, people on SSI must have limited assets. Generally, individuals with assets under $2,000, or couples with assets under $3,000, can qualify for SSI. However, when we figure your assets, we don't count such items as your home, your car (unless it's an expensive one) and most of your personal belongings.

Your Social Security office can tell you more about the income and asset limits.

How Does Social Security Define Disability?

The General Definition of Disability

Disability under Social Security is based on your inability to work. You will be considered disabled if you cannot do work you did before and we decide that you cannot adjust to other work because of your medical condition(s). Your disability also must last or be expected to last for at least a year or to result in death.

For children, we decide if the condition results in marked and severe functional limitations. The condition must have lasted or be expected to last for at least 12 months or be so severe that the child is not expected to live.

How This Definition of Disability Applies to People with HIV Infection

A person with symptomatic HIV infection is often severely limited in his or her ability to work. In other words, if the evidence shows that you have symptomatic HIV infection that severely limits your ability to work, and if you meet the other eligibility factors, the chances are very good that you will be able to receive Social Security or SSI benefits. On the other hand, some people with HIV infection may be less impaired and able to work, so they may not be eligible for disability.

How Does Social Security Evaluate Your Disability?

Social Security works with an agency in each state, usually called a Disability Determination Service (DDS), to evaluate disability claims. DDS staff follow a process that applies to all disability claims. It's a step-by-step process involving 5 questions. They are:

Step 1—Are you working? If you are and your earnings average more than $700 a month, you generally cannot be considered disabled. If you are not working, we go to the next step.

Step 2—Is your condition severe? Your condition must interfere with basic work-related activities for your claim to be considered.

If it does not, we will find that you are not disabled. If it does we will go to the next step.

Step 3—Is your condition found in the list of disabling impairments? For each of the major body systems, we maintain a list of impairments that are so severe they automatically mean you are disabled. If your condition is not on the list we have to decide if it is of equal severity to an impairment that is on the list. If it is, we will find that you are disabled. If it is not we will go to the next step.

Note: There is a complete list of impairments for HIV infections. This list includes many conditions associated with symptomatic HIV infection, including some that apply specifically to women and children with HIV infection.

Following is a list of some of the HIV-related conditions or impairments:

- Pulmonary tuberculosis resistant to treatment
- Kaposi's sarcoma
- *Pneumocystis carinii* pneumonia (PCP)
- Carcinoma of the cervix
- Herpes Simplex
- Hodgkin's disease and all lymphomas
- HIV Wasting Syndrome
- Syphilis and Neurosyphilis
- Candidiasis
- Histoplasmosis

Remember: These are just a few examples. You can see a complete list of HIV-related impairments at any Social Security office.

Step 4—Can you do the work you did previously? If your condition is severe, but not at the same or equal severity as an impairment on the list, then we must determine if it interferes with your ability to do the work you did previously. If it does not, your claim will be denied. If it does, we go to the next step.

Step 5—Can you do any other type of work? If you cannot do the work you did in the past, we see if you are able to adjust to other work. We consider you medical conditions and your age, education, past work experience, and any transferable skill you may have. If you cannot adjust to other work, your claim will be denied.

Remember, at all steps in the process, your impairment must be documented. Documentation includes medical records from your doctors, as well as laboratory test results, X-ray reports etc. The HIV infection itself—that is, the presence of the virus—must be documented as well as any HIV-related manifestations. It is important that we have evidence of signs, symptoms and laboratory findings associated with HIV infection, as well as information on how well you are able to function day-to-day. The signs and symptoms may include: repeated infections; fevers/night sweats; enlarged lymph nodes, liver or spleen; lower energy or generalized weakness; dyspnea on exertion; persistent cough; depression/anxiety; headache; anorexia; nausea and vomiting; and side effects of medication and/or treatment, as well as how your treatment affects your daily activities.

Evaluation of HIV Infection in Women

Statistics show that there is an increasing number of women with HIV diseases. Social Security's guidelines for the immune system recognize that HIV infection can show up differently in women than in men. In addition to the criteria outlined in the previous section, DDS disability evaluators consider specific criteria for diseases common in women. These include: vulvovaginal candidiasis (yeast infection); genital herpes; pelvic inflammatory disease (PID); invasive cervical cancer; genital ulcerative disease; and condyloma (genital warts caused by the human papilloma virus). The list of impairments describes the level of severity necessary for these impairments to be considered disabling.

Evaluation of HIV Infection in Children

We have separate listings for children with HIV infection. These guidelines recognize that the course of the disease in children can differ from adults. In order to be found disabled, a child must have a condition that exactly matches or is equal in severity to either the adult or childhood HIV listing or another impairment found in the list of impairments.

How Do You File for Disability Benefits?

You apply for Social Security and SSI disability benefits by calling or visiting any Social Security office. All Social Security files are kept strictly confidential. It would help if you have certain documents with you when you apply. But don't delay filing because you don't have all the information you need. We'll help you get the rest of it after you sign up. The information you'll need may include:

- your Social Security number and birth certificate;

- the Social Security numbers and birth certificates for family members signing up on your record; and

- a copy of your most recent W-2 form (or your tax return if you're self-employed).

If you're signing up for SSI, you will need to provide records that show that your income and assets are below the SSI limits. This might include such things as bank statements, rent receipts, car registration, etc.

You'll also need to give us information about how your condition affects your daily activities, the names and addresses of your doctors and clinics where you've received treatment and a summary of the kind of work you've done in the past. If you have medical evidence such as reports of blood tests, laboratory work or a physical, it would be helpful if you brought them with you. Following are some guidelines for providing us with medical and vocational information that will help speed up your claim. But first we want you to know what Social Security does to make the process work as smoothly as possible.

What Steps Has Social Security Taken to Ensure Prompt Processing and Payment of Disability Benefits?

All HIV infection claims receive prompt attention and priority handling. For many people applying for SSI with a medical diagnosis of symptomatic HIV infection, the law allows us to presume they are disabled. This permits us to pay up to six months of benefits pending a final decision on the claim. You will qualify for this immediate payment if:

- a medical source confirms that the HIV infection is severe enough to meet Social Security's criteria;

- you meet the other SSI nonmedical eligibility requirements; and

- you are not doing substantial work, i.e. your earnings are under $700 per month.

If you have symptomatic HIV infection but the local Social Security office cannot provide immediate payment, a disability evaluation specialist at the DDS may still make a presumptive disability decision at any point in the process where the evidence suggests a high likelihood that your claim will be approved. (If we later decide you are not disabled, you will not have to pay back the money you received.)

We have made special arrangements with a number of AIDS service organizations, advocacy groups and medical facilities to help us get the evidence we need to streamline the claims process. And many DDS's have Medical/Professional Relations Officers who work directly with these organizations to make this process work smoothly.

What You Can Do to Expedite the Processing of Your Claim

You can play an active and important role in ensuring that your claim is processed accurately and quickly. The best advice we can give you is to keep thorough records that document the symptoms of your illness and how it affects your daily activities, and then to provide all of this information to Social Security when you file your claim. Here are some guidelines you can follow:

- Document the symptoms of your illness early and often.

- Use a calendar to jot down brief notes about how you feel on each day. Record any of your usual activities you could not do on any given day. Be specific, and don't forget to include any psychological or mental problems.

- Help your doctor help you. Not all doctors may be aware of all the kinds of information we need to document your disability. Ask your doctor or other health care professional to track the course of your symptoms in detail over time and to keep a thorough record of any evidence of fatigue, depression, forgetfulness, dizziness and other hard-to-document symptoms.

- Keep records of how your illness affected you on the job. If you were working, but lost your job because of your illness, make notes that describe what it is about your condition that forced you to stop working.

- Give us copies of all these records when you file. In addition to these records, be sure to list the names, addresses and phone numbers of all the doctors, clinics and hospitals you have been to since your illness began. Include your patient or treatment identification number if you know it. Also include the names, addresses and phone numbers of any other people who have information about your illness.

Helping You Return to Work

If you return to work, Social Security has a number of special rules, called work incentives, that provide cash benefits and continued Medicare or Medicaid coverage while you work. They are particularly important to people with HIV disease who, because of the recurrent nature of HIV-related illnesses, may be able to return to work following periods of disability.

The rules are different for Social Security and SSI beneficiaries. For people getting Social Security disability benefits, they include a nine-month trial work period during which earnings, no matter how much, will not affect benefit payments; and a three-year guarantee that, if benefits have stopped because a person remains employed after the trial work period, a Social Security check will be paid for any month earnings are below the substantial level (generally $700). In addition, Medicare coverage extends through the three-year timeframe after the trial work period, even if your earnings are substantial.

SSI work incentives include continuation of Medicaid coverage even if earnings are too high for SSI payments to be made, help with setting up a plan to achieve self-support (PASS), and special consideration for pay received in a sheltered workshop so that SSI benefits may continue even though the earnings might normally prevent payments.

The ticket to Work and Work Incentives Improvement Act of 1999 substantially expands opportunities for people with disabilities who want to work.

- The law extends Part A premium—free Medicare coverage for seven years and nine months for Social Security disability beneficiaries who work, four-and-a-half years beyond the previous 39 months of extended coverage.

- States may now provide Medicaid coverage to people who are not yet too disabled to work and who have incomes above 250 percent of the federal poverty level.

- Starting early in 2001, Social Security and SSI beneficiaries may receive a ticket they may use to obtain vocational and rehabilitation and other employment support services from an approved provider of their choice. An individual using a ticket will not need to undergo the regularly scheduled disability reviews. The program will be phased in nationally over a three-year period.

- Also as of January 1, 2001, when a person's Social Security or SSI disability benefits have ended because of earnings from work, he or she can now request reinstatement of benefits without filing a new application.

What You Need to Know about Medicaid and Medicare

Medicaid and Medicare are our country's two major government-run health insurance programs. Generally, people on SSI and other people with low incomes qualify for Medicaid, while Medicare coverage is earned by working in jobs covered by Social Security, for a railroad or for the federal government. Many people qualify for both Medicare and Medicaid.

Medicaid Coverage

In most states, Social Security's decision that you are eligible for SSI also makes you eligible for Medicaid coverage. (Check with your local Social Security or Medicaid office to verify the requirements in your state.)

State Medicaid programs are required to cover certain services, including inpatient and outpatient hospital care and physician services. States have the option to include other services, such as intermediate care, hospice care, private duty nursing and prescribed drugs.

For more information about Medicaid, contact your local Medicaid agency.

Medicare Coverage

If you get Social Security disability, you will qualify for Medicare coverage 24 months after the month you became entitled to those benefits. Medicare helps pay for:

- inpatient and outpatient hospital care;
- doctor's services;
- diagnostic tests;
- skilled nursing care;

- home health visits;

- hospice care; and

- other medical services.

For more information about Medicare, call or visit your local Social Security office to ask for the booklet, *Medicare* (Publication No. 05-10043).

Help for Low-Income Medicare Beneficiaries

If you get Medicare and have low income and few resources, your state may pay your Medicare premiums and, in some cases, other out-of-pocket Medicare expenses such as deductibles and coinsurance. Only your state can decide if you qualify. To find out if you do, contact your state or local welfare office or Medicaid agency. For more general information about the program, contact Social Security and ask for the leaflet, *Medicare Savings for Qualified Beneficiaries* (HCFA Publication No. 02184).

For More Information Visit our Internet Website

If you have a computer and can access the Internet, check out Social Security Online, our Internet website at www.ssa.gov for a variety of information and services, including:

- Publications you can download on all aspects of Social Security programs

- Forms you can use to request various services, such as a Social Security Statement, a replacement Social Security or Medicare card, or benefit verification

- *Social Security eNews*, an electronic newsletter that you can receive by e-mail free-of-charge to help you keep up with the latest changes in Social Security programs

- A Retirement Planner, designed to help people of all ages plan their future financial security using their Social Security benefits as a base

If you don't have a personal computer, many libraries and other nonprofit organizations provide Internet access services to the public. Call your local library for more information.

Call Our 800 Number

You can get recorded information 24 hours a day, including weekends and holidays, by calling our toll-free number, 1-800-772-1213. You can speak to a service representative between the hours of 7 a.m. and 7 p.m. on business days. Our lines are busiest early in the week and early in the month so, if your business can wait, it's best to call at other times. Have your Social Security number handy when you call.

People who are deaf or hard of hearing may call our toll-free TTY number, 1-800-325-0778, between 7 a.m. and 7 p.m. on business days.

We treat all calls confidentially—whether they're made to our toll-free numbers or to one of our local offices. We also want to ensure that you receive accurate and courteous service. That is why we have a second Social Security representative monitor some incoming and outgoing telephone calls.

Part Five

Issues for Women
and Children with AIDS

Chapter 44

Women and AIDS

Menstrual Irregularity

Women have long reported menstrual irregularities associated with HIV infection, including shortened or lengthened time between menstruation, heavier or lighter flow of menstrual blood and other irregularities. Research findings, however, have been yielding conflicting results regarding the association between menstrual irregularity and HIV status. A new study confirms an association and observes that irregularities appear more frequently as HIV disease progresses.

Included in this report were 802 HIV-positive and 273 HIV-negative women from two large studies (HIV Epidemiology Study or HERS and Women's Interagency HIV Study or WIHS). Women self-reported information about their menstrual cycle over the course of six months. Overall, the study found that HIV-positive women, who were otherwise healthy, had high CD4+ cell counts, were not experiencing unwanted weight loss (wasting syndrome) and not using/abusing drugs were unlikely to have menstrual irregularities. As HIV disease progresses, however, there does appear to be some effect of HIV on hormones, as measured by increased incidence of menstrual irregularities. Women with lower CD4+ cell counts (below 200) were 50% more likely to have longer menstrual cycles (over 40 days) than women

From Project Inform: "Women and AIDS Update," © 1999 Project Inform, from *PI Perspective* #27, April 1999, reprinted with permission. For more information, contact the National NIV/AIDS Treatment Hotline, 800-822-7422, or visit our website, www.projectinform.org.

with counts above 200. Women with high HIV levels (above 150,000 copies/ml) had the most variability in their menstrual cycle, shorter and longer times between cycles with a large amount of unpredictability.

This study confirms a relationship between HIV infection and changes in the menstrual cycle, which becomes more pronounced as HIV disease progresses, CD4+ cell counts fall below 200 and HIV levels increase. The study confirms that other factors are important determinants of menstrual irregularity and should be considered when and if they occur. These include drug use, poor nutrition, severe medical illness and weight loss associated with chronic illness. A number of other factors have also been identified in other studies

Menstrual Irregularity Co-Factors

Age: Younger and older age are both associated with menstrual irregularities. Young women often have irregularities when first beginning to menstruate, sometimes lasting through puberty. Older women, especially those going through menopause, also commonly have irregularities. On either end of this age spectrum, hormone therapy (e.g. progesterone/estrogen) may help to regulate menstrual cycles. However, it is not known if trying to regulate these natural changes is helpful.

Body Mass Index: Women who are very thin, malnourished, or who generally have extremely low levels of body fat often have menstrual irregularities, particularly increased time between menstruation and/or very light bleeding during periods. For women who are thin because of malnutrition and unwanted weight loss issues, attention to treating unwanted weight loss can help to regulate the cycle.

Drug Use (substance use/abuse): Injection drug and other substance use are associated with changes in menstrual cycles.

Illnesses and Infections: Some illnesses, and side effects from drugs used to treat them, can influence menstrual cycles. Inflammatory and infectious conditions (e.g. vaginitis and pelvic inflammatory disease) can also affect regularity.

Dysplasia: Dysplasia (e.g. vulvar, vaginal, cervical and ovarian) is associated with changes in menstrual cycles.

Race: While this particular study only looked at whites, Latinos and African Americans, there did appear to be more menstrual irregularities among African Americans compared to the other groups. It may be, in this particular study, that other factors confounded the ability to truly isolate any differences caused by race difference. However, even this hint of a racial differential warrants further study.

Comments

It is not surprising that there is a relationship between HIV infection and menstrual irregularities. Male hormone irregularities (testosterone deficiencies) are associated with HIV disease progression, fatigue and wasting syndrome. Similarly, female hormone changes, as measured by increases in menstrual irregularities, are associated with advanced HIV-disease and wasting syndrome. The question now is what to do about these changes. Will hormone replacement therapy (e.g. estrogen/progesterone) help regulate menstrual cycles and/or improve symptoms associated with hormone imbalances such as fatigue and decreased sexual drive? Should women receive anabolic steroids (like testosterone) when they experience signs of unwanted weight loss and/or decrease in sexual energy? Now that menstrual irregularities have been documented, and the group of women likeliest to experience them have been defined, studies looking at therapies to intervene and correct these irregularities should proceed quickly. Activist attention is needed to make it happen.

Human Papillomavirus

Human papillomavirus (HPV) is a sexually transmitted disease that causes anal and genital warts and is associated with anal and cervical dysplasia. It is a common infection, particularly among women with HIV. Several studies confirm previous findings that women with HIV, particularly those with low CD4+ cell counts, have increased frequency and severity of HPV-associated cervical dysplasia.

One study examined the incidence of HPV-associated lesions in women without HPV who were enrolled in a study from 1991-98. Every six months, 369 HIV-positive and 334 HIV-negative volunteers had gynecological (GYN) exams and colposcopies. Thirty-one (8%) of HIV-infected and two (1%) of HIV-negative women developed HPV-related lesions throughout follow-up (3.3 years, 3.7 years, respectively). Not only were HIV-positive women more likely to develop HPV-related lesions, but the average time to lesion development was shorter (24 months, 44 months, respectively). Also, the majority (61%) who developed a lesion had a history of cervical intraepithelial neoplasia or CIN. (CIN—or cervical dysplasia—is a form of abnormal cell growth of which, at its most severe, is cervical cancer.) The study found that risk factors for lesion development included CD4+ cell counts below 500 and detection of HPV in cervico-vaginal lavage (CVL, a screening procedure).

Another study examined the relationship between incidence of HPV and immune suppression in 268 female intravenous drug users. In it, 814 HIV-positive and 84 HIV-negative women underwent an average of six HPV measurements. Among 187 women with follow-up visits subsequent to the first measurement, the probability of testing HPV-positive increased dramatically for HIV-positive (78.7%) compared to HIV-negative women (47.5%). It was high among HIV-positive women with CD4+ cell counts below 200 (92.9%). Also, of 107 women evaluated by colposcopies, eleven had biopsies confirming CIN. These results suggest that HIV-infection and its associated immunodeficiency is strongly related to the persistence of HPV which in turn is associated with CIN.

Another study characterized the incidence and progression of HPV in HIV-infected women with varying levels of immune suppression. Between 3/96 and 7/98, 112 women were evaluated by twice-yearly GYN exams, CVL and STD screenings. In the study, 112 women (63%) had detectable HPV at the initial exam, with another 77 (69%) testing HPV-positive during the course of the study. In addition, 23 (20.5%) were infected with two or more HPV types, and three were infected with a unique or previously unidentified type. These results demonstrate that HPV is highly prevalent and persistent among women with HIV. They demonstrate that HPV types may be distinct in women with HIV.

Comments on HPV

These studies confirm that HIV-related immune suppression is a co-factor for the development of HPV and HPV-associated cervical dysplasia. Other co-factors include smoking, age of first sexual intercourse and, possibly, hormonal issues. These studies underline the importance of careful and regular GYN screenings for women, particularly those with CD4+ cell counts below 500 (e.g. at least every six months).

Treatment of Recurrent Cervical Dysplasia (CIN)

Previous studies confirm that abnormal cell growth in the cervix (cervical dysplasia), associated with cervical cancer, is more common and potentially more aggressive among women living with HIV compared to uninfected women. Women with HIV have extremely high recurrence rates of cervical dysplasia after standard treatment (39-87% among HIV-positive women vs. 0-18% among HIV-negative women). A study of the AIDS Clinical Trials Group (ACTG 200) examined the safety and effectiveness of a therapy called 5-Fluorouracil (5-FU) for preventing recurrent cervical dysplasia (CIN). 5-FU has been successful in treating skin lesions in HIV-negative people as well as vaginal dysplasia in women with immune suppression not associated with HIV.

One hundred and one women who had received standard treatments for cervical dysplasia (CIN grades 2 or 3) received either 5% 5-FU or no therapy and were followed for a year and a half (18 months). Those receiving 5-FU received one 2-gram application intravaginally at bedtime every two weeks for six months. The medication was not administered during menstruation. Pap smears and colposcopies were scheduled at regular intervals during the 18 months of follow-up.

Of the 50 women who received 5-FU, 14 (28%) developed cervical dysplasia recurrence, compared to 24 (47%) of the 51 women in the observation arm. Most significantly, 5-FU therapy was significantly correlated to prolonged time to recurrence of CIN and decreased probability of developing high grade CIN, which requires more aggressive treatment. Additionally, 5-FU therapy reduced recurrent cervical dysplasia with minimal side effects (vaginal discharge was the most common, occurring in six women). These results suggest that this treatment should be offered to HIV-positive women after therapy for high-grade CIN.

Chapter 45

Gynecological Complications in Women with HIV

Gynecological (GYN) conditions are the most commonly reported complication of women living with HIV and AIDS. Many of the conditions HIV-positive women experience also affect women who are not living with HIV. However, GYN complications in women with HIV usually occur more frequently, are more serious and are more difficult to treat. They range from chronic, recurrent yeast infections to abnormal menstrual cycles (periods) and vaginal warts (caused by human papillomavirus, or HPV) to cervical cancer. For many women, recurrent GYN conditions are often the very first signs of HIV infection.

When monitoring and treating GYN conditions, it is important to consider what GYN health reveals about the status of a woman's immune system. What happens to the immune system, for instance, when a common GYN condition like vaginal candidiasis (yeast infections) becomes increasingly more difficult to treat? What does the absence of an HIV-infected woman's period (amenorrhea), a common menstrual abnormality in women with HIV, tell us about immune function? How does the increase in rates and severity of cervical abnormalities experienced in women with HIV relate to a weakening immune system?

From Project Inform: Excerpted from "GYN Conditions in Women with HIV," © 1999 Project Inform, reprinted with permission. For more information, contact the National NIV/AIDS Treatment Hotline, 800-822-7422, or visit our website, www.projectinform.org. Resources in this chapter were verified December 2002.

This chapter contains information on symptoms, tests and treatments for common GYN conditions. It should serve as a tool to enable routine self-monitoring and care for GYN health and to facilitate informed conversations with health care providers when GYN complications occur.

Vaginal Candidiasis

Vaginal candidiasis, or vaginal yeast infections (sometimes called vaginitis), is a fungal infection of the vulva and/or vagina common in many women. It is the most common initial symptom of HIV in women and is also the most common reason that HIV-infected women first seek medical attention. Recurrent vaginal yeast infections and/or yeast infections that become less responsive to treatment are a sign of a weakening immune system.

While a variety of factors, including antibiotic use and oral contraceptives, can result in recurrent vaginal yeast infections, they generally are not the underlying causes in women with HIV. Rather, recurrent vaginal candidiasis in women with HIV is most often associated with a decline of CD4+ cell counts. When CD4+ cell counts fall below 200, the risk of recurrent vaginal and oral (in the mouth) yeast infections increase. As the immune system is further weakened and damaged, yeast infections occur more frequently, becoming more aggressive and less responsive to therapy. Therefore, intervening and treating candidiasis is important. Moreover, halting the damage of the immune system through the treatment of HIV disease, and allowing the immune system to rebuild itself so that it can control candidiasis is key to a long-term solution to the problem of recurrent yeast infections.

Symptoms of vaginal candidiasis include itching and swelling of the vulva, thick white-yellow or cheesy discharge and burning upon urination. With increased immune suppression, the primary location of the candida infection may shift from the vagina to the mouth or esophagus, the tube leading from the mouth to the stomach.

There are several effective forms of treatment for vaginal candidiasis, including creams and suppositories such as clotrimazole (Gyne-Lotrimin) which are available over-the-counter and by prescription. If the candidiasis is unresponsive to local (i.e. at the site of the yeast infection) treatment, the antifungal drugs fluconazole (Diflucan) or ketoconazole (Nizoral) are usually effective. These are drugs taken orally, in a pill form, and treat fungal infections throughout the body (i.e. systemically). However, recent studies caution that women with very low CD4+ cell counts (less than 50) who have used fluconazole extensively are at increased risk of developing fluconazole-resistant candidiasis. Many researchers advise the use of local treatments as the first choice in treating candidiasis, reserving systemic therapies, such as fluconazole, as a back-up. Dietary modifications such as decreasing sugar intake, addition of lactobacillus-containing yogurt (it will be on the label) or acidophilus capsules (available in health food stores), may also help prevent recurrences of candidiasis.

More Tips Which May Help Prevent Recurrent Vaginal Yeast Infections

Don't douche! Douching changes the vagina's natural acid level (called pH level) and causes inflammation, both of which may increase the risk of further infection, including STDs. Your body has a natural douching system—let it work.

Avoid the use of scented soap, bleach and fabric softeners when doing laundry. Scented laundry soap contains chemicals which can aggravate a yeast infection. Residual bleach in your clothing may destroy healthy bacteria which help your body keep fungal infections at bay. Fabric softeners block moisture absorption, causing moist areas of the skin to stay damp, thus encouraging bacteria, etc.

Avoid tight fitting clothes. Tight clothing blocks air flow and yeast infections grow best in moist environments. Thus, loose fitting clothing, which allows airflow provides a dryer environment.

Wear cotton underwear. Unlike synthetic materials such as polyester, Lycra and nylon, cotton breathes better, which means it lets air in and doesn't trap moisture.

Avoid washing the vaginal area with deodorant soaps and soaps which are heavily scented or perfumed. Some women claim that when they stop using scented soaps in the shower or bath, yeast infections heal better and don't recur as often. This would include avoiding bubble baths.

Try a non-soap cleanser like unscented Nutribiotic Non-soap with aloe vera to slightly moisturize the skin and promote healing. Soap can have a drying effect on the skin and can further aggravate the vaginal area affected by a yeast infection. Non-soap cleansers can be obtained at most health food stores and many supermarkets.

HIV and STDs

There is some concern that sexually transmitted diseases (STDs) might speed up the rate of HIV progression. This is based on observations that infections activate the body's immune system which in turn increases HIV replication. When HIV replication increases, there is an increase in damage to the immune defenses as the virus infects and destroys important immune cells.

An increase in the amount of HIV in genital secretions has been noted with several STDs. In some instances, increases in HIV replication caused by STDs and other GYN infections may be restricted to the genital tract. This means that there might not be an increase in HIV in the blood, as measured during regular doctor visits, but there may be an increase in HIV in the genital tract, specifically. Increases in HIV replication may cause damage to the immune environment in the genital tract. Currently, it remains unknown what these increases in HIV in genital secretions mean over the long haul, but common sense suggests that damage to the immune environment in the genital tract will lead to increased GYN complications. Thus, more numerous STDs, or STDs left untreated, will probably contribute to increasing complications over time.

Untreated STDs assist the spread of HIV infection. For those who are HIV infected, an untreated STD increases the probability of passing HIV to their sex partners. An untreated STD also makes an HIV negative person more susceptible to acquiring HIV from an HIV positive sex partner. This relationship between HIV and STDs underlines the importance of early STD diagnosis and treatment.

Herpes Simplex Virus

Genital herpes is usually caused by herpes simplex virus 2 (HSV-2), but can also be caused by the same virus that causes cold sores (HSV-1). Once a person is infected with herpes, the infection remains present for life. Though it may be dormant for long periods, recurrent outbreaks of symptoms are also typically part of the disease. Several studies show that the sexually transmitted disease herpes simplex virus type 2 (HSV-2) may take an altered course in people with HIV-related immune suppression. For instance, the painful sores in and around the genitals and/or anus caused by herpes tend to be more frequent, persistent and require higher doses of treatment. The most common sites of recurrent herpes infection in women are the labia majora (the outer vaginal lips), the labia minora (the vagina's inner lips) and the buttocks.

It is important to remember that symptoms of herpes correlate with the severity of HIV-related immune deficiency. For example, HSV ulcers persisting for over one month are associated with severe immunosuppression and are considered an AIDS-defining illness.

Oral acyclovir (Zovirax) and famciclovir (Famvir) are used to treat herpes. For women with frequent HSV outbreaks, daily acyclovir therapy may be helpful in the prevention of outbreaks. If herpes stops responding to acyclovir (e.g. sores don't go away within two weeks after starting acyclovir therapy), a number of other therapies are available to treat acyclovir-resistant herpes. These include: intravenous foscarnet (Foscavir) and topical cidofovir (Vistide).

Syphilis

Syphilis is a progressive bacterial infection that is usually sexually transmitted. It is important to recognize and treat syphilis promptly because the disease may progress more rapidly due to immune suppression associated with HIV. Progression occurs in three stages: primary syphilis, characterized by painless ulcers or lesions; secondary syphilis, indicated by widespread lesions and swollen lymph glands; and tertiary syphilis, most often characterized by lesions in organs and tissues (sometimes called neurosyphilis as it often affects the central nervous system).

Standard treatment for syphilis is oral penicillin or ceftriaxone (Rocephin). Several studies report that treatment for primary staged syphilis—a single dose of penicillin G benzathine (Bicillin)—may fail in HIV-infected persons. Therefore, like herpes, it may be necessary to treat HIV positive people with syphilis using higher doses of standard antibiotic therapy or longer courses of treatment.

HIV in the Female Genital Tract

Inflammation of the vagina caused by unhealthy bacteria or physical trauma due to penetration, douching or other factors, can increase the risk of contracting HIV. When the vagina is inflamed, there are small breaks in the vaginal membranes, exposed blood cells and an increase in the vaginal acid level (called pH level). All of these factors can decrease the vagina's ability to defend against HIV and other STDs.

The role of HIV in the genital tract and how it promotes or worsens GYN conditions is only beginning to be understood. Some studies have shown that high levels of HIV in genital secretions (also called cervicovaginal secretions or CVS) correlate with high levels of HIV in the blood and/or GYN infections, swelling and tenderness. HIV interacts with other viral infections, such as herpes simplex virus (HSV) and human papilloma virus (HPV), the virus that causes genital warts. HIV and related immune suppression may also increase susceptibility to other infections, particularly vaginal candidiasis (yeast infections) and chlamydia. Finally, data from a recent study also show that, compared to HIV negative women, positive women have more chronic inflammation (including pain, itching and discharge) around the vagina and cervix without a causative STD.

Other Common STDs

Diseases such as chlamydia, gonorrhea, trichomonas and bacterial vaginosis commonly occur among women with HIV. Currently, standard treatment regimens are used to treat these conditions. These include antibiotics such as azithromycin (Zithromax), ceftriaxone or doxycycline (Vibramycin) to treat chlamydia and penicillin and/or tetracycline (Achromycin) to treat gonorrhea. Both bacterial vaginosis and trichomonas are treated with metronidazole (MetroGel, Flagyl).

When these diseases occur, the vaginal acid level (pH level) changes, making the GYN environment more welcoming to other infections (including HIV infection). Furthermore, untreated GYN complications, particularly chlamydia and gonorrhea, are the common cause of pelvic inflammatory disease (sometimes called PID) and cervicitis (tenderness and swelling of cervix). Thus, it is important to treat these common STDs in order to prevent further complications.

Pelvic Inflammatory Disease (PID)

Pelvic inflammatory disease (PID) represents a range of inflammatory disorders of the upper genital tract, including the fallopian tubes, the uterus, ovaries and, in advanced stages, the abdominal lining. Common symptoms of PID include chronic, moderate-to-severe pain; tenderness in the abdomen; irregular menstrual cycles; nonmenstrual bleeding and painful and frequent urination. Like other gynecological conditions, PID appears to be more prevalent, severe and resistant to treatment among women with HIV and especially women with AIDS. Indeed, the Centers for Disease Control and Prevention (CDC) recommend hospitalization and intravenous (directly into the vein) antibiotics for treating PID in women with HIV. Studies indicate that relapse of PID occurs more often in women with suppressed immunity.

Cervicitis

Inflammation of the cervix, known as cervicitis, is another symptom of PID. A number of conditions can lead to cervicitis. Chlamydia and gonorrhea infections can result in swelling of the cervix. Cervicitis may also result from untreated trichomonas or bacterial vaginosis. Cytomegalovirus (CMV), a virus in the herpes family which is also the leading cause of blindness among people with AIDS, can also be a GYN complication and may cause cervicitis as well. Cervicitis is often present without symptoms. When symptoms do occur, they include non-menstrual bleeding, bleeding after penetrative intercourse, painful urination and lower back pain. The treatment for cervicitis depends on the identified cause of the condition.

Human Papillomavirus and Cervical Disease

Human papillomavirus (HPV) is a sexually transmitted disease and the cause of genital warts. HPV primarily affects the cervix and plays a primary role in the development of cervical dysplasia (abnormal cells) and cervical cancer. Recent studies have demonstrated that women with HIV, particularly those with low CD4+ counts, have an increased frequency and severity of HPV-related cervical dysplasia. The outcome for HIV positive women with cervical cancer—the most severe form of cervical dysplasia and an AIDS-defining illness—is much graver than for women without HIV. However, if detected early, less severe grades of dysplasia (CIN I or II) are fairly easily treated which stresses the need for regular and timely GYN screening to catch pre-cancerous conditions before they become severe.

Women with HIV have high recurrence rates of cervical dysplasia after standard treatment (39-87% among HIV-positive women vs. 0-18% among HIV-negative women). A study of the AIDS Clinical Trial Group (ACTG 200) suggests that 5-Fluorouracil (5-FU) is safe and effective for preventing recurrent cervical dysplasia (CIN). Study participants who received one 2-gram application intravaginally at bedtime every two weeks for six months had reduced recurrent cervical dysplasia with minimal side effects.

In addition to cervical dysplasia, if symptoms of HPV infection occur, they often include multiple small warts on the vagina or around the anus. Many types of treatment are available when symptoms of HPV occur including surgical removal, electro-cautery (removal by electric current), chemical removal, laser removal and the topical cream imiquimod (Aldara). Unfortunately, treatment can be painful

317

and HPV-related warts commonly reoccur. Recent studies caution against the use a common treatment option called cryotherapy which involves freezing off the wart or abnormal cells. Cryotherapy can cause normal tissue to heal over deeper areas of dysplasia, causing future genital screenings to appear normal while abnormal tissue grows undetected beneath the surface. Also, many women report that the aftermath of cryotherapy can be very painful.

Menstrual Irregularities

Changes in periods (menstrual cycles) are common, regardless of HIV status. Many of the changes reported by HIV positive women include irregular periods, heavier or lighter periods, a worsening of symptoms associated with premenstrual syndrome (PMS) and a darkening of menstrual blood. Another common menstrual disorder among HIV positive women is the absence of menstruation altogether. This condition is called amenorrhea and it is defined as a history of no menstrual periods for more than 90 days. In some studies, amenorrhea has been more frequent among women with lower CD4+ counts (less than 50).

It is not known exactly how HIV disease affects the reproductive system and the menstrual cycle or how female hormones—estrogen and progesterone—interact with the immune system. Studies have shown that substance abuse, chronic illness and significant weight loss can lead to a dysregulation of the hypothalamus, the part of the brain that regulates sex hormone secretion and can affect menstruation. It is presumed that problems with the immune system due to HIV cause changes in female hormones and result in menstrual irregularities.

HIV-infected women with abnormal or changed menstrual bleeding should seek medical attention to determine the cause of the abnormality. Heavy bleeding or painful periods are associated with pelvic inflammatory disease, discussed above. They may also be explained by low platelets (the component of the blood involved in clotting and immune response) associated with HIV infection. A low platelet count is determined by a blood test called a complete blood count (CBC). If your platelet count is low (under 50,000), be sure to review your medications with your doctor because some of them (including aspirin and ibuprofen) may affect the body's blood clotting process. Several treatments are available for platelet counts below 20,000, including the anti-HIV drug zidovudine (AZT, Retrovir), corticosteroids, intravenous gamma globulins and platelet transfusions. In addition, alcohol should be avoided because it may block platelet production and interfere with normal blood clotting processes.

Heavy and/or frequent menstrual bleeding (dysmenorrhea) can cause anemia, or low red blood cells, which can also lead to amenorrhea. While the symptoms of dysmenorrhea and amenorrhea are opposing, they may both be caused by anemia. Anemia is also a common condition among HIV positive women and can cause fatigue. When severe, anemia can also lead to amenorrhea.

It is important to investigate all potential causes of amenorrhea. Aside from anemia, these may include pregnancy, ovarian cysts, opportunistic infections, menopause or other GYN conditions. Other factors may include the use of antiviral therapy and other medications (such as megestrol), street drugs (particularly heroin and/or marijuana use) and poor nutrition. Finally, body weight changes, stress and too much exercise can cause a defect in the secretion of a hormone necessary for normal menstruation to occur (called gonadotropin-releasing hormone or GnRH).

There are several ways to alleviate many of the GYN symptoms that accompany common menstrual problems. Premenstrual and menstrual cramping usually responds to over-the-counter medications including aspirin, ibuprofen (Motrin or Advil) or naproxen (Aleve). Some women experiencing menopausal symptoms choose to treat with hormone replacement therapy or herbal and nutritional therapies. Birth control pills which mimic normal menstrual cycles are also used to treat amenorrhea. Finally, stress reduction, vitamin supplementation (such as a regular One-A-Day vitamin), regular exercise and nutrition should always be incorporated into any treatment plan.

Menopause

Menopause—the end of menstruation—is a natural and universal phase for women. Menopause occurs because of natural changes which happen over time (usually 10-15 years) in a woman's reproductive system. These changes include declining production of the hormone estrogen. Without sufficient levels of estrogen, the uterine lining cannot thicken in preparation for an embryo. Thus, no ovulation occurs (the passing of an egg out of the fallopian tubes into the thickened uterus walls) and menstruation stops.

Women usually experience menopause between the ages of 38-58, with most women entering menopause around the age of 51. There is some evidence that women with HIV may experience menopause earlier. This may be due to many HIV-related factors such as anemia, reduced hormone production, chronic illness, weight loss, possible effects of antivirals, street drugs and smoking. Nevertheless, the symptoms of menopause appear to be the same for HIV positive and negative women alike. They include heavier, irregular or missed periods, hot flashes, vaginal dryness and other changes of the vagina.

Many women undergo hormone replacement therapy (HRT) in order to replace the estrogen lost during menopause. While HRT eliminates the hot flashes brought on by menopause, it is not without its own dangers and unknown risks. Menopausal women with a history of breast cancer should avoid estrogen replacement therapy because it may stimulate the growth of cancer cells. New research indicates that progesterone (megestrol acetate) may also be effective at decreasing hot flashes. Progesterone is increasingly prescribed to menopausal women with a history of breast cancer because it is not an estrogen. Unfortunately, there is not enough research to point to the dangers or benefits of HRT on women with HIV.

Screening

Since women with HIV have high rates and generally more severe cases of GYN complications, it is important to screen frequently and regularly. GYN screening is normally done with one of two diagnostic tools, the Pap smear and/or colposcopy.

Pap Smear

A Pap smear is a test used to detect cervical cancer and is a standard part of the routine gynecological examination. It involves inserting a long cotton swab into the vagina and swabbing ells from the cervix which are then examined under the microscope. While the Pap smear is relatively non-invasive, often only causing a sensation that feels like pressure on the cervix, the usefulness of the test is beginning to be called into question—especially when it is being used as a screening tool for cervical cancer in women with HIV. (NOTE: When there is tenderness or swelling, even a Pap smear, which is generally not painful, can cause discomfort).

The problem with Pap smears as a useful diagnosis procedure lies in the fact that 15-30% of Pap smears results that come back as normal are, upon subsequent colposcopy and biopsy, abnormal (called false negative results). In other words, abnormal pre-cancerous cell growth that may require further examination or immediate treatment pass undetected during the Pap test. The problem of false-negative Pap smears has lead some health care providers to suggest colposcopy as a more accurate screening procedure, particularly among HIV positive women where early detection is most critical.

Colposcopy involves the examination of the cervix for signs of cancerous growth by means of a flexible magnifying tube (called a colposcope) which is inserted in the vagina. While insertion of the colposcope into the vagina may cause discomfort, the actual procedure usually isn't painful. Still, colposcopy has its own drawbacks. Not only does it require management by a specialist but, coupled with biopsy, it can be a painful experience with some risk of infection and bleeding. At this point, it is difficult to say whether or not colposcopy screening is a necessary procedure for HIV-positive women without signs of an abnormal Pap smear.

Pap Plus Speculoscopy

A promising new screening tool called Pap Plus Speculoscopy (PPS) has recently gained FDA approval. It is almost as sensitive as a colposcopy plus biopsy, is less invasive and painful, and does not require a specialist to perform the procedure. PPS involves a standard Pap smear and the lighting of the cervix with a chemical light called a Speculite after the vinegar wash. The Speculite whitens abnormal tissues so a clinician may detect potential disease. This procedure feels like a regular Pap plus a tingly, sometimes stingy sensation due to the vinegar wash. The new test is becoming more widely available in STD, Planned Parenthood and other GYN health providing clinics.

Interactions between Anti-HIV Drugs and Oral Contraceptives

Several anti-HIV drugs are known to interfere with the way the body processes oral contraceptives (OC). The most commonly used oral (hormonal) contraceptive is called ethinyl-estradiol (estrogen and progesterone). The following is a list of known drug interactions:

Indinavir (Crixivan): moderately increases ethinyl-estradiol levels in the blood; dose change not necessary.

Nevirapine (Viramune): significantly decreases ethinyl-estradiol levels in the blood, making oral contraceptive less effective; increase in OC dose or additional method of birth control recommended.

Nelfinavir (Viracept): significantly decreases ethinyl-estradiol levels in the blood, making oral contraceptive less effective; increase in OC dose or additional method of birth control recommended.

Ritonavir (Norvir): significantly decreases ethinyl-estradiol levels in the blood, making oral contraceptive less effective; increase in OC dose or additional methods of birth control recommended.

Efavirenz (Sustiva): increases ethinyl-estradiol (estrogen and progesterone) levels in the blood. It is not yet known whether a dose modification is necessary.

Understanding Our Immune System

Our immune system is our body's defense against infections and diseases. Our skin—the body's largest organ—is the first line defense of our immune system. It creates a barrier which keeps disease-causing organisms away from our blood and organs. If an organism, like bacteria, fungus or virus, gets into our body, a variety of cells respond by fighting off and destroying the organism, or at least keeping it in check so that it doesn't cause disease. Understanding this response by the immune system helps us to better understand HIV, other diseases and GYN complications.

The immune system plays an important role in controlling symptoms of infection. In fact, you can have an infection without having a disease. A good example of this is herpes simplex virus (HSV). Many are infected with the herpes virus, but only when it becomes active and lesions (i.e. symptoms) are present does someone actually have the disease. Acyclovir, which is an anti-herpes drug, helps the immune system keep the herpes virus as inactive as possible. But drugs are not a substitute for the immune system. Drugs generally work with the immune system to prevent or treat disease. When a person has a weakened immune system, an anti-herpes drug alone will not work as well in controlling a herpes outbreak.

Another example of the immune system's role in controlling disease is cytomegalovirus (CMV). About 60-80% of adults are infected with CMV. The immune system does an incredible job of keeping CMV from causing any harm. When the immune system is weakened, however, CMV can cause serious and life-threatening disease. In fact, it is the leading cause of blindness in people with HIV and among the leading causes of death of people with AIDS. Although there are no cures for either HSV or CMV, an intact and healthy immune system can control these viruses from causing symptoms and disease.

In some ways, HIV is similar to HSV or CMV. As with HSV and CMV, you can be infected with HIV and not have any symptoms. The difference between HIV and these other viruses, however, is that even though you may not experience symptoms, HIV is slowly attacking and destroying your immune defenses. In other words, HIV destroys the very immune system that keeps you from getting many diseases. Thus, even though you might feel good and have no symptoms of HIV disease, a doctor might recommend that you start anti-HIV medications. This is because anti-HIV drugs will keep the virus from severely damaging your immune system, in essence preventing you from getting symptoms of HIV/AIDS.

So what does this have to do with GYN health? An increase in GYN complications could be a sign that your immune system is weakening and is beginning to lose its ability to keep viruses, fungi and bacteria under control in your vagina/genital tract. Recurring symptoms, such as vaginal or oral yeast infections, skin problems, bacterial infections or herpes, tell us that our immune system is damaged and the infections only worsen the situation. Preserving the immune system before these conditions occur is critical. And while it's important to treat the problem (e.g. treat the vaginal yeast infection, herpes, genital warts, etc.), it's also important to treat the real underlying problem—a weakened immune system. If damage to the immune system by HIV is allowed to continue, the GYN complications, as well as many other types of infections, will increasingly become more of a problem. Intervening when complications do occur by seeking treatment and care for all of HIV disease, including GYN complications, is key to preservation, promotion and enhancement immune health. It is never too early to take charge of your health. Knowledge of what it's telling you is the first step.

Stress and Its Affect on Our Immune System

When people are under stress they have a tendency to develop more infections, common colds, herpes outbreaks, vaginal yeast infections or other diseases. Why does this happen? Partly because the chemicals released in our body when we experience stress actually weaken our immune system. Moreover, the organ responsible for producing important immune cells, called the thymus, becomes damaged by these chemicals. In other words, both the cells, as well as the source for new cells, become damaged and weakened by the chemicals that our body produces when we feel stress. Finding ways to alleviate stress, such as going for a walk, talking about your feelings with a close friend, taking a bath, meditation or massage, can help to strengthen your immune system.

The ways in which stress affects other parts of our lives can also weaken the immune system. Sometimes when we feel stressed out we also get depressed, don't eat regularly, don't sleep well or find it difficult to take care of ourselves on a day-to-day basis. All of these things can further weaken the immune system. Understanding health as it pertains to the whole body, and including stress-reduction, improved diet, health-promoting exercise, normal sleep patterns and steps to improve general well being are important. Managing HIV disease is not just about anti-HIV drugs, viral load and GYN complications. It's a broader picture that's about many parts of life.

Conclusion

Many of the GYN complications HIV positive women experience also affect women who are not living with HIV. However, the same conditions tend to be more frequent and are more serious and difficult to treat in women with a compromised immune system. At the same time, GYN complications further compromise the immune system. Consequently, it is very important that GYN complications be diagnosed, monitored and treated under the guidance of a health care provider.

Since many of these complications lack obvious symptoms and can persist undetected, regular exams are crucial, even when feeling well. Like breast exams, Pap smears, colposcopies and PPS are designed to detect early, pre-cancerous conditions. Detection and treatment at these early stages is a critical step in preventing a GYN condition from progressing, as is monitoring your own GYN health and advocating for your own best behalf.

Abnormal GYN Screening Terms

Atypia: These cells show minimal changes. May be atypical due to the presence of a vaginal infection, the use of oral contraceptives or because the person doing the Pap smear may have not handled the cells properly.

Carcinoma-In-Situ (CIS): On a Pap smear, this report means the same thing as CIN 3, the entire sample shows dysplasia. However, the sample shows no sign of invasive cancer.

CIN 1: Cervical Intraepithelial Neoplasia. CIN means abnormal growth or tumor in the tissue covering or surrounding the cervix. CIN 1 means that one-third of the sample has dysplasia or pre-cancer. It is mild dysplasia.

CIN 2: CIN 2 means 2/3 of the sample has dysplasia. It is moderate dysplasia.

CIN 3: CIN 3 means the entire sample shows cells with dysplasia. It is severe dysplasia.

Dysplasia: Means abnormal development. Dysplasia is a pre-cancerous condition. Dysplasia is categorized as mild to severe by using CIN 1-3 and CIS to represent the extent of the problem.

SIL: Squamous Intraepithelial Lesions. SIL is another way to describe dysplasia by identifying lesions in the thin cellular layers of the vaginal tract. Again, SIL suggests a pre-cancerous condition.

Related Resources

The following list are national resources. For local and regional resources, contact your local AIDS service organization.

Women's Programs/Newsletters

Project WISE / WISE Words
205 13th Street, Suite 2001
San Francisco, CA 94103
Toll Free: 800-822-7422
Tel: 415-558-9051 or 415-558-8669
Fax: 415-558-0684
Internet: http://www.projectinform.org
E-Mail: info@projectinform.org

WISE Words is the free three-times yearly publication of Project WISE, Project Inform's program focusing on HIV/AIDS treatment information and advocacy for women.

Women Alive
1566 Burnside Avenue
Los Angeles, CA 90019
Toll Free: 800-554-4876
Tel: 213-965-1564
Fax: 323-965-9886
Internet: http://www.women-alive.org
E-Mail: info@women-alive.org

Women Alive publishes a quarterly newsletter and is active in policy and treatment issues affecting women living with HIV.

WORLD (Women Organized to Respond to Life-threatening Diseases)
414 Thirteenth Street, 2nd Floor
Oakland, CA 94612
Tel: 510-986-0340
Fax: 510-986-0341
Internet: http://www.womenhiv.org
E-Mail: info@womenhiv.org

WORLD publishes a monthly newsletter for women with HIV and has a peer advocate program, a treatment training program and retreats for HIV-positive women.

Teens

Bay Area Young Positives
518 Waller Street
San Francisco, CA 94117
Tel: 415-487-1616
Fax: 415-487-1617
Internet: http://www.baypositives.org

BAY Positives is a national organization by and for youths living with HIV disease.

Pediatrics

Pediatric AIDS Foundation
2950 31st Street, #125
Santa Monica, CA 90405
Toll Free: 888-499-4673
Tel: 310-314-1459
Fax: 310-314-1469
Internet: http://www.pedaids.org
E-Mail: info@pedaids.org

The Pediatric AIDS Foundation advocates on behalf of and funds pediatric research in AIDS. This trial hotline gives listings of studies and provides information for children with HIV/AIDS.

Chapter 46

Women Over 50 Living with HIV: Menopause and Hormone Replacement Therapy

This chapter focuses on women over 50 who are living with HIV. There are many health concerns related to aging that may or may not impact HIV. This chapter highlights the research that has been done on aging and HIV; discusses what happens to your immune system as you get older and how HIV can impact that process; and discusses HIV and menopause, treatments for menopause and what you can do to relieve symptoms. Finally, it provides some resources and a screening chart that you can take to the doctor to help guide you in your healthcare.

As you age your body undergoes many changes. Some are related to genetics—if your father or grandfather had cardiovascular disease, then you're at more risk for developing this condition. Other changes are a natural and normal result of your body merely getting older and slowing down. Also, you're more at risk for developing a variety of conditions, like diabetes.

Some of the health changes we experience as we age are similar to some symptoms of HIV infection. The process of aging varies for everyone, but it's not unusual for people to experience fatigue, suppressed immunity, skin conditions and nutritional problems. Some HIV side effects, like loss of fat in the face and arms, also occur naturally in some people as they age.

From Project Inform: Excerpted from "HIV and Older Age," from *Wise Words,* Number 10, July 2002, © 2002 Project Inform; reprinted with permission. For more information, contact the National NIV/AIDS Treatment Hotline, 800-822-7422, or visit our website, www.projectinform.org.

For someone who is aging with HIV, these changes make knowing the cause and treating these conditions more difficult. For women over 50 living with HIV, there are many unique questions and concerns. Whether you're a woman over 50 who recently found out you were HIV-positive or you've been living with HIV for many years, these years can be very challenging.

What does the research show?

Very little research has been done on HIV and older age; however, there are some answers. A large study to assess HIV, immunology and aging is ongoing and more information will likely be available in the coming years. Even less research and information is available for older women living with HIV. This too is beginning to change as larger studies of women begin to yield information.

Some data suggest that older and younger people do equally well when responding to anti-HIV medications and experiencing side effects or risk of HIV disease progression. However, older people on therapy were less likely to see as large and increase in CD4+ cell counts. For women, questions around HIV and menopause, or taking hormone replacement therapy (HRT), have not been well studied.

One study suggests that women over 40 are at a higher risk for developing changes in body composition, called lipodystrophy. It is unclear whether this is related to gender, age or a combination. Another study looked at 40 pre- and postmenopausal women, 19 HIV-positive women and 21 HIV-negative women. The study looked at how often reduced bone mineral density occurred in older pre- and postmenopausal HIV-positive women. Bone density on the lower spine, hip and total body was measured.

This study showed that women living with HIV who had used a protease inhibitor had reduced bone density compared both to HIV-negative and HIV-positive women who had never taken protease inhibitors. Several observations have been made about bone problems associated with using various anti-HIV therapies. Whether this impacts women more than men is unknown, but even older women without HIV are at increased risk for bone mineral loss. This information is important especially for older women who have other known risks for bone mineral loss. For more information on lipodystrophy and bone problems associated with HIV, call Project Inform's hotline at 1-800-822-7422.

There are conflicting data around older age and HIV disease progression. One study found that older and younger people had similar rates of viral suppression. However, older people on similar therapies had weaker CD4+ cell count responses. Another study found that people older than 60 at the time of HIV diagnosis have a shorter survival time than younger people at their time of HIV diagnosis. Finally, another study found that older age might be associated with a higher rate of disease progression. This study observed that an older person with HIV is likely to progress to AIDS at a faster rate than younger people at the same CD4+ cell count. Many of these studies are small, however, and many factors besides age could have influenced these observations.

On a positive note, a retrospective study looking at 84 older women with HIV found that women on HRT had a higher survival rate. In addition, researchers found lower rates of cervical dysplasia (abnormal cell changes associated with pre-cancerous conditions) and chlamydia in the older women than the younger women.

The lack of research and information on aging and HIV can be discouraging. However, it is important that we continue to advocate for research, to include older people living with HIV, especially women, and make our voices heard.

Menopause and HIV

Often called the change of life, menopause is a natural event that happens to every woman, but affects each woman uniquely. Menopause can happen naturally or be induced through surgery or therapy. At menopause, several changes happen to the female reproductive system:

1. The ovaries stop producing the female sex hormone, estrogen;

2. a woman stops menstruating (her period stops);

3. a woman can no longer bear children.

Menopause can begin anywhere between 40 and 55. It is a slow and gradual process, occurring over 3-5 years. During this time you may have infrequent and/or inconsistent periods. Pre-menstrual symptoms (PMS) may intensify or change. Menopause is complete when you have not menstruated for 12 months in a row. Women living with HIV may experience irregularities in their cycles, even if they're not going through menopause. It's important you discuss this with your doctor, so you can tell if the changes are related to HIV, menopause or some combination.

The body changes that occur and the decrease in estrogen during menopause express themselves in many ways. For some women the physical signs are mild and they are able to cope with them. For others, menopausal symptoms are very severe and difficult to cope with. The decision to take treatment is yours. It may or may not be the right choice for you. Discuss your concerns and questions with your doctor. He or she can help you weigh the risks and the benefits.

Any type change in life can be difficult on you and those around you. For women with HIV, many of these life changes from aging are similar to the impact that HIV can have on your physical and emotional health. Take time to make yourself aware of these possible changes and encourage others to do the same.

The following information can help you understand menopause symptoms, how they're similar to HIV, the treatments and how to relieve symptoms.

Memory Loss or Lack of Concentration

You may have trouble remembering things like what you just did, or what you said to someone. It may be difficult for you to concentrate on one thing for long periods of time.

HIV Connection

Dementia is a brain disorder that affects a person's ability to think clearly and can impact his or her daily activities. AIDS dementia complex (ADC)—dementia caused by HIV infection—is a complicated syndrome made up of different nervous system and mental symptoms. These symptoms are somewhat common in people with HIV disease.

Studies show that older HIV-positive people experience AIDS dementia more frequently than younger people.

Some symptoms resembling forms of dementia can also be side effects of certain anti-HIV drugs.

Other Things You Can Do

- Make lists of things to do and cross them out as you complete them.

- Ask a friend, family member or someone you trust to remind you about appointments, meds, etc.

- Do things that you do everyday at the same time.

- Talk with your doctor about getting tested for ADC.

- Read "AIDS Dementia Complex," available at www.projectinform.org or 1-800-822-7422.

Hot Flashes

A hot flash is a sensation of heat in the face or moving across the upper half of the body. They last 30 seconds to several minutes and often times hot flashes are accompanied by a rapid heart beat. Your skin may have a tingly sensation and you may experience chills, sweats or be unable to breathe well.

HIV Connection

- Night sweats are associated with HIV and HIV-related conditions.

- Side effects caused by HRT/ERT are also side effects caused by anti-HIV medications particularly nausea, bloating, headaches, dizziness and depression.

- Lipodystrophy affects many people living with HIV. Lipodystrophy refers to changes in fat distribution in the body and irregularities in certain blood tests (increase in triglycerides, bad cholesterol levels, risk of diabetes and elevated blood pressure). Discuss the risks and benefits of HRT and ERT with your doctor if you are experiencing lipodystrophy.

Treatment

Hormone Replacement Therapy (HRT) is the combination of estrogen and progestin (a synthetic form of progesterone). Progesterone can protect against developing endometrial cancer (cancer of the uterine lining). HRT relieves hot flashes and night sweats.

There are different schedules for taking HRT in pill form. You could take estrogen every day for a set number of days, add progestin for 10-14 days, and then stop taking one or both for a specific period of time. You would repeat the same pattern monthly. This cyclic schedule can cause light menstrual bleeding.

You can take estrogen and progestin together every day of the month without any break. This continuous pattern can stop monthly bleeding after about six months of treatment. However, problem spotting may continue for longer. Talk with your doctor about the schedule that is best for you.

Estrogen Replacement Therapy (ERT) is estrogen alone. Take as pill or tablet, vaginal creams, vaginal ring inserts, implants, shots or patches that stick to the skin and the body absorbs estrogen.

Depending on your symptoms your doctor will suggest a certain form.

Things to Know

- Women who have NOT had a hysterectomy (removal of uterus, including ovaries) can take HRT.

- HRT is known to worsen liver disease in some cases. Depending on the severity of liver damage, HRT may or may not be an option for you if you have liver disease. Discuss this with your doctor.

- Women with these conditions can talk with their doctors about the risks and benefits of HRT/ERT: high levels of triglycerides (fat in the blood), a personal or family history of blood clots and/ or breast cancer and abnormal uterine bleeding.

- Side effects for both HRT/ERT include: vaginal bleeding, breast tenderness (this will go away after several months), nausea, bloating, headaches, dizziness and depression.

- Depending on the form, HRT/ERT can be stopped and started again. If you stop, their protective effects will stop and the side effects may continue.

- Your decision about hormone therapy should be reviewed each year with your doctor at your annual checkup.

Other Things You Can Do

- Avoid small spaces, caffeine, alcohol, spicy foods and hot humid weather.

- Vitamin E helps to relieve hot flashes.

- Drink plenty of water (at least eight cups a day).

- Women living with HIV often experience abnormal uterine bleeding. Talk with your doctor if you are having uterine bleeding and find out what the cause may be. It could be an infection that needs to be treated immediately.

- Read "Dealing with Drug Side Effects," "Lipodystrophy," and "GYN Conditions," available at 1-800-822-7422 or www.projectinform.org.

Fatigue

Fatigue is a feeling of being constantly tired or having low energy even with enough rest. Activities like climbing stairs may be difficult. Fatigue can also be psychological, like having a hard time concentrating.

HIV Connection

- A very common symptom of HIV.

- A side affect of anti-HIV meds.

- Associated with anemia, also side effect of anti-HIV meds.

Other Things You Can Do

- Try going to sleep at night and waking in the morning at the same time.

- A little exercise can ease stress and make you feel stronger and more energetic.

- Keep easy-to-prepare foods on hand for times when you're too tired to cook.

Insomnia

Insomnia and night sweats can be very uncomfortable, making it difficult to sleep at night.

HIV Connection

- Insomnia is very common with HIV for many reasons. Receiving an HIV diagnosis can be overwhelming, making it difficult to sleep well.

- Insomnia has also been associated with anti-HIV meds, like d4T (Zerit) and saquinavir (Fortovase).

Other Things You Can Do

- Wear clothes that are made with breathable fabric (cotton, linen) and are cooler to sleep in.

- Avoid flannel sheets.

- Keep the window slightly open or keep a fan the room.

- Drink at least eight cups of water a day and keep a glass by the bed.

Emotional Changes/Mild Depression

You may experience highs and lows in your moods: one minute you're happy and the next you're irritable or feeling anxious.

HIV Connection

Depression is associated with HIV and some specific anti-HIV meds and anti-hepatitis therapy. Women living with HIV experience more depression than men.

Treatment

HRT/ERT may improve mood and psychological well-being.

Other Things You Can Do

- Let your family and friends know that you may not always feel good.

- Exercise can help ease and improve your mood swings.

- Meditation can also help.

Skin and Hair Changes

The skin becomes less firm and drier. Hair becomes thinner and more brittle.

HIV Connection

- Sudden or abnormal hair loss can result from taking anti-HIV meds, for example, indinavir (Crixivan).

- Other medications to treat cancers, circulatory disorders, ulcers and arthritis can also cause hair loss.

Other Things You Can Do

- Avoid excessive hair dyeing, perming, straightening, braiding, and using hair dryers.

- Stress can also affect your hair growth and the health of your hair. Take steps to reduce stress and anxiety.

- B-complex vitamins can help relieve dry skin and hair.

Osteoporosis

Osteoporosis is a disorder where a significant amount of bone mineral decreases, causing a loss of bone mass and strength. This loss is referred to as low bone mineral density. The bones become thinner and more likely to break from a fall or minor stress. Postmenopausal osteoporosis is very common in women. Estrogen protects your bones; so with the decrease in estrogen production, there is less protection of your bones. This puts you at risk for having weak bones.

HIV Connection

Recent studies have found that people living with HIV have low bone mineral density. However, the causes and significance of lower bone mineral density for HIV-positive people remains unclear. The data are conflicting as to whether this is related to specific anti-HIV treatments or all of them.

Similar side effects are caused by anti-HIV meds.

Treatment

HRT/ERT can reduce the risk of osteoporosis. Treatments for osteoporosis include: Alendronate Sodium (Fosamax), Risedronate (Actonel), Raloxifene (Evista), and Calcitonin (Miacalcin). Calcitonin is available as a nasal spray or injection.

Things to Know

Side effects for osteoporosis meds can include: Fosamax can cause abdominal or musculoskeletal pain, nausea, heartburn, irritation of the esophagus; Actonel can cause stomach upset, constipation, diarrhea, bloating, gas and headaches; and Miacalcin can cause an allergic reaction, skin rash and runny nose.

Other Things You Can Do

- Get a bone mineral density test to measure the density of your bones (bone mass). It can determine whether you need medication to help maintain your bone mass, prevent further loss and reduce fracture risk. The test is painless and non-invasive.

- Weight-bearing exercises.

Urinary Tract Infections

The walls of the urethra become thin which increases the chance of urinary tract infections. As the muscles, which support the bladder and the urethra weaken, urine leakage is more common.

HIV Connection

None.

Treatment

ERT vaginal ring (see Hot Flashes).

Heart Palpitations

Heart palpitations occur when the heart beats irregularly or misses one or two beats.

HIV Connection

None.

Other Things You Can Do

- Discuss this with your doctor; to be sure, be screened for heart disease.

- Entering menopause, women are at higher risk for heart disease. This symptom may be related to menopause or another cause.

Vaginal Dryness

The vagina becomes dry and the vaginal walls become thin causing pain. Intercourse may be painful.

HIV Connection

None.

Treatment

ERT vaginal cream (see Hot Flashes).

Other Things You Can Do

Use water-based lubricant during intercourse. While not proven, vaginal gels containing wild yams have been used to relieve vaginal dryness. What ERT and these gels will do to HIV levels in the vagina is unknown.

A Personal Journey

Following is a discussion with Hulda—an older women living with HIV—whose strength and courage can be an inspiration to us all. Hulda was diagnosed when she was 47 years old and is now 58.

How was it when you were diagnosed?

I was diagnosed in 1991. It felt like a death sentence. Both of my sons were in the service, and I felt very guilty. My only prayer was that they come home safe and whole. I was more concerned about them than I was about myself.

As an older woman living with HIV, how are things different for you?

As an older woman it is harder to get around. My body gets more tired-fatigue. You have to accept the fact that you're getting older. Your immune system is weakening as you get older.

For the older community, HIV is a taboo subject. A lot of older people feel like they're immune to HIV. We are not immune to it.

How do you take care of yourself?

I take a lot of vitamins and minerals. I do acupuncture, chiropractor, massage. I am taking anti-HIV meds. The way I look at it, you either live with it or die with it. What I do is focus on how I am going to live.

What services do older women need?

Counseling groups for older people—get them to talk about their HIV. Studies on HIV meds and how they work with anti-aging meds. Older people on the corner let us be seen and heard, going into community and senior centers and churches and older people talking to older people.

We are vulnerable—first we need to get this message out to the older community. Then we can go to the community and senior centers and churches and increase awareness.

What are some of the difficulties and challenges of being an older woman living with HIV?

Losing my friends, not being recognized by family members and community members, the medical community. Counselors burn out—they are there for you and then they leave. It's not easy being an older person in your community. There's no community for older persons, there's a stigma. A lot of older people think they're too old to have another mate, too old to exercise; and it doesn't make sense to take meds cause you are going to die anyway.

It's not always about HIV issues; it's about companionship, becoming older, children, having to tell family, the stigma.

What and/or who has been helpful and supportive for you?

My sons make me feel more human, their support is crucial. The WORLD retreat in 1992—I looked around and realized, "Hmm, that is happening to me." Eventually I got the courage to talk. I started listening to people, and realized that maybe there is some help out there for me. I could not do it without other people. I'm not ashamed to talk with older people. I want to make people smile because it makes me feel good.

Any final words of wisdom for women like yourself who may be reading this?

Old is not dead. We still have a place in this community. We are the caregivers, before we take care of everyone else we must take care of ourselves. You may go forward and fall into the next step; but that's okay, you'll get there.

Chapter 47

Gender Difference in Viral Load

In current medical practice, HIV levels and CD4+ cell counts are measured and interpreted and help guide anti-HIV therapy decision-making without regard to gender. Two recently reported studies are giving pause to this standard of practice. They suggest that women have progression of HIV disease at lower viral levels than men. A Federal Guidelines Panel, which provides guidance on the use of anti-HIV therapy in adults, recently held a meeting to review new information on gender differences in viral load. It concluded that presently these new data are not different enough to warrant recommendations for a different standard of care for women with HIV, nor should they be cause for alarm for women living with HIV. Nevertheless, women and their doctors should be aware of these data which may support initiating and switching therapy at a lower HIV levels than what is currently recommended in the Federal Guidelines document.

The A.L.I.V.E. Study Results

The first of two studies was presented at the 1998 World AIDS Conference in Geneva, Switzerland and was recently summarized in the scientific journal, *The Lancet*. Based on a large group of HIV-positive men and women with a history of injection drug use, involved in the

From Project Inform: "Gender Difference in Viral Load," from *PI Perspective* #27, April 1999, © 1999 Project Inform; reprinted with permission. For more information, contact the National NIV/AIDS Treatment Hotline, 800-822-7422, or visit our website, www.projectinform.org.

A.L.I.V.E. study. It compared blood samples collected and stored from 527 participants since the late 1980s with 285 blood samples collected at least three years later.

HIV levels, CD4+ cell counts and information about the general health of the study participants at both time points were examined to see if there were unique differences according to gender and/or race. Differences based on gender did come forward. Women in the study had HIV levels 38 to 65% lower than what was observed in men. In general, women's HIV levels were half that of men in the study.

Viral load was consistently lower in women than men even after adjustments for CD4+ cell count differences were made. This difference persisted after accounting for other factors that the researchers felt could possibly influence the lower viral levels seen in women, such as race, current and previous use of anti-HIV therapy and use of street drugs. None of these factors explained the gender difference in HIV viral levels.

Researchers also looked at the association of viral load, CD4+ cell count and time to AIDS between men and women. They found that women and men with similar CD4+ cell counts had a similar progression time to AIDS. In addition, the differences in viral levels among men and women suggest that women appear to progress to AIDS with about half the viral load as men. In other words, women with half the viral load as men had a similar time to AIDS. Respectively, women with the same viral load as men had a higher risk of AIDS. What this probably means in is that for women with low CD4+ cell counts (e.g. below 200), CD4+ cell count is a more reliable indicator of general health and overall risk of HIV disease progression than is HIV levels. It also suggests that increases in HIV levels that are sustained, even modest ones, might be slightly more of concern to women than their male counterparts.

The WIHS Study Results

Similar findings were presented at the recent Conference on Retroviruses and Opportunistic Infections from a second study. Stored blood samples in 1984-85 from 1,511 HIV-positive men enrolled in the Multicenter AIDS Cohort Study (MACS) were compared with blood samples obtained in 1994-95 from 1,262 HIV-positive women enrolled in the Women's Interagency HIV Study (WIHS). When the original blood samples were collected, no one from either group was using anti-HIV therapies.

Like the ALIVE study, differences in viral load emerged. The degree of difference, however, was less dramatic. Also, differences were associated with specific CD4+ cell count levels. HIV levels were not different among men and women with CD4+ cell counts below 200. However, women whose CD4+ cell counts were 200-500 had a 40% lower viral level compared to men with the same CD4+ cell count. For CD4+ cell counts above 500, viral levels were 24% lower for women than for men. Thus, according to the WIHS/MACS comparison, women's overall viral load was approximately 20% lower than men's, with significant differences in the two CD4+ cell groupings shown in Table 47.1.

Table 47.1. Differences in Viral Load According to CD4+ Cell Count (WIHS/MACS)

CD4+ Cell Count	% Lower Viral Level in Women
Less than 200	56%
200-500	67%
Above 500	71%

Researchers from the WIHS/MACS cohort conclude that HIV load is lower in women than men, but only at CD4+ cell counts above 200. They suggest that the use of the viral load tests, particularly when used as a starting point for beginning anti-HIV therapy, may need to be adjusted for gender to account for this difference. The largest impact of these findings is probably on how they affect women with CD4+ cell counts in the 200 to 500 range who are making decisions about therapy changes based on viral load.

Commentary on These Findings

While these findings are far from confirmed, they do raise important questions with regard to viral load in women and related risks of disease progression. These studies also remind us of two other points. CD4+ cell counts provide useful measures of the risk of disease progression and their meaning is not influenced by gender. Moreover, the decision to start, add or change therapy should never be decided solely on the basis of one laboratory measure (e.g. just viral load, just CD4+ cell counts, etc.).

Treatment decisions should factor in trends in viral load, trends in CD4+ cell counts, the number of available future options, side effects, ease of adherence, how one feels about anti-HIV therapy and measures of overall general health. Whether or not viral load differences according to gender should be considered a treatment decision point demands further study.

Chapter 48

Pregnancy and HIV

Recent studies show that HIV-positive women who get pregnant do not get any sicker than those who are not pregnant. That is, becoming pregnant does not appear to be dangerous to the health of an HIV-infected woman.

However, although AZT by itself can help protect newborns from HIV, it is not the best choice for the mother's health. Combination therapies using at least three drugs are the standard treatment. If a pregnant woman takes AZT by itself, she may get less benefit from combination therapy in the future.

On the other hand, combination therapy might cause birth defects, especially during the first three months. For example, pregnant women should not use the drug efavirenz (Sustiva). Preliminary studies of pregnant women who used protease inhibitors show good results, with virtually no HIV-infected newborns and no unusual birth defects.

A pregnant woman should consider all of the possible side effects of antiviral medications. Some of them could be worse for pregnant women. For example, in January 2001, the FDA warned pregnant women not to use both ddI and d4T in their antiviral treatment due to a high rate of a dangerous side effect called lactic acidosis.

If you have HIV and you are pregnant, or if you want to become pregnant, talk with your doctor about your options for taking care of

Fact Sheet Number 611, © 2002 New Mexico AIDS InfoNet; reprinted with permission. Fact sheets are regularly updated; check the website, www.aidsinfonet.org for the most recent information.

343

yourself and reducing the risk of HIV infection or birth defects for your new child.

The Bottom Line

An HIV-infected woman who becomes pregnant needs to think about her own health and the health of her new child. The risk of transmitting HIV to a newborn can be cut to just 2% if the mother takes AZT during the last 6 months of her pregnancy, delivers her child by Cesarean section, and the newborn takes AZT for six weeks.

Pregnancy does not seem to make the mother's HIV disease any worse. However, some medications used to fight HIV or to treat opportunistic infections might cause birth defects. This is especially true during the first 3 months of pregnancy. If a mother chooses to stop taking some medications during pregnancy, her HIV disease could get worse.

Any woman with HIV who is thinking about getting pregnant should carefully discuss treatment options with her doctor.

How Do Babies Get AIDS?

The virus that causes AIDS, HIV, can be transmitted from an infected mother to her newborn child. Without treatment, about 20% of babies of infected mothers get infected. Mothers with higher viral loads are more likely to infect their babies. However, no viral load is low enough to be safe. Infection can occur any time during pregnancy, but usually happens just before or during delivery. The baby is more likely to be infected if the delivery takes a long time. During delivery, the newborn is exposed to the mother's blood. Drinking breast milk from an infected woman can also infect babies. Mothers who are HIV-infected should not breast-feed their babies.

How Can We Prevent Infection of Newborns?

Mothers can reduce the risk of infecting their babies if they:

- Use antiviral medications,
- Keep the delivery time short, and
- Don't breast-feed the baby

Use antiviral medications: The risk of transmitting HIV drops from 20% to 8% or less if antiviral medications are used. Transmission rates are lowest if the mother takes AZT during the last six months of her pregnancy, and the newborn takes AZT for six weeks after birth. Even if the mother does not take antiviral medications until she is in labor, the transmission rate can be cut by almost half. Two methods have been studied:

- AZT and 3TC during labor, and for both mother and child for one week after the birth.

- One dose of nevirapine during labor, and one dose for the newborn, 2 to 3 days after birth. Although these shorter treatments do not work as well, they are less expensive and might be helpful in developing countries.

Keep delivery time short: The risk of transmission increases with longer delivery times. If the mother uses AZT and delivers her baby by cesarean section (C-section), she can reduce the risk of transmission to about 2%.

Do not breast-feed the baby: There is about a 14% chance that a baby will get HIV infection from infected breast milk. This risk can be eliminated if HIV-infected women do not breast-feed babies. Baby formulas should be used.

In developing countries, however, there might not be clean water to prepare baby formulas. The World Health Organization believes that the risk of transmitting HIV is less than the health risk of using contaminated water.

How Do We Know If a Newborn Is Infected?

Most babies born to infected mothers test positive for HIV. Testing positive means you have HIV antibodies in your blood. Babies get HIV antibodies from their mother even if they aren't infected with the virus.

If babies are infected with HIV, their own immune systems will start to make antibodies. They will continue to test positive. If they are not infected, the mother's antibodies will gradually disappear and the babies will test negative after about 6 to 12 months.

Another test, similar to the HIV viral load test, can be used to find out if the baby is infected with HIV. Instead of antibodies, these tests detect the HIV virus in the blood.

Chapter 49

Status of Perinatal HIV Prevention

During the early 1990s, before perinatal preventive treatments were available, an estimated 1,000-2,000 infants were born with HIV infection each year in the United States. Today, the United States has seen dramatic reductions in mother-to-child, or perinatal, HIV transmission rates. These declines reflect the widespread success of Public Health Service (PHS) recommendations made in 1994 and 1995 for routinely counseling and voluntarily testing pregnant women for HIV, and for offering zidovudine (AZT) to infected women during pregnancy and delivery, and for the infant after birth.

Perinatal Prevention Saves Lives and Dollars

On a national level, HIV/AIDS surveillance and other studies continue to demonstrate that perinatal HIV prevention is making a difference, both in terms of lives and resources saved:

- Between 1992 and 1997, perinatally acquired AIDS cases declined 66% in the United States.

- A study conducted in four states (Michigan, New Jersey, Louisiana, and South Carolina) found that the proportion of pregnant

---

"Status of Perinatal HIV Prevention: U.S. Declines Continue," National Center for HIV, STD and TB Prevention, Centers for Disease Control and Prevention (CDC), updated November 1999; available online at http://www.cdc.gov/hiv/pubs/facts/perinatl.htm.

women voluntarily tested for HIV increased from 68% in 1993 to 79% in 1996. The percentage of women offered AZT increased from 27% in 1993 to 85% in 1996. However, the study also found that 15% of HIV-infected pregnant women in these states did not receive prenatal care and therefore could not be offered this intervention.

- Among women in CDC's Perinatal AIDS Collaborative Transmission Study (PACTS), AZT use increased following the publication of PHS guidelines, and the rate of perinatal transmission dropped from 21% to 11%. The PACTS study includes women from four cities—New York City, Newark, Atlanta, and Baltimore.

- Prenatal care that includes HIV counseling and testing and AZT treatment for infected mothers and their children saves lives and resources. Without intervention, a 25% mother-to-infant transmission rate would result in the birth of an estimated 1,750 HIV-infected infants annually in the United States, with lifetime medical costs of $282 million.

- The estimated annual cost of perinatal prevention in the United States is $67.6 million. This investment prevents 656 HIV infections and saves $105.6 million in medical care costs alone—a net cost-savings of $38.1 million annually.

HIV transmission from mother to child during pregnancy, labor, and delivery or by breast-feeding has accounted for 91% of all AIDS cases reported among U.S. children. The best ways to prevent infection in children are to prevent infection in women and to encourage early prenatal care that includes HIV counseling and testing.

Perinatal HIV Transmission Heavily Affects Communities of Color

Women of color and their children have always been disproportionately affected by the HIV epidemic. In 1998, of the 10,998 total AIDS cases reported among U.S. women, 8,830 (80%) were among African American and Hispanic women. Of the 382 children reported with AIDS in 1998, 321 (84%) were African American and Hispanic (see chart below). We must continue to improve HIV prevention efforts for women of color and ensure that interventions provide the information, skills, and support needed to reduce their HIV-related risks.

What Else Is Needed?

Perinatal HIV prevention activities must help ensure that all HIV-infected women are reached early in pregnancy with prenatal care and with the opportunity to learn their HIV status. If infected, they should be offered preventive therapy to improve the chances that their children will be born free of infection and to ensure quality HIV care and treatment for mothers and their babies. Achieving this goal will require increased access to and use of prenatal care.

Women who use drugs during pregnancy are the least likely to get prenatal care. Increased efforts are needed at all levels (community, state, national) to integrate substance abuse and HIV prevention activities and assist pregnant women in accessing needed services to improve their own health and the health of their babies.

Chapter 50

Pediatric AIDS

HIV infection is often difficult to diagnose in very young children. Infected babies, especially in the first few months of life, often appear normal and may exhibit no telltale signs that would allow a definitive diagnosis of HIV infection. Moreover, all children born to infected mothers have antibodies to HIV, made by the mother's immune system, that cross the placenta to the baby's bloodstream before birth and persist for up to 18 months. Because these maternal antibodies reflect the mother's but not the infant's infection status, the test is not useful in newborns or young infants.

In recent years, investigators have demonstrated the utility of highly accurate blood tests in diagnosing HIV infection in children 6 months of age and younger. One laboratory technique called polymerase chain reaction (PCR) can detect minute quantities of the virus in an infant's blood. Another procedure allows physicians to culture a sample of an infant's blood and test it for the presence of HIV.

Currently, PCR assays or HIV culture techniques can identify at birth about one-third of infants who are truly HIV-infected. With these techniques, approximately 90 percent of HIV-infected infants are identifiable by 2 months of age, and 95 percent by 3 months of age. One innovative new approach to both RNA and DNA PCR testing uses

Excerpted from "Backgrounder: HIV Infection in Infants and Children," National Institute of Allergy and Infectious Disease (NIAID), updated July 31, 2000; available online at http://www.niaid.nih.gov/newsroom/simple/background.htm.

dried blood spot specimens, which should make it much simpler to gather and store specimens in field settings.

Progression of HIV Disease in Children

Researchers have observed two general patterns of illness in HIV-infected children. About 20 percent of children develop serious disease in the first year of life; most of these children die by age 4 years.

The remaining 80 percent of infected children have a slower rate of disease progression, many not developing the most serious symptoms of AIDS until school entry or even adolescence. A recent report from a large European registry of HIV-infected children indicated that half of the children with perinatally acquired HIV disease were alive at age 9. Another study, of 42 perinatally HIV-infected children who survived beyond 9 years of age, found about one-quarter of the children to be asymptomatic with relatively intact immune systems.

The factors responsible for the wide variation observed in the rate of disease progression in HIV-infected children are a major focus of the NIAID pediatric AIDS research effort. The Women and Infants Transmission Study, a multisite perinatal HIV study funded by NIH, has found that maternal factors including Vitamin A level and CD4 counts during pregnancy, as well as infant viral load and CD4 counts in the first several months of life, can help identify those infants at risk for rapid disease progression who may benefit from early aggressive therapy.

Signs and Symptoms of Pediatric HIV Disease

Many children with HIV infection do not gain weight or grow normally. HIV-infected children frequently are slow to reach important milestones in motor skills and mental development such as crawling, walking and speaking. As the disease progresses, many children develop neurologic problems such as difficulty walking, poor school performance, seizures, and other symptoms of HIV encephalopathy.

Like adults with HIV infection, children with HIV develop life-threatening opportunistic infections (OIs), although the incidence of various OIs differs in adults and children. For example, toxoplasmosis is seen less frequently in HIV-infected children than in HIV-infected adults, while serious bacterial infections occur more commonly in children than in adults. Also, as children with HIV become sicker, they may suffer from chronic diarrhea due to opportunistic pathogens.

Pneumocystis carinii pneumonia (PCP) is the leading cause of death in HIV-infected children with AIDS. PCP, as well as cytomegalovirus (CMV) disease, usually are primary infections in children, whereas in adults these diseases result from the reactivation of latent infections.

A lung disease called lymphocytic interstitial pneumonitis (LIP), rarely seen in adults, also occurs frequently in HIV-infected children. This condition, like PCP, can make breathing progressively more difficult and often results in hospitalization.

Children with HIV suffer the usual childhood bacterial infections—only more frequently and more severely than uninfected children. These bacterial infections can cause seizures, fever, pneumonia, recurrent colds, diarrhea, dehydration and other problems that often result in extended hospital stays and nutritional problems.

HIV-infected children frequently have severe candidiasis, a yeast infection that can cause unrelenting diaper rash and infections in the mouth and throat that make eating difficult.

Treatment of HIV-Infected Children

NIAID investigators are defining the best treatments for pediatric patients. Currently there are 16 drug products approved by the FDA for the treatment of adult HIV infection. Through major contributions by the Pediatric ACTG, 10 antiretroviral agents have pediatric label information, including 3 protease inhibitors.[1] While the basic principles that guide treatment of pediatric HIV infection are the same as for any HIV-infected person, there are a number of unique scientific and medical concerns that are important to consider in the treatment of children with HIV infection.

These range from differences from adults in age-related issues such as CD4 lymphocyte counts and drug metabolism to requirements for special formulations and treatment regimens that are appropriate for infants through adolescents. As in adults, treatment of HIV-infected children today is a complex task of using potent combinations of antiretroviral agents to maximally suppress viral replication.

Researchers supported by NIAID are focusing not only on the development of new antiretroviral products but also on the critical question of how to best use the treatments that are currently available. Treatment strategy questions designed to identify what the best initial therapy is, when failing regimens should be switched and strategies for how to address the antiretroviral needs of children with advanced disease are examples. Long-term assessment of these children is also a high priority to assess sustained antiretroviral benefits as well as to monitor for potential adverse consequences of treatment.

Problems of Families

A mother and child with HIV usually are not the only family members with the disease. Often, the mother's sexual partner is infected, and other children in the family may be infected as well. Frequently, a parent with AIDS does not survive to care for his or her HIV-infected child.

In the countries hardest hit by the AIDS epidemic, some 8.2 million children under 15 around the world have been orphaned by AIDS—90 percent of them in sub-Saharan Africa alone.[2] The rate is expected to increase. One in three of these orphans is under age five.[3] Communities and extended families are struggling with and often overwhelmed by the vast number of AIDS orphans. Many orphans and other children from families devastated by AIDS face multiple risks, such as forced relocation, violence, living on the streets, drug use, and even commercial sex. Other children suffer because sex education and services are not available to them or do not communicate effectively to them. Living in a country undergoing political turmoil or where fathers migrate for work can also raise the risk of a child becoming HIV-infected.

In the U.S., most children living with HIV/AIDS live in inner cities, where poverty, illicit drug use, poor housing and limited access to and use of medical care and social services add to the challenges of HIV disease.

One encouraging note is that, according to UNAIDS, where information, training, and services to help prevent HIV infection are made available and affordable to young people, they are more likely to make use of them than their elders are.[4]

Management of the complex medical and social problems of families affected by HIV requires a multidisciplinary case management team, integrating medical, social, mental health and educational services. NIAID provides special funding to many of its clinical research sites to provide for services, such as transportation, day care, and the expertise of social workers, crucial to families devastated by HIV.

References

1. Riley, L.E. and Green, M.F. Elective caesarean delivery to reduce the transmission of HIV. 1999. *N Engl J Med* 340:13, 1032.

2. UNAIDS, Report, p. 9.

3. Centers for Disease Control and Prevention. National Center for HIV, STD, and TB Prevention. Divisions of HIV/AIDS. International Projections/Statistics. Web: http://www.cdc.gov/hiv/stats.htm#international.

4. UNAIDS, Update, p. 9.

Chapter 51

Guidelines for the Use of Antiretroviral Agents in Pediatric HIV Infection

Guidelines

In 1993, the Working Group on Antiretroviral Therapy and Medical Management of HIV-Infected Children, composed of specialists caring for human immunodeficiency virus (HIV)-infected infants, children, and adolescents, was convened by the National Pediatric and Family HIV Resource Center (NPHRC). On the basis of available data and a consensus reflecting clinical experience, the Working Group concluded that antiretroviral therapy was indicated for any child with a definitive diagnosis of HIV infection who had evidence of substantial immunodeficiency (based on age-related CD4+ T-cell count thresholds) and/or who had HIV-associated symptoms. ZDV monotherapy was recommended as the standard of care for initiation of therapy. Routine antiretroviral therapy for infected children who were asymptomatic or had only minimal symptoms (i.e., isolated lymphadenopathy or hepatomegaly) and normal immune status was not recommended.

Since the Working Group developed the 1993 recommendations, dramatic advances in laboratory and clinical research have been made. The

This chapter includes excerpts from "Guidelines for the Use of Antiretroviral Agents in Pediatric HIV Infection," National Institutes of Health, December 14, 2001, available online at http://www.aidsinfo.nih.gov/guidelines/pediatric/html; and "Pediatric Antiretroviral Drug Information," National Institutes of Health, December 14, 2001, available online at http://www.aidsinfo.nih.gov.

rapidity and magnitude of HIV replication during all stages of infection are greater than previously believed and account for the emergence of drug-resistant viral variants when antiretroviral treatment does not maximally suppress replication. New assays that quantitate plasma HIV RNA copy number have become available, permitting a sensitive assessment of risk for disease progression and adequacy of antiretroviral therapy. A new class of antiretroviral drugs, protease inhibitors, has become available; these agents have reduced HIV viral load to levels that are undetectable and have reduced disease progression and mortality in many HIV-infected persons. Therefore, therapeutic strategies now focus on early institution of antiretroviral regimens capable of maximally suppressing viral replication to reduce the development of resistance and to preserve immunologic function. Additionally, the results of Pediatric AIDS Clinical Trials Group (PACTG) protocol 076 have demonstrated that the risk for perinatal HIV transmission can be substantially diminished with the use of a regimen of ZDV administered during pregnancy, during labor, and to the newborn.

These advances in HIV research have led to major changes in the treatment and monitoring of HIV infection in the United States. A summary of the basic principles underlying therapy of HIV-infected persons has been formulated by the National Institutes of Health (NIH) Panel to Define Principles of Therapy of HIV Infection. Treatment recommendations for infected adults and post-pubertal adolescents have been updated by the U.S. Department of Health and Human Services Panel of Clinical Practices for Treatment of HIV Infection.

Although the pathogenesis of HIV infection and the general virologic and immunologic principles underlying the use of antiretroviral therapy are similar for all HIV-infected persons, there are unique considerations needed for HIV-infected infants, children, and adolescents. Most HIV infections in children are acquired perinatally, and most perinatal transmission occurs during or near the time of birth, which raises the possibility of initiating treatment in an infected infant during the period of initial (i.e., primary) HIV infection (if sensitive diagnostic tests are used to define the infant's infection status early in life). Perinatal HIV infection occurs during the development of the infant's immune system; thus, both the clinical manifestations of HIV infection and the course of immunologic and virologic markers of infection differ from those for adults. Treatment of perinatally infected children will occur in the context of prior exposure to ZDV and other antiretroviral drugs used during pregnancy and the neonatal period, for maternal treatment, to prevent perinatal transmission, or both. Additionally, drug pharmacokinetics change during the transition from the newborn period to adulthood, requiring specific evaluation of drug dosing and toxicity in infants and children. Finally, optimizing adherence to therapy in children and adolescents requires specific considerations.

To update the 1993 antiretroviral treatment guidelines for children and to provide guidelines for antiretroviral treatment similar to those for HIV-infected adults, NPHRC, the Health Resources and Services Administration (HRSA), and NIH reconvened the Working Group on Antiretroviral Therapy and Medical Management of HIV-Infected Children, consisting of experts caring for HIV-infected children and adolescents, family members of HIV-infected children, and government agency representatives. The Working Group met in June 1996 and again in July 1997 to establish and finalize new guidelines for the treatment of HIV-infected infants, children, and adolescents. These were initially published in 1998 both in *MMWR* which is periodically updated and as a supplement to the journal *Pediatrics*. The supplement included both antiretroviral therapy as well as management of complications of HIV infection.

The treatment recommendations provided in this chapter are based on published and unpublished data regarding the treatment of HIV infection in adults and children and, when no definitive data were available, the clinical experience of the Working Group members. The Working Group intended the guidelines to be flexible and not to supplant the clinical judgment of experienced health-care providers. These guidelines will be modified by the Working Group as new information and clinical experience become available. The most recent information is available on the HIV/AIDS Treatment Information Service Website (http://aidsinfo.nih.gov).

Concepts Considered in the Formulation of Pediatric Treatment Guidelines

The following concepts were considered in the formulation of these guidelines:

1. Identification of HIV-infected women before or during pregnancy is critical to providing optimal therapy for both infected women and their children and to preventing perinatal transmission. Therefore, prenatal HIV counseling and testing with consent should be the standard of care for all pregnant women in the United States.

2. Enrollment of pregnant HIV-infected women; their HIV-exposed newborns; and infected infants, children, and adolescents into clinical trials offers the best means of determining safe and effective therapies.

3. Pharmaceutical companies and the federal government should collaborate to ensure that drug formulations suitable for administration to infants and children are available at the time that new agents are being evaluated in adults.

4. Although some information regarding the efficacy of antiretroviral drugs for children can be extrapolated from clinical trials involving adults, concurrent clinical trials for children are needed to determine the impact of the drug on specific manifestations of HIV infection in children, including growth, development, and neurologic disease. However, the absence of clinical trials addressing pediatric-specific manifestations of HIV infection does not preclude the use of any approved antiretroviral drug in children.

5. All antiretroviral drugs approved for treatment of HIV infection may be used for children when indicated—irrespective of labeling notations.

6. Management of HIV infection in infants, children, and adolescents is rapidly evolving and becoming increasingly complex; therefore, wherever possible, management of HIV infection in children and adolescents should be directed by a specialist in the treatment of pediatric and adolescent HIV infection. If this is not possible, such experts should be consulted regularly.

7. Effective management of the complex and diverse needs of HIV-infected infants, children, adolescents, and their families requires a multidisciplinary team approach that includes physicians, nurses, social workers, psychologists, nutritionists, outreach workers, and pharmacists.

8. Determination of HIV RNA copy number and CD4+ T-cell levels is essential for monitoring and modifying antiretroviral treatment in infected children and adolescents as well as adults; therefore, assays to measure these variables should be made available.

9. Health-care providers considering antiretroviral regimens for children and adolescents should consider certain factors influencing adherence to therapy, including a) availability and palatability of pediatric formulations; b) impact of the medication schedule on quality of life, including number of medications, frequency of administration, ability to co-administer with other prescribed medications, and need to take with or without food; c) ability of the child's caregiver or the adolescent to administer complex drug regimens and availability of resources that might be effective in facilitating adherence; and d) potential for drug interactions.

10. The choice of antiretroviral regimens should include consideration of factors associated with possible limitation of future treatment options, including the presence of or potential for the development of antiretroviral resistance. HIV resistance assays may prove useful in guiding initial therapy and in changing failing regimens but their value in children has not been established and expert clinical interpretation is required. These assays should be made available for perinatally infected children.

11. Monitoring growth and development is essential for the care of HIV-infected children. Growth failure and neurodevelopmental deterioration may be specific manifestations of HIV infection in children. Nutritional-support therapy is an intervention that affects immune function, quality of life, and bioactivity of antiretroviral drugs.

Identification of Perinatal HIV Exposure

Appropriate treatment of HIV-infected infants requires HIV-exposed infants to be identified as soon as possible, which can be best accomplished through the identification of HIV-infected women before or during pregnancy. Universal HIV counseling and voluntary HIV testing with consent are recommended as the standard of care for all pregnant women in the United States by the Public Health Service (PHS), the American Academy of Pediatrics, and the American College of Obstetricians and Gynecologists and are endorsed by the Working Group.

Early identification of HIV-infected women is crucial for the health of such women and for care of HIV-exposed and HIV-infected children. Knowledge of maternal HIV infection during the antenatal period enables: a) HIV-infected women to receive appropriate antiretroviral therapy and prophylaxis against opportunistic infections for their own health; b) provision of antiretroviral chemoprophylaxis with ZDV during pregnancy, during labor, and to newborns to reduce the risk for HIV transmission from mother to child; c) counseling of infected women about the risks for HIV transmission through breast milk and advising against breast feeding in the United States and other countries where safe alternatives to breast milk are available; d) initiation of prophylaxis against *Pneumocystis carinii* pneumonia (PCP) in all HIV-exposed infants beginning at age four to six weeks in accordance with PHS guidelines; and e) early diagnostic evaluation of HIV-exposed infants to permit early initiation of aggressive antiretroviral therapy in infected infants.

If women are not tested for HIV during pregnancy, counseling and HIV testing should be recommended during the immediate postnatal period. When maternal serostatus has not been determined during the prenatal or immediate postpartum period, newborns should undergo HIV antibody testing with counseling and consent of the mother unless state law allows testing without consent. The HIV-exposure status of infants should be determined rapidly because the neonatal component of the recommended ZDV chemoprophylaxis regimen should begin as soon as possible after birth and because PCP prophylaxis should be initiated at age four to six weeks in all infants born to HIV-infected women. Those infants who have been abandoned, are in the custody of the state, or have positive toxicology screening tests should be considered at high risk for exposure to HIV, and mechanisms to facilitate rapid HIV screening of such infants should be developed.

Diagnosis of HIV Infection in Infants

HIV infection can be definitively diagnosed in most infected infants by age one month and in virtually all infected infants by age six months by using viral diagnostic assays. A positive virologic test (i.e., detection of HIV by culture or DNA or RNA polymerase chain reaction [PCR]) indicates possible HIV infection and should be confirmed by a repeat virologic test on a second specimen as soon as possible after the results of the first test become available. Diagnostic testing should be performed before the infant is age 48 hours, at age one to two months, and at age three to six months. Testing at age 14 days also may be advantageous for early detection of infection. HIV-exposed infants should be evaluated by or in consultation with a specialist in HIV infection in pediatric patients.

Specific Issues in Antiretroviral Therapy for HIV-Infected Adolescents

Adult guidelines for antiretroviral therapy are appropriate for post-pubertal adolescents because HIV-infected adolescents who were infected sexually or through injecting-drug use during adolescence follow a clinical course that is more similar to that of adults than to that of children. The immunopathogenesis and virologic course of HIV infection in adolescents is being defined. Most adolescents have been infected during their teenage years and are in an early stage of infection, making them ideal candidates for early intervention. A limited but increasing number of HIV-infected adolescents are long-term survivors of HIV infection acquired perinatally or through blood products as young children. Such adolescents may have a unique clinical course that differs from that of adolescents infected later in life. Because many adolescents with HIV infection are sexually active, issues associated with contraception and prevention of HIV transmission should be discussed between the health-care provider and the adolescent.

Dosage for medications for HIV infection and opportunistic infections should be prescribed according to Tanner staging of puberty and not on the basis of age. Adolescents in early puberty (i.e., Tanner Stage I and II) should be administered doses using pediatric schedules, whereas those in late puberty (i.e., Tanner Stage V) should follow adult dosing schedules. Youth who are in their growth spurt (i.e., Tanner Stage III in females and Tanner Stage IV in males) should be closely monitored for medication efficacy and toxicity when using adult or pediatric dosing guidelines.

Puberty is a time of somatic growth and sex differentiation, with females developing more body fat and males more muscle mass. Although these physiologic changes theoretically could affect drug pharmacokinetics (especially for drugs with a narrow therapeutic index that are used in combination with protein-bound medicines or hepatic enzyme inducers or inhibitors), no clinically consequential impact has been noted with nucleoside analogue reverse transcriptase inhibitor (NRTI) antiretroviral drugs. Clinical experience with PIs and non-nucleoside reverse transcriptase inhibitor (NNRTI) antiretroviral drugs is more limited.

Specific Issues of Adherence for HIV-Infected Children and Adolescents

Lack of adherence to prescribed regimens and subtherapeutic levels of antiretroviral medications may enhance the development of drug resistance. Data indicate that the development of resistance to one of the available PI antiretrovirals may reduce susceptibility to some or all of the other available PI drugs, thus substantially reducing subsequent treatment options. Similarly, the development of resistance to one of the available NNRTIs may be associated with resistance to the other members of the NNRTI class of drugs. Therefore, education of infected children and/or their caregivers regarding the importance of compliance with the prescribed drug regimen is necessary when therapy is initiated and should be reinforced during subsequent visits. Many strategies can be used to increase medication adherence, including intensive patient education over several visits before therapy is initiated, the use of cues and reminders for administering drugs, development of patient-focused treatment plans to accommodate specific patient needs, and mobilization of social and community support services.

Adherence to drug regimens is especially problematic for children. Infants and young children are dependent on others for administration of medication; thus, assessment of the capacity for adherence to a complex multi-drug regimen requires evaluation of the caregivers and their environments and the ability and willingness of the child to take the drug. Liquid formulations or formulations suitable for mixing with formula or food are necessary for administration of oral drugs to young children. Lack of palatability of such formulations can be problematic depending on the child's willingness and ability to accept and retain the medication. Absorption of some antiretroviral drugs can be affected by food, and attempting to time the administration of drugs around meals can be difficult for caregivers of young infants who require frequent feedings. Many other barriers to adherence to drug regimens exist for children and adolescents with HIV infection. For example, unwillingness of the caregivers to disclose their child's HIV infection status to others may create specific problems, including reluctance of caregivers to fill prescriptions in their home neighborhood, hiding or relabeling medications to maintain secrecy within the home, reduction of social support (a variable associated with diminished treatment adherence), and a tendency to eliminate midday doses when the parent is away from the home or the child is at school.

A comprehensive assessment of adherence issues should be instituted for all children in whom antiretroviral treatment is considered; evaluations should include nursing, social, and behavioral assessments. Intensive follow-up is required particularly during the critical first few months after therapy is started; patients should be seen frequently to assess adherence, drug tolerance, and virologic response. Coordinated, comprehensive, family-centered systems of care often can address many of the daily problems facing families that may affect adherence to complex medical regimens. For some families, certain issues (i.e., a safe physical environment and adequate food and housing) may take priority over medication administration and need to be resolved. Case managers, mental-health counselors, peer educators, outreach workers, and other members of the multidisciplinary team often may be able to address specific barriers to adherence.

HIV-infected adolescents have specific adherence problems. Comprehensive systems of care are required to serve both the medical and psychosocial needs of HIV-infected adolescents, who are frequently inexperienced with health-care systems. Many HIV-infected adolescents face challenges in adhering to medical regimens for reasons that include a) denial and fear of their HIV infection; b) misinformation; c) distrust of the medical establishment; d) fear and lack of belief in the effectiveness of medications; e) low self-esteem; f) unstructured and chaotic lifestyles; and g) lack of familial and social support. Treatment regimens for adolescents must balance the goal of prescribing a maximally potent antiretroviral regimen with realistic assessment of existing and potential support systems to facilitate adherence.

Developmental issues make caring for adolescents unique. The adolescent's approach to illness is often different from that of an adult. The concrete thought processes of adolescents make it difficult for them to take medications when they are asymptomatic, particularly if the medications have side effects. Adherence with complex regimens is particularly challenging at a time of life when adolescents do not want to be different from their peers. Further difficulties face adolescents who live with parents to whom they have not yet disclosed their HIV status and those who are homeless and have no place to store medicine.

Treatment Recommendations

General Considerations

Issues associated with adherence to treatment are especially important in considering whether and when to initiate therapy. Antiretroviral therapy is likely to be most effective in patients who are naive to treatment and who therefore are less likely to have antiretroviral-resistant viral strains. Lack of adherence to prescribed regimens and subtherapeutic levels of antiretroviral medications, particularly protease inhibitors, may enhance the development of drug resistance and like-lihood of virologic failure. Participation by the caregivers and child in the decision-making process is crucial, especially in situations for which definitive data concerning efficacy are not available.

HIV-Infected Children with Immunologic or Clinical Symptoms of Infection

Antiretroviral therapy has provided substantial clinical benefit to HIV-infected children with immunologic or clinical symptoms of HIV infection, particularly as more potent therapies have become available. Initial clinical trials of monotherapy with ZDV, didanosine (ddI), lamivudine (3TC), or stavudine (d4T) demonstrated substantial improvements in neurodevelopment, growth, and immunologic and/or virologic status. Subsequent pediatric clinical trials in symptomatic, antiretroviral-naive children have demonstrated that combination therapy with either ZDV and 3TC or ZDV and ddI is clinically, immunologically, and virologically superior to monotherapy with ddI or ZDV as initial therapy. In clinical trials in antiretroviral-experienced children, combination therapy that included a protease inhibitor was shown to be virologically and immunologically superior to dual nucleoside combination therapy.

The recognition of the enhanced potency of combination therapy and the identification of new viral targets and classes of antiretroviral agents has led to improvements in antiretroviral therapy that have been accompanied by enhanced survival of HIV-infected children and a reduction in opportunistic infections and other complications of HIV infection. This was demonstrated in a prospective longitudinal cohort study, PACTG 219 that started enrollment prior to the availability of protease inhibitor therapy. The increased use of protease inhibitor-containing highly active combination therapy (from 0% prior to 1996 to over 70% by 1998) was accompanied by a substantial decrease in mortality: mortality was only 1% in 1997/1998 compared to 5% in 1995/1996. A similar reduction in mortality with introduction of combination therapy in HIV-infected children in Italy has also been reported.

Asymptomatic HIV-Infected Children

When to initiate therapy for asymptomatic infants and older children with normal immune function is less certain. Phase III clinical trial data to address the effectiveness of antiretroviral therapy in this group are not available. However, it is known that control of viral replication is particularly poor in perinatally infected infants, as demonstrated by the high levels of HIV RNA that are observed during the first 1-2 years of life following perinatal infection. Initiation of aggressive antiretroviral therapy during this early period of viral replication could theoretically preserve immune function, diminish viral dissemination, lower the steady state viral load, and result in improved clinical outcome. Preliminary data from clinical trials of early antiretroviral therapy with three- and four-drug combinations in antiretroviral-naive HIV-infected children under two years of age (some as young as 15 days) indicate that initiation of therapy early in the course of HIV infection, including during the period of primary infection in the neonate, may be able to produce long-term suppression of viral replication and preservation of immune function in some children. However, the proportion of children who achieve HIV RNA levels below the limits of detection with potent therapy may be lower among young infants than older children and adults, in part because virologic response is related to viral load at the time therapy is initiated and young infants have substantially higher viral loads. Although a complete virologic response may not be attained in all children, some studies have suggested that immunologic and clinical benefit may be observed in individuals who are partial responders to therapy.

The potential problems with early therapy include the risk of short- and long-term adverse effects, particularly for drugs given to very young infants, where there are only limited data on pharmacokinetics, drug dosing, and safety. These concerns are particularly relevant because life-long administration of therapy may be necessary, and studies in both adults and children have suggested that optimal benefit may be achieved with the first regimen. Additionally, if viral replication is not suppressed, ongoing viral mutation is likely to result in the development of antiretroviral resistance, curtailing the duration of benefit that early therapy might confer and potentially limiting future treatment options.

When to Initiate Therapy

Before antiretroviral therapy is initiated, it is critical that caregivers and patients (when age-appropriate) are counseled regarding the importance of adherence to the prescribed treatment regimen. Potential problems should be identified and resolved prior to starting therapy, even if this delays initiation of therapy. Additionally, frequent follow-up is important to provide assessment of virologic response to therapy, drug intolerance, viral resistance, and adherence.

HIV-Infected Children with Immunologic or Clinical Symptoms of Infection

Antiretroviral therapy is recommended for all HIV-infected children with clinical symptoms of HIV infection (i.e., those in clinical categories A, B, or C) (Table 51.2) or evidence of immune suppression (i.e., those in immune categories 2 or 3) (Table 51.1)—regardless of the age of the child or viral load. Clinical trial data from both adults and children have demonstrated that antiretroviral therapy in symptomatic patients slows clinical and immunologic disease progression and reduces mortality.

Asymptomatic HIV-Infected Children under Age 12 Months

Ideally, antiretroviral therapy should be initiated in all HIV-infected infants aged <12 months as soon as a confirmed diagnosis is established—regardless of clinical or immunologic status or viral load. HIV-infected infants aged <12 months are considered at high risk for disease progression, and the predictive value of immunologic and virologic parameters to identify infants who will have rapid progression is less than that for older children. Identification of infection during the first few months of life permits clinicians to initiate antiretroviral therapy or intensify ongoing antiretroviral therapy used for chemoprophylaxis of perinatal transmission during the initial phases of primary infection.

However, definitive clinical trial data documenting therapeutic benefit from this approach are not currently available. Additionally, information on drug dosing in infants under age 3-6 months is limited. Hepatic and renal functions are immature in the newborn, undergoing rapid maturational changes during the first few months of life. This can result in substantial differences in antiretroviral dose requirements between young infants and older children; for example, data from clinical trials indicate that higher nelfinavir and ritonavir doses are required in infants to achieve therapeutic drug levels. Because resistance to antiretroviral drugs (particularly protease inhibitors) can develop rapidly when drug concentrations fall below therapeutic levels (either as a result of inadequate dosage or incomplete adherence), issues associated with adherence should be fully assessed and discussed with the HIV-infected infant's caregivers before the decision to initiate therapy is made.

368

Asymptomatic HIV-Infected Children Age 12 Months or Older

Two general approaches for initiating therapy in asymptomatic children aged >1 year were outlined by the Working Group. The first approach would be to initiate therapy in all HIV-infected children, regardless of age or symptom status. Such an approach would ensure: a) treatment of infected children as early as possible in the course of disease and b) intervention before immunologic deterioration. Data from prospective cohort studies indicate that most HIV-infected infants will have clinical symptoms of infection by age one year. Most asymptomatic infected children aged >1 year also have CD4+ T-cell percentages of <25%, which is indicative of immunosuppression (Table 51.1) and warrants antiretroviral therapy.

An alternative approach would be to defer treatment in asymptomatic children aged >1 year with normal immune status in situations in which the risk for clinical disease progression is low (i.e., low viral load) and when other factors (i.e., concern for adherence, safety, and persistence of antiretroviral response) favor postponing treatment. In such cases, the health-care provider should regularly monitor virologic, immunologic, and clinical status. Factors to be considered in deciding when to initiate therapy include a) high or increasing HIV

Table 51.1. 1994 Revised Human Immunodeficiency Virus Pediatric Classification System: Immune Categories Based on Age-Specific CD4+ T-Cell and Percentage*

	<12 mos		1-5 yrs		6-12 yrs	
Immune category	*No./mm³*	*(%)*	*No./mm³*	*(%)*	*No./mm³*	*(%)*
Category 1: no suppression	≥1,500	(≥25%)	≥1,000	(≥25%)	≥500	(≥25 %)
Category 2: Moderate suppression	750-1,499	(15%-24%)	500-999	(15%-24%)	200-499	(15%-24%)
Category 3: Severe suppression	<750	(<15%)	<500	(<15%)	<200	(<15%)

* Modified from: CDC. 1994 Revised classification system for human immunodeficiency virus infection in children less than 13 years of age. *MMWR* 1994; 43 (No. RR-12): p. 1-10

RNA levels, b) rapidly declining CD4+ T-cell count or percentage to values approaching those indicative of moderate immune suppression (i.e., immune category 2 [Table 51.1]), or c) development of clinical symptoms.

Issues associated with adherence to treatment are especially important in considering whether and when to initiate therapy. Antiretroviral therapy is most effective in patients who have never received therapy and who therefore are less likely to have antiretroviral-resistant viral strains. Lack of adherence to prescribed regimens and subtherapeutic levels of antiretroviral medications, particularly PIs, may enhance the development of drug resistance. Participation by the

Table 51.2. 1994 Revised Human Immunodeficiency Virus Pediatric Classification System: Clinical Categories*(continued on next page)

Category N: Not Symptomatic
Children who have no signs or symptoms considered to be the result of HIV infection or who have only one of the conditions listed in category A.

Category A: Mildly Symptomatic
Children with two or more of the following conditions but none of the conditions listed in categories B and C:

Lymphadenopathy (>0.5 cm at more than two sites; bilateral = one site)

Hepatomegaly

Splenomegaly

Dermatitis

Parotitis

Recurrent or persistent upper respiratory infection, sinusitis, or otitis media

Category B: Moderately Symptomatic (continued on next page)
Children who have symptomatic conditions, other than those listed for category A or category C, that are attributed to HIV infection. Examples of conditions in clinical category B include but are not limited to the following:

Anemia (<8 gm/dL), neutropenia (<1,000/mm3), or thrombocytopenia (<100,000/mm3) persisting >30 days

Bacterial meningitis, pneumonia, or sepsis (single episode)

Candidiasis, oropharyngeal (i.e., thrush) persisting for >2 months in children aged >6 months

Cardiomyopathy

Cytomegalovirus infection with onset before age one month

caregivers and child in the decision-making process is crucial, especially in situations for which definitive data concerning efficacy are not available.

Choice of Initial Antiretroviral Therapy

Based on clinical, immunological and virological data from clinical trials in adults and children, antiretroviral drug regimens are listed as *Strongly Recommended*, *Recommended as an Alternative*, *Offered in Special Circumstances* or *Not Recommended*.

Table 51.2. 1994 Revised Human Immunodeficiency Virus Pediatric Classification System: Clinical Categories* (continued)

Category B: Moderately Symptomatic (continued from previous page)
Diarrhea, recurrent or chronic

Hepatitis

Herpes simplex virus (HSV) stomatitis, recurrent (i.e., more than two episodes within one year)

HSV bronchitis, pneumonitis, or esophagitis with onset before age one month

Herpes zoster (i.e., shingles) involving at least two distinct episodes or more than one dermatome

Leiomyosarcoma

Lymphoid interstitial pneumonia (LIP) or pulmonary lymphoid hyperplasia complex

Nephropathy

Nocardiosis

Fever lasting >1 month

Toxoplasmosis with onset before age one month

Varicella, disseminated (i.e., complicated chickenpox)

Category C: Severely Symptomatic
Children who have any condition listed in the 1987 surveillance case definition for acquired immunodeficiency syndrome, with the exception of LIP (which is a category B condition).

*Centers for Disease Control and Prevention. 1994 revised classification system for human immunodeficiency virus infection in children less than 13 years of age. *MMWR*, 1994. 43 (No. RR-12): p. 1-10.

Combination therapy is recommended for all infants, children, and adolescents who are treated with antiretroviral agents. When compared with monotherapy, combination therapy a) slows disease progression and improves survival, b) results in a greater and more sustained virologic and immunologic response, and c) delays development of virus mutations which confer resistance to the drugs being used. Monotherapy with the currently available antiretroviral drugs is no longer recommended to treat HIV infection. Use of ZDV as a single agent is appropriate only when used in infants of indeterminate HIV status during the first 6 weeks of life to prevent perinatal HIV transmission. Infants who are confirmed as being HIV-infected while receiving ZDV chemoprophylaxis should be changed to a recommended standard combination antiretroviral drug regimen or, if immediate treatment is deferred, have single agent ZDV discontinued pending therapeutic decisions.

When to Change Antiretroviral Therapy

The following three reasons warrant a change in antiretroviral therapy: a) failure of the current regimen with evidence of disease progression based on virologic, immunologic, or clinical parameters; b) toxicity or intolerance to the current regimen; and c) new data demonstrating that a drug or regimen is superior to the current regimen. When therapy must be changed because of treatment failure or suboptimal response to treatment, clinicians should work with families to assess the possible contribution of adherence problems to the failure of the current regimen. Issues regarding adherence should be addressed to increase the likelihood of a successful outcome when initiating a new therapy. These issues are best addressed before therapy is instituted and need to be reinforced during therapy.

Intensive family education, training in the administration of prescribed medications, and discussion of the importance of adherence to the drug regimen should be completed before initiation of new treatment. In addition, frequent patient visits and intensive follow-up during the initial months after a new antiretroviral regimen is started are needed to support and educate the family and to monitor adherence, tolerance, and virologic response to the new regimen.

Pediatric Antiretroviral Drug Information

As of February 2001, there were 15 antiretroviral drugs approved for use in HIV-infected adults and adolescents; 11 of these have an approved pediatric treatment indication. These drugs fall into three major classes, NRTIs, NNRTIs and protease inhibitors.

Nucleoside Analogue Reverse Transcriptase Inhibitors

Abacavir (ABC, Ziagen®)

In December of 1998, abacavir (ABC) was approved by the FDA for combination therapy in adults and children age 3 months or older, based on controlled trials in adults and children.

Adverse Effects: A potentially fatal hypersensitivity reaction occurs in approximately 5% of adults and children receiving ABC. Symptoms include flu-like symptoms, respiratory symptoms, fever, rash, fatigue, malaise, nausea, vomiting, diarrhea, and abdominal pain. Patients developing these symptoms should have ABC stopped and not restarted, since hypotension and death have occurred with rechallange. In a randomized study comparing ABC/ZDV/3TC to ZDV/3TC alone, 4 of 146 children receiving ABC and 2 of 44 children in the ZDV/3TC group who switched to open-label ABC therapy developed a hypersensitivity reaction, which resolved upon discontinuation of therapy. Onset of the hypersensitivity reaction occurred between 1 to 2 weeks after ABC was started. Nausea and vomiting alone may occur in as many as one-third of children receiving ABC in combination with other antiretroviral agents.

When using ABC, parents and patients must be cautioned about the risk of a serious hypersensitivity reaction; a medication guide and warning card should be provided to parents. Patients should also be advised to consult their physician immediately if signs or symptoms consistent with a hypersensitivity reaction occur. Children experiencing a hypersensitivity reaction should be reported to the Abacavir Hypersensitivity Registry (1-800-270-0425). While ABC may be included as a component of a treatment regimen for children who have failed prior antiretroviral therapy, it should be recognized that it is less likely to be active in children with extensive prior treatment with NRTIs. Lactic acidosis and severe hepatomegaly with steatosis, including fatal cases, have been reported with the use of nucleoside analogues alone or in combination, including ABC.

Didanosine (ddI, Videx®)

Didanosine (ddI) received FDA approval in 1991 for adults and pediatric patients older than 6 months of age with advanced HIV infection who were intolerant to or deteriorating on ZDV. Since that time the indications have been broadened and dosage recommendations reduced. In October 2000 a new delayed-release formulation of enteric-coated beadlets was approved for use in adults allowing for once-daily ddI administration in selected patients.

Adverse Effects: Fatal and nonfatal pancreatitis has occurred during therapy with this agent used alone or in combination regimens in both treatment-naive and treatment-experienced patients, regardless of degree of immunosuppression. Didanosine should be suspended in patients with suspected pancreatitis and discontinued in patients with confirmed pancreatitis. Pancreatitis appears to be more common in adult patients and may be dose-related. It has occurred more commonly in patients with predisposing factors, including a prior history of pancreatitis, baseline elevation of serum transaminases, and concurrent administration of other drugs known to cause pancreatitis, such as pentamidine and d4T. Hydroxyurea appears to increase the risk of pancreatitis when co-administered with ddI. Didanosine may cause peripheral sensory neuropathy. Asymptomatic peripheral retinal depigmentation has been observed in <5% of children receiving ddI, is not associated with loss of vision, and appears to reverse with discontinuation of therapy. Diarrhea has been reported, and may be more related to the antacid/buffer with which the drug is formulated than to ddI itself. Lactic acidosis and severe hepatomegaly with steatosis, including fatal cases, have been reported with the use of nucleoside analogues alone or in combination, including didanosine.

Lamivudine (3TC, Epivir®)

Lamivudine (3TC) was approved in November 1995 for use in infants greater than 3 months of age and children based on efficacy studies in adults in conjunction with safety and pharmacokinetic studies in children. In September 1997, it was approved as a fixed combination of 3TC/ZDV for adults and adolescents greater than 12 years old. In November 2000, it was approved as a fixed-dose combination of 3TC/ZDV/abacavir for adolescents and adults weighing greater than 40 kg.

Adverse Effects: 3TC is very well tolerated. The major reported toxicities are pancreatitis and peripheral neuropathy. Headache, fatigue and gastrointestinal upset have also been described. Lactic acidosis and severe hepatomegaly with steatosis, including fatal cases, have been reported with the use of nucleoside analogues alone or in combination, including 3TC.

Stavudine (d4T, Zerit®)

Stavudine (d4T) was approved in September 1996 for use in infants and children greater than six months of age based on evidence from controlled trials in adults and on safety and pharmacokinetic data from children.

Adverse Effects: d4T's most significant toxicity is peripheral neuropathy, but this appears to be less common in children than adults. Elevated hepatic transaminases are seen in about 11% and pancreatitis in 1% of adults enrolled in clinical trials of d4T. d4T has been studied in pediatric patients in combination with ddI; no pharmacokinetic interactions were observed and there were no cases of peripheral neuropathy. Lactic acidosis and severe hepatomegaly with steatosis, including fatal cases, have been reported with the use of nucleoside analogues alone or in combination, including d4T. ZDV is a potent inhibitor of the intracellular phosphorylation of d4T in vitro, and at least one adult clinical trial indicates that there may also be in vivo antagonism associated with this combination. Therefore, d4T and ZDV should not be co-administered.

Zalcitabine (ddC, Hivid®)

In August 1994 zalcitabine (ddC) was approved for use in adults and adolescents older than 13 years of age. It is not FDA-approved for use in pediatric patients.

Adverse Effects: Although uncommon, peripheral neuropathy was observed in some children in PACTG 138. ddC has similar toxicities as ddI; combination with ddI is not recommended due to overlapping genotypic resistance mutations and enhanced risk of peripheral neuropathy and pancreatitis. Rashes and oral ulcerations have also been reported with ddC therapy in children. Lactic acidosis and severe hepatomegaly with steatosis, including fatal cases, have been reported with the use of nucleoside analogues alone or in combination, including ddC.

Zidovudine (ZDV, AZT, Retrovir®)

Zidovudine (ZDV) was the first NRTI studied in adult and pediatric clinical trials and the first antiretroviral agent approved for therapy of HIV infection. ZDV first received FDA approval for the treatment of HIV infection in adults in 1987. It was approved for use in children ages 3 months to 12 years in May 1990. Perinatal trial PACTG 076 established that a ZDV prophylactic regimen given during pregnancy, labor and to the newborn reduced the risk of perinatal HIV transmission by nearly 70%. Zidovudine received FDA approval for that indication in August 1994.

Adverse Effects: ZDV is generally well tolerated in children with its major toxicities being macrocytic anemia and neutropenia. Dose reduction and hematopoietic growth factors such as erythropoietin and filgrastim (NEUPOGEN, G-CSF) have been used to mitigate these toxicities. ZDV has also been associated with reversible myopathy and cardiomyopathy. Other reported toxicities of ZDV include fatigue, headache, and nausea. Lactic acidosis and severe hepatomegaly with steatosis, including fatal cases, have been reported with the use of nucleoside analogues alone or in combination, including ZDV.

Non-Nucleoside Analogue Reverse Transcriptase Inhibitors

Delavirdine (DLV, Rescriptor®)

Delavirdine (DLV) was approved in April 1997 for use in adolescents 16 years and older and adults in combination with other antiretroviral agents. This agent, similar to others in its class has no activity against HIV-2 but is specific for HIV-1. This NNRTI has had very limited study in pediatric patients under age 13 years.

Adverse Effects: Skin rash is the most common toxicity observed with DLV, as observed with the other NNRTIs. Skin rash attributable to DLV was observed in 18% of all adults receiving combination regimens with DLV in phase II and III trials; an incidence rate as high as 50% was reported in some trials (Rescriptor label). Dose titration did not significantly reduce the incidence of rash, but the rash was more common in adults with lower CD4+ cell counts and typically appeared within one to three weeks of treatment. Severe rash such as Stevens Johnson Syndrome, while rare, does occur; like the other NNRTIs, DLV should be discontinued if severe rash or severe rash with constitutional findings occurs. Other toxicities were uncommon; elevated liver transaminases were observed in 2-7% of adults receiving DLV but did not differ from comparison groups receiving regimens not including DLV. In the one phase I study involving children, the most frequently reported adverse effects were rash in 40% (all grade 1 or 2) and vomiting in 40%.

Efavirenz (DMP-266, EFV, Sustiva™)

Efavirenz (EFV) was approved in September 1998 for children older than 3 years of age, adolescents and adults.

Adverse Effects: The toxicity profile for efavirenz differs for adults and children. In adults, a central nervous system (CNS) complex of confusion, agitation, sleep disturbance, nightmares, hallucinations or other symptoms has been reported in more than 50% of patients. These symptoms usually occur early in treatment and rarely require drug discontinuation. Bedtime dosing, particularly during the first several weeks of therapy appears to decrease the occurrence and severity of this side effect. Adverse CNS effects occurred in 14% of children receiving EFV in clinical studies. The principal side effect of EFV seen in children is rash, which was seen in up to 40% of children compared to 27% of adults. The rash is usually maculopapular, pruritic, and mild to moderate in severity and rarely requires drug discontinuation. Onset is typically in the first 2 weeks of treatment. While severe rash and Stevens Johnson Syndrome have been reported, this is rare. Other reported adverse events include diarrhea, nausea, and increased aminotransferase levels.

Nevirapine (NVP, Viramune®)

Nevirapine (NVP) is approved for use in children greater than 2 months old. NVP is a dipyridodiazepinone derivative and is specific for HIV-1. It does not inhibit any of the human cellular DNA polymerases.

Adverse Effects: The most common adverse events reported in adults include headache, nausea, fever, and skin rashes. In initial clinical trials of NVP treatment in HIV-infected children, rash was observed in 24%. When a 2-week lower dose lead in period was used, the incidence of rash is decreased. In a study of 4-drug therapy including nevirapine (given with 2 week lead in), rash was observed in only 6% of children. Granulocytopenia was the second most frequent adverse event, seen in 16%. However, it should be noted the children were also receiving ZDV, a known cause of granulocytopenia. The skin rash typically presents in the first 28 days after initiating therapy and in rare cases has progressed to Stevens-Johnson syndrome, toxic epidermal necrolysis, a severe skin rash accompanied by hypersensitivity reactions (characterized by rash, constitutional symptoms such as fever, arthralgia, myalgia, and lymphadenopathy, and visceral involvement such as hepatitis, eosinophilia, granulocytopenia, and renal dysfunction) or death. NVP should be discontinued if severe rash or severe rash with constitutional findings occurs. Patients experiencing rash during the 14-day lead-in period should not have their NVP dose increased until the rash has resolved. Severe, life-threatening and in some cases fatal hepatotoxicity, including fulminant and cholestatic hepatitis, hepatic necrosis and hepatic failure, has been reported in NVP-treated patients. Increased serum transaminases levels or a history of hepatitis B or C infection prior to starting nevirapine are associated with higher risk for hepatic adverse events. The majority of cases has occurred during the first 12 weeks of NVP therapy, and frequent and intensive clinical and laboratory monitoring, including liver function tests, is important during this time period. However, about one third of cases occurred after 12 weeks of treatment, so continued periodic monitoring of liver function tests is needed. In some cases, patients presented with non-specific prodromal signs or symptoms of hepatitis and progressed to hepatic failure; patients with symptoms or signs of hepatitis should have liver function tests performed. NVP should be permanently discontinued and not restarted in patients who develop clinical hepatitis (FDA 12/00).

Protease Inhibitors

Amprenavir (APV, Agenerase®)

The Food and Drug Administration in April 1999 approved amprenavir (APV) for use in combination with other antiretrovirals in adults and children over 4 years of age. This approval was based upon the results of controlled trials of up to 24 weeks duration in treatment naive and experienced adults. Pediatric approval was based upon analysis of two open label trials in treatment experienced children, one after 8 weeks of therapy and one after 4 weeks of therapy. APV is available in both liquid and solid formulations.

Adverse Effects: Data compiled from 30 phase I-III studies of amprenavir in 1330 adult and pediatric patients revealed the following most frequently reported adverse events: nausea, diarrhea, rash, headache, oral paresthesia, and fatigue. The majority of adverse events were mild to moderate. Nausea, rash, including Stevens-Johnson Syndrome, and vomiting were the most common adverse events associated with discontinuation of treatment. The most common drug related adverse events in trials of pediatric patients are vomiting, nausea, diarrhea, and rash. APV should be discontinued for severe rash, including Stevens-Johnson Syndrome, or moderate rash with systemic symptoms. APV is related to the sulfonamides and the potential for cross-sensitivity of sulfonamides and APV is unknown. APV should therefore be used with caution in patients with sulfona-mide allergy. Signs of lipodystrophy have been reported in a few patients on amprenavir. As with all agents in this class, new onset diabetes mellitus, exacerbation of pre-existing diabetes mellitus, hyperglyce-mia, and diabetic ketoacidosis may occur.

Indinavir (IDV, Crixivan®)

Indinavir (IDV) was approved in 1996 for use in adolescents and adults older than 18 years of age. Like the other PIs, IDV is prone to multiple drug interactions due to its interaction with the cytochrome P450 system (see product label). A liquid formulation is not yet avail-able. Administration of IDV with a meal high in calories, fat and protein results in a reduction in plasma IDV concentrations; administration with lighter meals (e.g. dry toast with jelly, apple juice and coffee with skim milk and sugar) results in little to no change in IDV pharmaco-kinetics.

Adverse Effects: The most serious side effect observed in both adults and children is nephrolithiasis. In double-blind clinical trials in adults, the incidence of nephrolithiasis was 9.3% in IDV-containing groups. Abnormal renal function (including acute renal failure) has been observed in a small number of patients with nephrolithiasis; abnormal renal function was generally transient and temporally re-lated to the acute episode. Interstitial nephritis has also been observed in patients receiving IDV. If signs and symptoms such as flank pain with or without hematuria occur, temporary interruption of therapy (for 1-3 days) during the acute episode may be considered. Adequate hydration is essential when IDV is administered. Nephrolithiasis may be somewhat more frequent among children, likely due to the diffi-culty in maintaining adequate hydration; in an IDV study in fifty-four children, 13% developed hematuria.

Lopinavir / Ritonavir (LPV / RTV, ABT-378 / r, Kaletra™)

Lopinavir/Ritonavir (LPV/RTV) is a fixed combination of these two protease inhibitors (133.3 mg of lopinavir plus 33.3 mg of ritonavir). LPV/RTV received FDA approval in 2000 for combination with other antiretroviral agents for the treatment of HIV-1 infection in adults and pediatric patients age six months and older. It is available in both liquid and solid formulations.

Adverse Effects: The most common side effects associated with LPV/RTV have been diarrhea, asthenia, and triglyceride and cholesterol elevations. Pancreatitis has been reported in adult patients taking LPV/RTV. High triglyceride levels may be a risk factor for pancreatitis to develop. As with all agents in this class, new onset diabetes mellitus, exacerbation of pre-existing diabetes mellitus, hyperglycemia, and diabetic ketoacidosis may occur.

Nelfinavir (NFV, Viracept®)

Nelfinavir (NFV) is approved for use in children over two years of age in combination with NRTIs and NNRTIs. It is available in both oral powder and tablet formulations. Like other agents in this class it is an inhibitor of the HIV-1 protease enzyme, which results in preventing cleavage of the gag-pol polyprotein. This inhibits viral replication by producing and releasing immature, non-infectious virions. NFV is active against HIV-1 and HIV-2 strains. Oral bioavailability of NFV has been reported to be 70-80% when administered with food; bioavailability is significantly reduced when the drug is taken in a fasting state. Like other PIs, NFV is metabolized by the cytochrome P450 enzyme system in the liver, inhibits CYP3A4 and is associated with a number of clinically significant pharmacologic drug interactions (see product label).

Adverse Effects: NFV in children has been relatively well tolerated, even when dosing schemes exceed adult recommended amounts. The most common adverse effects include diarrhea, abdominal pain, flatulence and rash. As with other protease inhibitors, new onset diabetes mellitus and exacerbations of previous hyperglycemia have been reported, as has the occurrence of the lipodystrophy syndrome. The long-term safety, durability of virologic efficacy, and the feasibility of children taking this drug for long periods of time is still under investigation.

Ritonavir (RTV, Norvir®)

Ritonavir (RTV) is approved for use in children over the age of 2 years in combination with other antiretroviral agents. It was the first

PI approved for use in children and is available as liquid and capsule formulations. It has specific activity for HIV-1, and to a lesser extent, HIV-2.

Adverse Effects: One small phase I study in children demonstrated a high rate of gastrointestinal intolerance. However, larger studies (e.g., PACTG 338) have shown better tolerance of the drug, particularly when dose escalation is used when initiating therapy. In PACTG 338, approximately 80% of children were able to tolerate RTV at 24 weeks of therapy. Circumoral paresthesia and taste perversion have been reported in adults receiving the drug. Hepatic transaminase elevations exceeding 5 times the upper limit of normal, clinical hepatitis and jaundice have been reported in adults receiving RTV alone or in combination with other antiretroviral drugs. There may be an increased risk for transaminase elevation in patients with underlying hepatitis B or C virus infection. Caution should be exercised when administering RTV to patients with pre-existing liver disease.

Saquinavir (SQV, hard gel capsule, Invirase®); soft gel capsule, Fortovase®)

In 1995, saquinavir (SQV) became the first protease inhibitor approved for use in adolescents and adults older then 16 years, in combination therapy with NRTIs. In its original formulation, as a hard gel capsule (Invirase), it had very limited bioavailability (~ 4%) following oral administration. In 1997, the FDA approved a soft gel capsule preparation (Fortovase) with significantly enhanced oral bioavailability. SQV has not been formally approved for use in children and is not yet available in a liquid preparation. Absorption of SQV soft gel capsule is enhanced by food.

Adverse Effects: The drug appears to be well tolerated, with mild gastrointestinal disturbances (diarrhea, nausea, abdominal pain) and reversible elevations in liver function tests being the most common side effects reported in adults. As with all agents in this class, new onset diabetes mellitus, exacerbation of pre-existing diabetes mellitus, hyperglycemia, and diabetic ketoacidosis have been reported.

Chapter 52

Preventing Pneumocystis Carinii *Pneumonia (PCP) in Children*

Pneumocystis carinii (NEW-mo-SIS-tis CA-RIN-nee-eye) pneumonia, or PCP, is a severe illness that adults and children with HIV or AIDS may get. It is caused by a germ called *Pneumocystis carinii*. Most children infected with this germ don't get pneumonia because their immune systems are normal. Children whose immune systems are badly damaged by HIV can get PCP. Children with HIV are less likely to get PCP today than in earlier years. However, PCP is still the most common serious infection among children with AIDS in the United States.

How do I know if my child has PCP?

If your child has PCP, he or she probably will have fever, cough, or trouble breathing. Children with PCP may die if the infection is not treated quickly. See your doctor immediately if your child has these symptoms. PCP can be diagnosed only by laboratory tests of fluid or tissue from the lungs.

How could my child catch PCP?

Most scientists believe PCP is spread in the air, but they don't know if it lives in the soil or someplace else. The PCP germ is very common.

"You Can Prevent PCP in Children: A Guide for People with HIV Infection," National Center for HIV, STD and TB Prevention, Centers for Disease Control and Prevention, updated September 1999; available online at http://www.cdc.gov/hiv/pubs/brochure/oi_pcpkidz.htm.

Since it is difficult to prevent exposure to PCP, you should get medical care for your child to prevent PCP.

How can I prevent PCP in my child?

The best way to prevent PCP in children is to prevent HIV in children. Pregnant women with HIV should speak with their doctors about taking antiretroviral treatments to prevent passing their HIV infection to their unborn child. Children whose mothers have HIV also can take anti-viral treatments and medicine to prevent PCP. The best drug for preventing PCP is trimethoprim-sulfamethoxazole (try-METH-o-prim - sul-fa-meth-OX-uh-sole), or TMP-SMX.

What is TMP-SMX?

TMP-SMX is a combination of two medicines. It has many different brand names, such as Bactrim, Septra, and Cotrim. Older children can take TMP-SMX in tablet form. You can also get TMP-SMX as a liquid for babies and young children.

What children should get treatment to prevent PCP?

All babies born to mothers with HIV should get TMP-SMX starting at 4 to 6 weeks old, even if it isn't known yet if they have HIV. This will help prevent PCP infection before it starts. If HIV tests later show that your baby does not have HIV, the TMP-SMX treatment can be stopped. If your baby has HIV, he or she should continue to get TMP-SMX treatment until reaching the age of 1 year. Your doctor will then decide if your child needs to continue the treatment, based on your baby's CD4 cell (sometimes called T-cell) count.

Babies don't get TMP-SMX treatment until they are at least 4 weeks old because most children will be taking zidovudine (also called AZT), and small children shouldn't take the two drugs together. Also, TMP-SMX can cause liver damage in babies younger than 4 weeks old. Babies don't usually get PCP until they are at least 8 weeks old.

What are the side effects of TMP-SMX?

TMP-SMX can make some people have a rash or feel sick. If the drug reaction is not severe, TMP-SMX should be continued because it works so much better than any other medicine to prevent PCP.

Are there other medicines to prevent PCP?

Yes. Check with your doctor about the possibility of other treatments. Your child should take all of his or her medicines as prescribed by your doctor. Don't lower the dosage without speaking with your doctor.

Can my child get PCP more than once?

Yes. If your child has already had PCP, he or she can get it again. TMP-SMX can prevent second infections with PCP. Therefore, treatment should be used even after your child has had PCP to prevent getting it again.

Part Six

Prevention and Research

Chapter 53

Combating Complacency in HIV Prevention

In the United States, complacency about the need for HIV prevention may be among the strongest barriers communities face as they plan to meet the next century's prevention needs. The great success that many people, but not all, have had with new highly active antiretroviral therapies (HAART, also known as drug cocktails) and the resulting decline in the number of newly reported AIDS cases and deaths are indeed good news. The underlying reality, however, is that the HIV epidemic in our country is far from over. This is true not only for the nation, but for the continuing number of HIV-infected individuals who now must face years—perhaps a lifetime—of multiple daily medications, possible unpleasant or severe side effects, and great expense associated with the medicines needed to suppress HIV and prevent opportunistic infections.

The success of HAART is good news for the people living longer, better lives because of it, but the availability of treatment may lull people into believing that preventing HIV infection is no longer important. This complacency about the need for prevention adds a new dimension of complexity for both program planners and individuals at risk.

National Center for HIV, STD and TB Prevention, Centers for Disease Control and Prevention (CDC), June 1998; available online at http://www.cdc.gov/hiv/pubs/facts/combat.pdf. Despite the age of this document, the issues raised are still pertinent in the fight against HIV/AIDS.

While the number of AIDS cases is declining, the number of people living with HIV infection is growing. This increased prevalence of HIV in the population means that even more prevention efforts are needed, not fewer. For individuals at risk, increased prevalence means that each risk behavior carries an increased risk for infection. This makes the danger of relaxing preventive behaviors greater than ever.

Past prevention efforts have resulted in behavior change for many individuals and have helped slow the epidemic overall. However, many studies find that high-risk behaviors, especially unprotected sex, are continuing at far too high a rate. This is true even for some people who have been counseled and tested for HIV, including those found to be infected.

The long-term effectiveness of HAART is unknown. Further, HIV may develop resistance to these drugs. The powerful treatments are complicated and involve taking large numbers of pills. Even the most motivated patients may forget to take all their medications or skip doses.

Some patients have been known to take drug holidays, completely stopping their medications for a number of days or weeks. These drug treatments are less effective when treatment schedules are not followed. Diversions from the prescribed treatment regimen increase the possibility of drug resistance developing, which would greatly narrow future treatment options for those infected with a drug-resistant strain of HIV. And, if the development of drug-resistance is coupled with a relaxation in preventive behaviors, resistant strains could be transmitted to others and spread widely.

Research among gay and bisexual men suggests that some individuals are less concerned about becoming infected than in the past and may be inclined to take more risks. This may be equally true in other groups at risk who might believe they no longer need to use condoms because protease inhibitors are so effective in treating HIV disease. The truth is, despite medical advances, HIV remains a serious and usually fatal disease that requires complex, costly, and difficult treatment regimens. These treatments don't work for everyone. Sometimes when they do work, they have unpleasant or intolerable side effects. Some people can't take them because the interaction with their other drugs causes serious problems.

Still others find it extremely difficult to maintain the drug treatment schedules. As we continue working to develop better treatment options, we must not lose sight of the fact that preventing HIV infection in the first place precludes the need for people to follow these difficult regimens.

The Challenge of Monitoring the HIV/AIDS Epidemic

The treatment effect on trends in the AIDS epidemic not only increases our need for combating complacency, but means that we have never been closer to losing our ability to monitor the epidemic.

Until recently, AIDS cases provided a reliable picture of trends in the HIV epidemic. Before highly effective treatments were available, researchers could take into account the time between HIV infection and progression to AIDS and estimate where and how many new infections were occurring based on observed cases of disease. Today, trends in AIDS cases and deaths may provide a valuable measure of groups for whom highly effective treatment is not available or has not succeeded. However, they no longer tell us enough about where and how many new infections are occurring—information critical for addressing the increasing need for prevention and treatment services. To allow the U.S. to target programs and resources most effectively, we must be able to keep pace with where the epidemic is going.

This means we need to improve our ability to track early HIV infections, before they progress to AIDS.

Pay Attention to Prevention—It Works

Sustained, comprehensive prevention efforts begun in the 1980s have had a substantial impact on slowing the HIV/AIDS epidemic in our country. While it is difficult to measure prevention—or how many thousands of infections did not occur as a result of efforts to date—we know the epidemic was growing at rate of over 80% each year in the mid-1980s and has now stabilized. While the occurrence of approximately 40,000 new infections annually is deeply troubling, we have made tremendous progress. We also have more scientific evidence than ever before on which prevention programs are most effective. There is no question that prevention works and remains the best and most cost-effective approach for bringing the HIV/AIDS epidemic under control and saving lives.

HIV prevention programs have been proven effective. Many studies indicate that prevention programs can contribute to changes in personal behavior that reduce risks of infection, and these changes are sustained over time. A 1997 scientific consensus conference sponsored by the National Institutes of Health that reviewed existing data on the effectiveness of HIV behavioral interventions concluded that behavioral interventions to reduce risk for HIV/AIDS are effective and should be disseminated widely.

Comprehensive school-based HIV and sex education programs have been shown to delay the initiation of sexual intercourse, reduce the frequency of intercourse, reduce the number of sex partners, or increase the use of condoms or other contraceptives.

Efforts to reduce risks of injection drug users through policy changes also have been evaluated and found to be very effective. For example, both New York and Connecticut reported significant reductions in the sharing of drug injection equipment after implementation of programs and policies that increased access to sterile injection equipment.

Perinatal prevention programs that identify and treat pregnant women who are HIV infected have shown dramatic success in reducing HIV transmission to their babies.

Screening the blood supply for HIV and heat-treating blood products for the treatment of hemophilia have nearly eliminated HIV transmission through these early transmission routes.

Postexposure prophylaxis for health care workers has shown some success in reducing HIV transmission rates among those with occupational exposure to HIV-infected blood.

Numerous HIV prevention programs have been shown to be cost-effective when compared against the resources required to treat and deliver HIV medical care to a person over the remaining years of their life. With the rising costs of lifetime treatment of HIV, effective prevention has become even more cost effective. New CDC estimates find that if only 1,255 infections are prevented each year, CDC's federally funded HIV prevention efforts in the United States are cost effective. If only 3,995 infections are prevented, our nation's investment in HIV prevention has actually saved money.

Comprehensive HIV Prevention Programs Work Best

People with HIV risk behaviors need an array of prevention messages, skills, and support to help them reduce sexual and drug-related risks. Drug injectors, for example, not only need strategies to help them stop using drugs or sharing needles, but also need to learn ways to protect themselves from sexual transmission if their partner has ever injected drugs and may have shared needles.

Substance use is a major problem in this country, and the intersection of substance use and sexual HIV transmission cannot be overlooked. Ideally, everyone who abuses any drug (including alcohol) should be offered counseling and treatment to help them stop using drugs and prevent HIV infection. HIV prevention interventions for the vast majority of substance users who are not in treatment also must address the sexual risks that are common among people who use drugs, including crack cocaine, marijuana, and alcohol.

Each and every generation of young people needs comprehensive, sustained health information and interventions that help them develop life-long skills for avoiding behaviors that could lead to HIV infection. Such comprehensive programs should include the involvement of parents as well as educators. The most effective programs start at an early age and are designed to encourage the adoption of healthy behaviors, such as exercising and eating a healthy diet, and to prevent the initiation of unhealthy ones, such as drug use, excessive alcohol consumption, smoking, and premature sexual activity, before they start.

Scientific studies show that treatment of other sexually transmitted diseases can greatly reduce the risk of transmitting and acquiring HIV.

The Many Dimensions of Prevention Provide Multiple Opportunities for Intervention

Primary HIV prevention means keeping people from becoming infected with HIV in the first place. Interventions must focus not only on uninfected populations—there also is a major role for preventing further infections by focusing on infected individuals and helping them develop skills for reducing the risk of infecting others.

Secondary HIV prevention means keeping people who already are HIV-infected safe and healthy by helping them avoid opportunistic infections and stopping the infection from progressing to AIDS.

In all prevention efforts, there is a growing need to address the link between HIV treatment and prevention. In some cases, such as preventing perinatal transmission to infants by providing antiretroviral drugs to the mother, treatment is prevention. We also know that the treatment of other STDs can greatly reduce a person's risk for sexually acquired HIV infection. And, scientists even now are exploring the possibility that combination drug therapies may reduce infectivity. With the lines between prevention and treatment beginning to fade, ongoing services for people who are HIV positive must balance medical advances with the behavioral and social support needed to preserve their quality of life and prevent the spread of infection.

We must maintain a focus on behavioral strategies. Even a vaccine doesn't stop a disease unless people use it—and in the case of HIV, a vaccine is unlikely to confer 100% lifelong immunity. Because no medical advance can succeed on its own, people must adapt their behaviors to work in tandem with it. To do this, they need several things:

- Access to prevention services and new medical treatments. For example, pregnant women who may not know they are infected with HIV cannot reduce the risk of transmission to their children unless they first get prenatal care that includes routine HIV counseling and voluntary testing. Those found to be infected then must have access to antiretroviral drugs.

- Assistance in developing skills to use new medical treatments. HAART, for example, involves complex treatment regimens and may require the development of compliance-related skills. For example, people may need to learn how to deal with side effects, what drug interactions might occur, how to lessen the risk of developing drug resistance, or how to cope with complicated schedules.

- Support and encouragement from family, friends, care providers, and the community at large will help people make and sustain behavioral changes in their lives.

Today, more than ever, we must recognize that medical advances do not negate the need for preventing disease—in fact, the availability of newer and better treatments often increases the need for prevention. How well we continue our work to develop integrated approaches to prevention and treatment may well define the future course of the HIV pandemic.

Chapter 54

Prevention and Treatment of Sexually Transmitted Diseases as an HIV Prevention Strategy

The interconnectedness of HIV and other sexually transmitted diseases (STDs) grows increasingly apparent as biomedical and behavioral scientists learn more about people's susceptibility and risks. CDC is applying new research to the prevention of all major STDs, including HIV infection, and is working to ensure communities have the information they need to design, implement, and evaluate comprehensive approaches to HIV and STD prevention.

The Parallel Epidemics of HIV Infection and Other STDs

Globally, an estimated 333 million new cases of curable STDs occur each year among adults, according to 1995 estimates by the World Health Organization. STDs in the United States have reached epidemic proportions with an estimated 12 million new cases each year. Of these, 3 million occur among teenagers, 13 to 19 years old. STDs are the most common reportable diseases in the United States.

The sexual spread of HIV in the United States has paralleled that of other STDs. For example, the geographic distribution of heterosexual HIV transmission closely parallels that of other STDs. Most of the health districts with the highest syphilis and gonorrhea rates in the United States are concentrated in the South, the same part of

National Center for HIV, STD and TB Prevention, Centers for Disease Control and Prevention (CDC), updated July 24, 1998; available online at http://www.cdc.gov/hiv/pubs/facts/hivstd.htm. Despite the older date of this document, the issues are still relevant.

the nation with the highest HIV prevalence among childbearing women. Researchers have long recognized that the risk behaviors which place individuals at risk for other STDs also increase a person's risk of becoming infected with HIV. STD surveillance can provide important indications of where HIV infection may spread, and where efforts to promote safer sexual behaviors should be targeted.

Other STDs Facilitate HIV Transmission

There is now strong evidence that other STDs increase the risk of HIV transmission and, conversely, that STD treatment reduces the spread of HIV.

- *Epidemiological studies:* Studies have repeatedly demonstrated that people are 2-5 times more likely to become infected with HIV when other STDs are present.

- *Biological studies:* Biological studies suggest both increased susceptibility to HIV infection and increased likelihood of infecting other people when other STDs are present.

Increased susceptibility: STDs that cause genital lesions can create a portal of entry for HIV. And even without lesions, STDs increase the number of HIV target cells (CD4 cells) in cervical secretions, thereby likely increasing HIV susceptibility in women.

Increased infectiousness: Studies have demonstrated that co-infection with HIV and other STDs results both in more shedding of HIV and in greater concentrations of HIV being shed. For example, in African studies, co-infection with gonorrhea and HIV more than doubles the proportion of HIV-infected individuals with HIV RNA detectable in genital secretions. Furthermore, the median concentration of HIV RNA in semen is dramatically increased in co-infected men compared with men infected with HIV alone.

New Evidence of the Effectiveness of STD Treatment in HIV Prevention

Intervention studies: New evidence indicates that STD detection and treatment can substantially reduce HIV transmission. For example:

- STD treatment reduces the prevalence and magnitude of HIV shedding. Treatment of gonorrhea in HIV-infected men resulted in a reduction in the number of men who shed HIV, as well as a lower concentration of HIV shed. With STD treatment, the level of shedding among co-infected men returns to the level seen in men who are not co-infected.

- STD treatment reduces the spread of HIV infection in communities. A community-level, randomized trial in a rural African community in Tanzania demonstrated a 42% decrease in new, heterosexually transmitted HIV infections in communities with improved STD treatment. An ongoing study in Uganda is further exploring the impact of mass STD treatment in slowing the spread of HIV. These studies will be critical in more clearly defining the role STD treatment can play in HIV prevention efforts in the developing world and in industrialized nations.

Making the Numbers Count: Turning What We Have Learned into Prevention

CDC has a wide range of initiatives to reduce the spread of STDs and the attendant increased risk of HIV transmission. Some of these include:

- Guidelines development. During the summer of 1998, CDC's Advisory Committee for HIV and STD Prevention (ACHSP) issued guidelines for local jurisdictions on the use of STD testing and treatment as an effective HIV prevention strategy in the United States.

- STD/HIV demonstration projects. CDC has awarded funds for demonstration projects in three areas of the country (North Carolina, Baltimore, and Louisiana) to provide on-site STD screening and treatment and related services in settings serving HIV-infected and at-risk individuals.

- Syphilis elimination. A national syphilis elimination effort will target the same areas of the country with increasing rates of heterosexually transmitted HIV infection. Because syphilis facilitates the transmission of HIV infection, syphilis elimination can have a significant effect on HIV transmission in many communities.

- STD-related Infertility Prevention Program. In 1998, the U.S. Congress allocated $17.5 million for infertility prevention. This program seeks to reduce infertility by improving the detection and treatment of chlamydia in women and their sexual partners. Chlamydia is a common STD that frequently goes undiagnosed in women, resulting in severe reproductive problems including infertility.

- Training programs. State training programs for STD and HIV staff are being targeted to areas with high rates of syphilis and gonorrhea. The training focuses on lessons learned from HIV community planning and the most effective use of STD screening and treatment.

- Comprehensive STD Prevention Systems (CSPS). Beginning in 1999, the CSPS Project Grants expanded requirements for comprehensive state and local STD programs. These state and local plans will: concentrate on collaboration between public and private sectors; seek community involvement to accomplish STD prevention goals; focus on issues related to quality, access, and assurance; and harness recent advances in clinical, epidemiologic, behavioral, and health services research. All programs are required to address the intersection of HIV with other STDs.

Chapter 55

Preventive Therapy for Non-Occupational Exposures to HIV

In recent years, the Public Health Service (PHS) has recommended the use of antiretroviral drugs to reduce the risk of occupational HIV transmission following workplace exposures (e.g., health care workers exposed through accidental needle-sticks). Scientific studies have shown the drugs to be both safe and effective for this use. While this type of therapy is not 100% effective, it has been found to significantly reduce the risk of HIV infection among health care workers following percutaneous (through the skin) exposures.

Questions have arisen about whether similar therapy should be offered to people with unanticipated sexual or drug injection-related exposures to HIV. However, researchers do not know if findings among health care workers are applicable in other settings where therapy may not be initiated as quickly, where the HIV status of the source may not be known, where the regimen cannot be closely monitored, and where repeated exposures may occur. To consider these questions, PHS convened scientific experts from across the nation to review all available data. The September 25, 1998, issue of the *Morbidity and Mortality Weekly Report* summarizes the data considered and the outcomes of this consultation.

PHS has concluded that there are no conclusive data on the effectiveness of antiretroviral therapy in preventing HIV transmission after non-occupational exposures. It is therefore not possible to make

National Center for HIV, STD and TB Prevention, Centers for Disease Control and Prevention (CDC), updated February 4, 2002; available online at http://www.cdc.gov/hiv/pubs/facts/petfact.htm.

definitive recommendations regarding its use. Because the therapy remains unproven and can pose risks, physicians should consider its use only in individual circumstances when the probability of HIV infection is high, the therapy can be initiated promptly, and adherence to the regimen is likely. It should not be used routinely and should never be considered a form of primary prevention.

Decisions regarding use should be made by physicians, in consultation with their patients and, as needed, an expert in the use of antiretroviral drugs. To help guide these discussions, the PHS report provides physicians a summary of available data and outlines factors that should be considered before prescribing therapy. The following factors should be evaluated in considering the potential benefit of therapy:

- Is there convincing evidence that the reported source of exposure is infected? Is the HIV-status of the source known?

- Is there a high risk of transmission from the exposure reported? This depends on the specifics of the risk event (e.g. no condom, torn condom, type of sex, receptive or insertive partner, injection before or after others, number of people sharing injection equipment) and the presence or absence of factors that would modify risk (e.g. vaginal or anal tears, bleeding, visible genital ulcers or other evidence of an active STD, bleach treatment of injection equipment).

- How much time has elapsed between exposure and presentation for medical care? While the interval during which postexposure antiretroviral therapy for non-occupational exposure can be beneficial in humans is unknown, animal studies suggest that the therapy is most effective when started with 1-2 hours of exposure and is probably not effective when started later than 24-36 hours after exposure.

- What is the frequency of this type of exposure? Antiretroviral treatment should not be used for repeated exposures.

Potential benefits must be weighed against the risks of drug toxicity, the difficulty of compliance with the regimen, and the potential for individuals at risk to abandon more effective prevention strategies. Because post exposure is an experimental therapy of unproven efficacy, it should only be prescribed with the informed consent of the patient, after explanation of the potential benefits and risks. Antiretroviral therapy should never be used routinely and should not be used when there is a low risk of transmission or when people seek care too late to anticipate an interruption in transmission.

The report also requests that physicians notify CDC of all cases in which postexposure therapy is prescribed for non-occupational exposures. Data collected through the CDC reporting system on the utilization, effectiveness, and toxicity of this therapy may provide the information needed to refine future recommendations.

Primary conclusions of the report include:

- Physicians and individuals at risk for HIV infection should remember that the most effective methods for preventing HIV remain those that prevent exposure to HIV in the first place. Attempting to prevent HIV infection by taking postexposure antiretroviral therapy should never take the place of adopting and maintaining behaviors that prevent HIV exposure. These include sexual abstinence, having sex only with an uninfected partner, consistent condom use, abstinence from injection drug use, and consistent use of clean equipment for those who are unable to cease injection drug use.

- There are no human data on the effectiveness of postexposure therapy in reducing HIV infection following sexual or drug-related exposures. While some animal studies suggest potential benefits of its use, it is not known how applicable these data are for humans.

- We do know that the therapy is not 100% effective. Even under ideal circumstances following an occupational exposure in a health care setting, where treatment is typically started within hours and can be closely monitored, infection has occurred despite therapy.

- There is no such thing as a morning after pill to prevent HIV infection. Postexposure antiretroviral therapy involves multiple drugs, taken several times a day, for at least 30 days. This is an extremely difficult and expensive regimen which can have severe side effects and costs $600 to $1000.

- Adherence to the regimen is critical, both to provide the best chance of effectiveness and to prevent the emergence of drug-resistant HIV. Several studies indicate that adherence to this lengthy regimen is difficult. Among rape victims in New York City, for example, only 16% of patients are known to have completed the regimen as prescribed. Among health care workers in the United States, just over 60% complete the regimen. Many report stopping the regimen because of side effects.

- If individuals at risk rely on this less effective strategy instead of maintaining consistently safe behaviors, they may be placing themselves in significant danger. Postexposure therapy should never be considered a form of primary HIV prevention.

Chapter 56

Prevention among Men Who Have Sex with Men

In the United States, HIV-related illness and death historically have had a tremendous impact on men who have sex with men (MSM). Even though the toll of the epidemic among injection drug users (IDUs) and heterosexuals has increased during the last decade, MSM continue to account for the largest number of people reported with AIDS each year. In 2000 alone, 13,562 AIDS cases were reported among MSM, compared with 8,531 among IDUs and 6,530 among men and women who acquired HIV heterosexually.

Overall, the number of MSM of all races and ethnicities who are living with AIDS has increased steadily, partly as a result of the 1993 expanded AIDS case definition and, more recently, of improved survival.

Continuing Risk among Young MSM

Abundant evidence shows a need to sustain prevention efforts for each generation of young gay and bisexual men. We cannot assume that the positive attitudinal and behavioral change seen among older men also applies to younger men. Recent data on HIV prevalence and risk behaviors suggest that young gay and bisexual men continue to

---

"Need for Sustained HIV Prevention among Men Who Have Sex with Men," National Center for HIV, STD and TB Prevention, Centers for Disease Control and Prevention (CDC), updated March 11, 2002; available online at http://www.cdc.gov/hiv/pubs/facts/msm.htm.

place themselves at considerable risk for HIV infection and other sexually transmitted diseases (STDs).

Ongoing studies show that both HIV prevalence ratio (the proportion of people living with HIV in a population) and prevalence of risk behaviors remain high among some young MSM. In a sample of MSM 15-22 years old in seven urban areas, CDC researchers found that, overall, 7% already were infected with HIV. Higher percentages of African Americans (14%) and Hispanics (7%) were infected than were whites (3%).

In the 34 areas with confidential HIV reporting, data show that substantial numbers of MSM still are being infected, especially young men. In 2000, 59% of reported HIV infections among adolescent males aged 13-19 and 53% of cases among men aged 20-24 were attributed to male-to-male sexual contact.

Research among gay and bisexual men suggests that some individuals are now less concerned about becoming infected than in the past and may be inclined to take more risks. This is backed up by reported increases in gonorrhea among gay men in several large U.S. cities between 1993 and 1996. Despite medical advances, HIV infection remains a serious, usually fatal disease that requires complex, costly, and difficult treatment regimens that do not work for everyone. As better treatment options are developed, we must not lose sight of the fact that preventing HIV infection in the first place precludes the need for people to undergo these difficult and expensive therapies.

These data highlight the need to design more effective prevention efforts for gay and bisexual men of color. The involvement of community and opinion leaders in prevention efforts will be critical for overcoming cultural barriers to prevention, including homophobia. For example, there remains a tremendous stigma to acknowledging gay and bisexual activity in African American and Hispanic communities.

Need to Combat Other STDs

Studies among MSM who are treated in STD clinics have shown consistently high percentages of HIV infection, ranging from nearly 4% in Seattle to a high of almost 36% in Atlanta. Some studies have shown that the likelihood of both acquiring and spreading HIV is 2-5 times greater in people with STDs, and that aggressively treating STDs in a community may help to reduce the rate of new HIV infections. Along with prompt attention to and treatment of STDs, efforts to reduce the behaviors that spread STDs are critical.

Prevention Services Must Reach Both Uninfected and Infected

Research has shown that high-risk behavior is continuing in some populations of MSM, including those who are infected with HIV. Because HIV-infected gay and bisexual men are living longer and healthier lives, greater efforts must be made to reach them with behavioral interventions that can help them protect their own health and prevent transmission to others.

Chapter 57

Prevention among Women Who Have Sex with Women

Female-to-female transmission of HIV appears to be a rare occurrence. However, case reports of female-to-female transmission of HIV and the well documented risk of female-to-male transmission of HIV indicate that vaginal secretions and menstrual blood are potentially infectious and that mucous membrane (e.g., oral, vaginal) exposure to these secretions have the potential to lead to HIV infection.

What do surveillance tools tell us about transmission between women?

Through December 1998, 109,311 women were reported with AIDS. Of these, 2,220 were reported to have had sex with women; however, the vast majority had other risks (such as injection drug use, sex with high-risk men, or receipt of blood or blood products). Of the 347 (out of 2,220) women who were reported to have had sex only with women, 98% also had another risk—injection drug use in most cases.

Note: information on whether a woman had sex with women is missing in half of the 109,311 case reports, possibly because the physician did not elicit the information or the woman did not volunteer it.

"HIV/AIDS and U.S. Women Who Have Sex with Women (WSW)," National Center for HIV, STD and TB Prevention, Centers for Disease Control and Prevention (CDC), updated August 1999; available online at http://www.cdc.gov/hiv/pubs/facts/wsw.htm.

What do investigations of female-to-female transmission show?

Women with AIDS whose only reported risk initially is sex with women are given high priority for follow-up investigation. As of December 1998, none of these investigations had confirmed female-to-female HIV transmission, either because other risks were subsequently identified or because, in a few cases, women declined to be interviewed. A separate study of more than 1 million female blood donors found no HIV-infected women whose only risk was sex with women. These findings suggest that female-to-female transmission of HIV is uncommon. However, they do not negate the possibility because it could be masked by other behaviors.

What are the behaviors that place WSW at risk of HIV infection?

Surveys of risk behaviors have been conducted in groups of WSW. These surveys have generally been surveys of convenient samples of WSW that differ in sampling, location, and definition of WSW. As a result, their findings are not generalizable to all populations of WSW. These surveys suggest that some groups of WSW have relatively high rates of high-risk behaviors, such as injection drug use and unprotected vaginal sex with gay/bisexual men and injection drug users.

What can WSW do to reduce their risk of contracting HIV?

Although female-to-female transmission of HIV apparently is rare, female sexual contact should be considered a possible means of transmission among WSW. These women need to know:

- that exposure of a mucous membrane, such as the mouth, (especially non-intact tissue) to vaginal secretions and menstrual blood is potentially infectious, particularly during early and late-stage HIV infection when the amount of virus in the blood is expected to be highest.

- that condoms should be used consistently and correctly each and every time for sexual contact with men or when using sex toys. Sex toys should not be shared. No barrier methods for use during oral sex have been evaluated as effective or approved by the FDA. However, women can use dental dams, cut-open condoms, or plastic wrap to help protect themselves from contact with body fluids during oral sex.

- their own and their partner's HIV status. This knowledge can help uninfected women begin and maintain behavioral changes that reduce their risk of becoming infected. For women who are found to be infected, it can assist in getting early treatment and avoiding infecting others.

Health professionals also need to remember:

- that sexual identity does not necessarily predict behavior, and that women who identify as lesbian may be at risk for HIV through unprotected sex with men.

- that prevention interventions targeting WSW must address behaviors that put WSW at risk for HIV infection, including injection drug use and unprotected vaginal-penile intercourse.

Chapter 58

Condom Use and HIV Prevention

What do condoms have in common with toothpaste and toilet paper? Not enough, according to Adam Glickman, owner of the Condomania stores in New York and Los Angeles. Glickman, who has sold condoms by the millions to individuals and organizations such as the Peace Corps and Planned Parenthood, says condoms should be viewed as ordinary, like toothpaste and toilet paper. "People have gotten past asking, 'Isn't brushing my teeth every morning a hassle?' Given the world we live in, wearing condoms is something you just have to do, like brushing your teeth. The stakes are too high."

Luis Lopez knows first-hand what's at stake. About 10 years ago, Lopez, now 31 and a health educator with the People with AIDS Coalition of New York, became infected with the HIV virus, which causes AIDS, during a casual sexual encounter. "I thought people with AIDS had purple spots or looked really skinny," Lopez says. "I thought by being discriminating about who I slept with, I could keep myself safe. We know now that makes no sense."

We know now that abstaining from sex is the only foolproof protection from the sexual passage of HIV and other sexually transmitted diseases (STDs). We know, too, that for those who choose to have sex with someone who has any chance of being infected, using a latex condom during every sexual encounter can significantly reduce

"Condoms: Barriers to Bad News," by Tamar Nordenberg, U.S. Food and Drug Administration (FDA), *FDA Consumer* magazine, March-April 1998, updated May 2001.

the risk of HIV and other sexually transmitted diseases, while protecting against pregnancy.

For those who can't or won't use latex condoms, the Food and Drug Administration has cleared two alternative barrier methods of birth control, a male condom made of polyurethane and a condom that is worn by the woman. Both help protect against pregnancy and may provide some level of protection from STDs.

Life-Saving Barrier

A male condom, sometimes called a rubber or prophylactic, is a sheath that fits snugly over a man's erect penis, with a closed end to catch the sperm and stop them from entering the woman's vagina. No prescription is needed to buy a condom.

Data show that if a condom is used correctly with every act of sexual intercourse for one year, about three out of every 100 women are expected to get pregnant.

Besides sperm, latex condoms act as a barrier to a wide variety of viruses, bacteria, and other infectious particles. By preventing contact with many sores and minimizing the exchange of infectious fluids, condoms can help prevent the transmission of sexually transmitted diseases, including HIV, gonorrhea, chlamydia, syphilis, herpes infection, and genital ulcers. Even though sperm are enormous compared to HIV, both are much too small to see. But even HIV, which is among the tiniest of STD organisms, cannot pass through a latex condom.

Millions of Americans are infected with these diseases each year, and hundreds of thousands of them become seriously ill or die as a result. According to the Centers for Disease Control and Prevention, in the United States, someone is infected with HIV every 13 minutes. CDC estimates that 65 percent of these AIDS cases can be attributed to sexual contact.

The best protection from such diseases is to not have sex or to have a mutually monogamous relationship with someone who is known to be uninfected. However, for those who are sexually active, studies have shown that proper and consistent use of latex condoms is the best defense.

A 1994 European study published in the *New England Journal of Medicine* looked at HIV transmission rates of heterosexual couples with one HIV-infected partner. The study compared the transmission rates for couples who used condoms consistently to those who didn't. Of the 123 couples who consistently used condoms, none of the HIV-free partners became infected during the study, whereas 12 of the 122

412

partners who didn't consistently use condoms became infected. "The scientific evidence is compelling," says Herbert Peterson, M.D., chief of CDC's women's health and fertility branch. "We're not guessing about this."

The spermicide nonoxynol-9, used in some condoms, has been shown to be effective as a contraceptive, and may reduce the risk of transmitting certain STDs. But the spermicide has not been proven to prevent sexual transmission of HIV.

Similarly, lambskin (or natural membrane) condoms, while effective for contraception, should not be used for disease protection because the naturally occurring pores in lambskin are large enough to allow some viruses to pass through.

Hole Check

Since 1976, FDA has regulated condoms to ensure their safety and effectiveness. Currently, manufacturers of American-made and imported condoms electronically test each condom for holes and other defects. Also, before distributing the condoms to retailers, manufacturers perform additional testing on random condoms from each batch, usually involving a water leak test to find holes and an air burst test to check condom strength.

FDA oversees the testing procedures by periodically inspecting the manufacturing facilities, and the agency tests some condoms in its own laboratories to confirm their quality.

Condoms are sold in various colors, shapes or packaging to suit different personal preferences. But, whether they glow in the dark or taste like strawberries, products that sufficiently resemble a condom must comply with FDA's requirements, even if they are labeled as novelties. The only condom-like products that need not comply are those that can't be used like condoms. For example, some novelty products have the closed end removed or are sealed so they can't be unrolled.

Correct and Consistent

Although condoms are generally expected to break less than 2 percent of the time—with more than half of the breakages occurring before ejaculation—real-life pregnancy rates over a year of condom use may be as high as 15 percent.

Inconsistent or incorrect use of condoms explains the discrepancy, according to Lillian Yin, director of the division in FDA that regulates condoms and other reproductive devices. One national survey of heterosexual adults with multiple sex partners found that only 17 percent used a condom every time they had sex.

"People say they use condoms," Yin says, "but do they use them each and every time and use them correctly? That's another ballgame. We hear it all the time—'We tried to use it, but ....'" But what? Partner trust was the most-cited reason for not wearing condoms in a recent study sponsored by the National Institutes of Health. But be careful, CDC cautions, because even a trustworthy partner could unknowingly have a sexually transmitted disease.

Many participants in the NIH study said they didn't always wear a condom because sex feels better without them. Lopez responds, "If you don't use them, you run the risk of something that feels much worse."

Sometimes a couple can't use a latex condom because one partner is allergic to latex. For these people, FDA has approved condoms made from polyurethane.

If a man objects to wearing a condom for some other reason, Planned Parenthood suggests possible replies. For example, to the partner who says, "I guess you don't really love me," the organization suggests responding, "I do, but I'm not risking my future to prove it." If the man still chooses not to wear a condom, the Reality female condom cleared by FDA in 1993 offers an alternative.

Using condoms consistently is a start, but using them correctly is another key to protecting oneself. User error, not poor condom quality, leads to most breakages. But a few simple rules can minimize breaks and leaks.

Even when used correctly, condoms aren't perfect, CDC acknowledges, comparing them to other important safety-enhancing behaviors like wearing seatbelts and bicycle helmets. Imperfect as they are, condoms can significantly reduce the rates of unintended pregnancies and sexually transmitted diseases.

"Correct and consistent condom use," says CDC's Peterson, "could break the back of the AIDS epidemic."

Handle with Care

To get the maximum protection against pregnancy and sexually transmitted diseases, remember the following things when using condoms:

- Store condoms in a cool, dry place out of direct sunlight. Don't make the common mistake of storing them in a glove compartment, wallet or purse.

- Don't use a condom if the package is damaged or the rubber material is sticky, brittle, discolored, or otherwise deteriorated. Don't use a condom after the expiration date or more than five years after the manufacturing date.

- Never reuse a condom. Use a new condom with each sexual act that involves contact with the penis.

- Handle a condom carefully to avoid damaging it with fingernails, teeth, or other sharp objects.

- Put on the condom after the penis is erect and before intimate contact. Place the condom on the head of the penis and unroll it all the way to the base. Leave an empty space at the end of the condom to collect semen. Remove any air remaining in the tip by gently pressing the air out toward the base of the penis.

- Ensure adequate lubrication during intercourse. When needed with latex condoms, use only water-based lubricants such as K-Y jelly or glycerin. Don't use oil-based lubricants such as baby oil, petroleum jelly, massage oil, body lotion, or cooking oil because they can weaken the latex. Oil-based lubricants may be used with polyurethane, however, without damaging the material.

- After ejaculation, hold onto the rim of the condom and carefully withdraw the penis while it is still erect.

For the Female

The pouch-shaped Reality female condom enables women to protect themselves against pregnancy and AIDS and other sexually transmitted diseases.

The female condom is made from polyurethane and, like the male condom, is a nonprescription barrier method of birth control. The device has a closed end that is inserted deep inside the vagina to catch the sperm and an open end that remains outside the body. A female condom should not be used with a male condom because the devices will not stay in place.

Over the course of a year, between 5 percent and 21 percent of women who use the female condom are expected to get pregnant, depending on whether the condom is used correctly with every act of vaginal intercourse. The female condom also provides some level of protection against STDs.

As with other condoms, follow label directions carefully to ensure that the material is not deteriorated or torn.

Chapter 59

Centers for Disease Control and Prevention (CDC) HIV/ AIDS Prevention Activities

As a part of its overall public health mission, CDC provides national leadership in helping control the HIV epidemic by working with community, state, national, and international partners in surveillance, research, prevention and evaluation activities. These activities are critically important, as CDC estimates that between 800,000 and 900,000 Americans currently are living with HIV. Also, the number of people living with AIDS is increasing, as effective new drug therapies are keeping HIV-infected persons healthy longer and dramatically reducing the death rate.

What is CDC's HIV/AIDS prevention strategy?

CDC employs a comprehensive approach to preventing further spread of HIV and AIDS. Strategies include monitoring the epidemic to target prevention and care activities, researching the effectiveness of prevention methods, funding local prevention efforts for high-risk communities, and fostering linkages with care and treatment programs. CDC is working in collaboration with many other governmental and nongovernmental partners at all levels to implement, evaluate,

"CDC's HIV/AIDS Prevention Activities," National Center for HIV, STD and TB Prevention (NCHSTP), Centers for Disease Control and Prevention (CDC), updated April 2, 2002, available online at http://www.cdc.gov/hiv/pubs/ facts/cdcprev.htm; and, "CDC's International Activities Support Global HIV Prevention Efforts," NCHSTP, CDC, March 2001, available online at http:// www.cdc/gov/hiv/pubs/facts/intrnatl.htm.

and further develop and strengthen effective HIV prevention efforts nationwide. CDC also is providing financial and technical support for disease surveillance; HIV antibody counseling, testing, and referral services; partner counseling and referral services; street and community outreach; risk-reduction counseling; prevention case management; prevention and treatment of other sexually transmitted diseases that can increase risks for HIV transmission; public information and education; school-based education on AIDS; international research studies; technology transfer systems; organizational capacity building; and program-relevant epidemiologic, socio-behavioral, and evaluation research.

How are CDC funds distributed?

In fiscal year 2001, nearly 80 percent of CDC's HIV prevention funds were distributed externally through cooperative agreements, grants, and contracts, primarily to state and local agencies. The largest portion of CDC's HIV prevention resources is awarded to state, local, and territorial health departments. Some of these funds support more than 200 local and regional HIV Prevention Community Planning groups.

How are prevention activities organized?

The National Center for HIV, STD and TB Prevention, Division of HIV/AIDS Prevention: The Division of HIV/AIDS Prevention is the primary division charged with CDC's HIV mission of preventing HIV infection and reducing the incidence of HIV-related illness and death, in collaboration with community, state, and national partners. Its nine branches oversee a variety of activities in support of this mission.

The Behavioral Intervention Research Branch applies current theory, practice, and empirical findings in designing and conducting research on state-of-the-art interventions to prevent HIV infection. Characteristics of the research include the use of formative studies to develop interventions, such as the examination of psychosocial and cultural determinants of risk behaviors, the collection and analysis of process and outcome data that includes both qualitative and quantitative measures, and the use of rigorous study designs to examine intervention effectiveness. Further, branch staff members assist in translating and replicating research findings for use in HIV prevention programs.

The Program Prevention Branch works with State and local public health departments, nongovernmental national/regional and local partners, and others to develop and implement programs, policies, and activities that mobilize affiliates and communities to become involved with and support local and statewide HIV prevention programs and activities. It plans, implements, and manages strategies and resources for HIV prevention in State and local health departments, community-based organizations, and other nongovernmental organizations to build comprehensive public health/private sector partnerships to prevent HIV/AIDS; provides technical consultation and program oversight to State and local health departments, community planning groups, and nongovernmental partners in operational aspects of HIV prevention; establishes guidelines and policies for implementation and continuation of State and local HIV prevention programs; and develops new operational programs and program announcements for HIV prevention.

The Program Evaluation Research Branch evaluates the processes, outcomes, and impacts of CDC HIV prevention programs, activities, and policies for their improvement and accountability; develops and enhances evaluation methods and systems; and serves as a resource for building evaluation capacity.

The Technical Information and Communications Branch uses both electronic media and printed materials to communicate scientific, statistical, programmatic, and technical information on HIV/AIDS to health care professionals, public health officials, prevention partners, federal government officials, and the general public.

The Capacity Building Branch assists providers in enhancing the capacity of individuals, organizations, and communities to conduct more effective and efficient HIV and AIDS prevention services.

The Epidemiology Branch's mission is to conduct biomedical and behavioral epidemiologic research to reduce HIV infection and disease progression. Accordingly, scientists in the Epidemiology Branch design and conduct studies in the United States and internationally to determine risk factors for HIV infection and disease, and to evaluate innovative biomedical and behavioral interventions in adults and children for preventing HIV infection and HIV-related disease. These studies are conducted by four research Sections including the HIV Vaccine Section, the Mother-Child Transmission & Pediatric and Adolescent Studies Section, the Clinical Epidemiology Section, and the Sexual Transmission and Injection Drug Use Studies Section. Domestically, the Epidemiology Branch is currently collaborating with partners in 25 states, and internationally is working with partners in Thailand, Côte d'Ivoire, Kenya, Botswana, Uganda, and Russia.

The Prevention Services Research Branch conducts research to develop and improve HIV prevention strategies. This includes conducting studies (1) to identify and evaluate specific at-risk populations, (2) of the determinants of risk for HIV infection in specific populations, (3) of HIV counseling and testing activities, and (4) of HIV genotypic variations and antiretroviral drug resistance. This branch also is responsible for collecting data on the extent of HIV prevalence and incidence in the United States, for assisting other Centers within CDC to evaluate new HIV-related tests, and for maintaining a repository of stored sera and cells for studies of HIV infection.

The Statistics and Data Management Branch provides statistical support, software systems design, and data management support for HIV/AIDS surveillance, HIV serosurveys, epidemiologic studies, and other studies conducted within the division; develops methods and coordinates efforts by statisticians to estimate the incidence of HIV infection; participates in the design, data analysis, and manuscript preparation for epidemiologic and behavioral studies and clinical trials; and conducts data analyses required by law for the allocation of HIV/AIDS prevention and treatment funds. The branch also provides national leadership in the development of statistical and data management planning, policy, implementation, and evaluation.

The Surveillance Branch conducts a national program of surveillance and research to monitor and characterize the HIV/AIDS epidemic, and its determinants and impact, to guide public health action at federal, state, and local levels. This includes surveillance of HIV infection and AIDS in collaboration with State and local health departments to provide population-based data for research, evaluation, and prevention at the National, State, and local levels. The branch maintains, analyzes, and disseminates information from the national confidential registry of

HIV/AIDS cases; monitors HIV-related morbidity and mortality and the use of PHS recommendations for prevention and treatment of HIV infection and AIDS; and conducts population-based surveillance of HIV-related risk behaviors in collaboration with state and local health departments.

The National Center for HIV, STD and TB Prevention Global AIDS Program: The Global AIDS Program (GAP) exists to help prevent HIV infection, improve care and support and build capacity to address the global HIV/AIDS pandemic. GAP provides financial and technical assistance through partnerships with communities, governments, and national and international entities working in resource-constrained countries.

What other CDC offices conduct HIV prevention activities?

Additional HIV prevention, education, and research programs are conducted in other CDC centers, institutes, and offices.

The National Center for Infectious Diseases (NCID)

NCID's Division of AIDS, STD, and TB Laboratory Research provides laboratory research on HIV and laboratory support for the surveillance, epidemiologic, and clinical activities of NCHSTP. It also conducts laboratory and epidemiologic studies of HIV-infected and uninfected persons with hemophilia and assists in the design, implementation, and evaluation of prevention and counseling programs for them and their families.

The Division of Healthcare Quality Promotion, also located in NCID, assists the U.S. Public Health Service, state and local health departments, hospitals, and professional organizations worldwide in the prevention and control of nosocomially acquired HIV infection.

The National Center for Chronic Disease Prevention and Health Promotion (NCCDPHP)

The Division of Adolescent and School Health, NCCDPHP, provides support to national, state, and local education agencies and other organizations with the capacity to address adolescent health to assist them in identifying and preventing HIV risk behaviors among youth.

NCCDPHP's Division of Reproductive Health conducts epidemiologic, applied behavioral, and operations research on the prevention of HIV in women at risk for both HIV and unintended pregnancy.

421

The National Center for Environmental Health's Clinical Biochemistry Branch

This branch operates a multicomponent quality assurance program for laboratories testing dried blood spots for HIV antibodies, provides method development and analytical services for the measurement of zidovudine and other antiretroviral drugs in epidemiological studies, and provides consultative services for emerging concerns in laboratory quality assurance.

The National Center for Health Statistics

This branch collects HIV/AIDS-related data in many of its data systems, including HIV-related deaths from the National Vital Statistics System, use of health services from the National Health Care Surveys, and data on HIV-related knowledge and HIV testing behaviors from the National Health Interview Survey and the periodic National Survey of Family Growth.

The National Institute for Occupational Safety and Health

The activity of this branch focuses on developing, implementing, and evaluating strategies for the prevention of occupational transmission of HIV, with special emphasis on personal protective equipment, engineering controls, and evaluation of organizational and behavioral factors that influence prevention strategies.

The Public Health Practice Program Office

This branch strengthens the community practice of HIV/AIDS prevention by developing and delivering training, improving the quality of clinical laboratory testing, developing computing and telecommunications tools, and conducting research into effective public health practice.

CDC's International Activities Support Global HIV Prevention Efforts

The Centers for Disease Control and Prevention's (CDC) research program is dedicated to advancing biomedical and behavioral science that promotes HIV/AIDS prevention in the United States and worldwide. The focus is on research, technical assistance, and training aimed at understanding the dynamics of HIV transmission and on developing and improving prevention technologies and strategies to control the spread of HIV/AIDS and minimize its consequences.

The World Health Organization (WHO) and the Joint United Nations Program on HIV/AIDS (UNAIDS) estimate that, worldwide, as many as 42 million people have been infected with HIV since the pandemic's onset, and each day 16,000 more become infected. Recognizing the urgency of the pandemic, CDC is committed to HIV/AIDS research within, as well as outside of, U.S. borders. To understand AIDS on a global level, research must address issues and conditions unique to different countries and to communities within countries. Many developing nations severely affected by the epidemic lack the research capacity, public health infrastructure, and financial and human resources to respond effectively. CDC's international work underscores the importance of developing, implementing, and evaluating diverse interventions to address issues among varied populations and to do so quickly and cost-effectively.

Collaborative Efforts Yield Prevention Benefits

Through collaborative agreements with governments of Côte d'Ivoire (Project RETRO-CI), Thailand (HIV/AIDS Collaboration), and Uganda, as well as in multiple other settings, CDC supports HIV/AIDS research field stations and participates in studies designed to increase our understanding of the epidemiology of HIV-1 and HIV-2 infections and to facilitate prevention and care efforts in the host countries and the United States. Specific research areas include the following:

- Reducing mother-to-child (perinatal) HIV transmission in developing countries around the world, where 1,600 babies are born with HIV or infected through breast-feeding each day. Collaborative research by CDC, the Thai Ministry of Public Health, and Mahidol University demonstrated that a short course of zidovudine (also known as AZT) given late in pregnancy and during delivery reduced the rate of HIV transmission to infants of infected mothers by half in the absence of breast-feeding and is safe for use in the developing world. A one-third reduction in early transmission was found with the same regimen in a breast-feeding population in Abidjan. The findings offer real hope to many developing nations that previously had no realistic options for preventing HIV-infected pregnant women from transmitting infection to their babies. CDC is now working with host countries and public health agencies worldwide (including the U.N. International

Children's Emergency Fund, UNAIDS, WHO) to help implement the short-course AZT regimen as widely as possible and to examine even newer interventions, such as single dose treatment with nevirapine. Researchers also continue to study other factors of mother-to-child HIV transmission for example, breast-feeding's role in HIV transmission in developing countries, where breast-feeding is an important source of nutrition for newborns, and the benefit and feasibility of replacement feeding or early weaning for infants of HIV-infected mothers in different settings.

- Developing effective interventions for high-risk populations in Côte d'Ivoire and Thailand. Researchers have collaborated with host countries to implement and evaluate HIV prevention interventions among injection drug users, female sex workers, and other populations at risk to provide them with the knowledge and support needed to protect themselves from HIV infection. Many of these interventions have proven effective, particularly programs to increase condom use and treat sexually transmitted diseases among female sex workers.

- Identifying possible factors that may confer immunity to HIV. Collaborating researchers from CDC and the Thai and Ivorian Ministries of Public Health are working to determine how certain groups of female sex workers have remained uninfected despite numerous exposures to HIV. Initial research looked at possible genetic characteristics that might lead to immunity in certain individuals, and current research focuses on the role the immune response to HIV may play in protection from infection. Researchers believe this research could have important implications for the future development of an HIV vaccine.

- Working to reduce the impact of HIV/AIDS in developing countries through practical treatment regimens. A joint study by CDC and Côte d'Ivoire's Ministry of Public Health found the first evidence that trimethoprim/sulfamethoxazole (TMP/SMX) (commonly referred to as otrimoxazole, Bactrim, or Septra) can significantly reduce the rate of death among HIV-infected tuberculosis patients in Africa. Data from the study demonstrated a 48% reduction in mortality and a 44% reduction in hospitalizations among HIV-infected tuberculosis patients who took TMP/SMX in addition to TB medication. These dramatic findings offer a realistic option to help reduce the overwhelming death toll from HIV in the developing world.

- Conducting genetic analyses and collecting surveillance data on genetic variations and drug resistance of HIV strains in host countries. Because of the increasing spread of HIV subtypes across international borders, these data may have implications for developing HIV vaccines and for promptly detecting and treating different HIV strains worldwide.

- Gathering surveillance data on HIV/AIDS trends among sentinel groups such as female sex workers, pregnant women, STD patients, injection drug users, and children to use in targeting, developing, and evaluating new interventions.

- Evaluating how to improve survival and quality of care for HIV-infected people, thus diminishing the personal and societal costs of the epidemic.

- Investigating HIV-related diseases (for example, STDs and tuberculosis) to identify links between these illnesses and to develop effective prevention and treatment strategies that can be applied globally.

- Investigating factors associated with heterosexual transmission of HIV. Worldwide, more people have been infected through heterosexual contact than any other exposure and in the United States, heterosexual transmission accounts for a growing percentage of both HIV infections and AIDS cases. Understanding the biomedical and behavioral aspects of heterosexual transmission is the key to containing HIV in this country and around the world.

- Supporting an HIV vaccine trial in Thailand. CDC has two primary roles in an HIV vaccine trial being conducted among injection drug users in Thailand. First, through its long-standing research collaboration with Thailand, CDC has been working for several years to help Thai health officials prepare to implement vaccine studies. Since 1995, CDC has assisted in measuring the level of new infections in Thailand, identifying a group of individuals who are willing to participate in a trial and can be followed over time to evaluate risk behaviors and infection, and working with the community to build the understanding and support necessary to implement the trial. Second, CDC has worked, and will continue to work, with Thai health officials and the U.S. developers of the vaccine, VaxGen, to ensure that individuals in the trial receive appropriate risk-reduction counseling and are fully educated about how the trial works, the potential risks and benefits of participation, and the need for maintaining good behavioral risk-reduction practices during the trial. (CDC also is providing support for a similar efficacy trial sponsored by VaxGen in the United States.)

* Collaborating with developing countries on implementing HIV counseling and testing programs using rapid HIV testing technology. CDC assistance in the design and implementation of HIV counseling and testing programs includes (1) collaborating on the evaluation of various rapid HIV test kits to determine an appropriate testing algorithm to be used in service delivery settings, (2) assisting with the piloting of the algorithm chosen for service delivery, (3) collaborating on the development or modification of counseling protocols and guidelines used for providing same-day HIV test results, and (4) providing assistance with the development of HIV counselor training materials and courses.

Chapter 60

HIV/AIDS Research: Successes Bring New Challenges

Even as we approach the third decade of the HIV/AIDS epidemic, HIV is still considered a new and complex disease for which there is no cure. As such, it presents unique challenges for research. In recent testimony before Congress, the Director of the Office of AIDS Research at the National Institutes of Health called HIV the "great plague of the 20th century—an epidemic of biblical proportions."[1]

According to the World Health Organization, 16.3 million men, women, and children with AIDS have died since the AIDS pandemic began in the early 1980s—including more than 420,000 American men, women, and children. AIDS has now surpassed tuberculosis and malaria as the leading infectious cause of death worldwide. In 1999 alone, a record 2.6 million people died from AIDS.[2,3] Given the continuing impact of the epidemic in the U.S. and around the world, there remains a critical need for HIV research to continue to identify ways to prevent and treat HIV infection.

What Is the Focus of HIV/AIDS Research?

HIV/AIDS research consists of a multitude of activities that focus on basic and clinical science to understand and treat HIV infection and its related conditions; prevention science to track and prevent the spread of HIV, understand the behaviors that put people at risk for

From *Capitol Hill Briefing Series on HIV/AIDS,* June 2000, © 2000 Henry J. Kaiser Family Foundation; reprinted with permission. Available online at http://www.kff.org/content/2000/1600/research.pdf.

HIV infection, and develop interventions to change these behaviors; and health services research to address the nexus between scientific research and the application of that research into health care services.

Basic Research: Explores the body's immune system, the molecular structure of the human immunodeficiency virus (HIV) that causes AIDS, and the ways in which the virus attacks the human body.

Clinical Research: Examines the impact of HIV on the human body and helps to identify the various medical conditions that affect people living with HIV/AIDS. Clinical research includes research conducted through clinical trials.

Epidemiologic Research: Studies the distribution and control of HIV/AIDS within populations, population subgroups and communities. Epidemiologic research includes the study of HIV and AIDS incidence (current rate or number of new cases) and prevalence (proportion or number of people living with HIV or AIDS at a particular point in time).

Behavioral and Social Science Research: Investigates ways to understand and change behaviors that may lead to HIV infection (e.g., unprotected sexual intercourse and the use of HIV-contaminated injection drug equipment) as well as the factors that may lead to such behaviors (e.g., low self-esteem, poverty, and complacency).

Health Services Research: Addresses such issues as cost, access, quality, and outcomes of services and care, including disparities in access across different population groups.

Who Conducts HIV/AIDS Research?

HIV/AIDS research is conducted by government research agencies, private industry, including pharmaceutical companies, and academic research centers and other institutions and organizations. In the U.S., most HIV/AIDS research is sponsored by the Federal government, primarily by the National Institutes of Health (NIH). Federal HIV/AIDS research also is conducted and supported by the Department of Veterans Affairs (the largest direct provider of HIV care services), the Department of Defense, the Food and Drug Administration, the Centers for Disease Control and Prevention (which focuses primarily on prevention and epidemiological research), and the Agency for

Healthcare Research and Quality (which focuses on health services research). Other Department of Health and Human Services agencies also conduct some health services research on HIV/AIDS.

The Office of AIDS Research (OAR), created in 1988, directs the scientific, budgetary, legislative, and policy elements of the NIH AIDS research program. In 1993, Congress enacted the NIH Revitalization Act (P.L.103-43), which created a permanent OAR, an OAR Advisory Council (composed of 18 non-government experts), and a full-time OAR Director.

Under the statute, OAR is required to develop an annual comprehensive plan and budget for all NIH-supported HIV/AIDS research. HIV/AIDS research at the NIH is conducted both through the NIH's intramural research program and through its extramural grants programs to researchers in academic settings around the country.[4] While all of NIH's 25 Institutes and Centers (ICs) conduct or support HIV/AIDS research, most of the work is led by 7 IC's.

Private industry, including pharmaceutical and biotechnology companies, have also played an important role in converting scientific advances into the development of effective treatments for HIV infection and the various conditions that affect people living with HIV/AIDS. A total of 75 pharmaceutical and biotechnology companies are involved in HIV/AIDS research and, as of December 1999, 61 AIDS-related medicines had been approved for sale in the U.S. A 1999 drug industry survey indicated that 102 medicines were in development for AIDS and AIDS-related conditions including an anti-HIV fusion inhibitor, 11 preventive vaccines, a new protease inhibitor designed to overcome resistance, and a gene therapy that infuses healthy CD4 cells into a person with AIDS.[7]

Finally, academic institutions are a major source of HIV/AIDS research and treatment. Medical schools and their affiliated teaching hospitals perform more than 50% of all NIH-supported research in the U.S.[8] and provide a disproportionate share of AIDS care in the U.S. Because of their expertise, NIH has entered into agreements with numerous academic health centers to house and conduct ongoing HIV-related basic, clinical, and prevention research around the country, including some of the major national and international clinical trial networks.

How Much Is Spent on Federal HIV/AIDS Research?

In fiscal year (FY) 1999, federal spending on HIV/AIDS research totaled $1.9 billion across the federal agencies. Research comprised

19% of the $9.7 billion in total federal spending on AIDS-related programs in that year. Most federal HIV/AIDS research spending is for activities conducted and sponsored by the NIH, which totaled $1.8 billion in FY 1999 and $2 billion in FY 2000.[4,9] Approximately 68% of HIV/AIDS research funding at NIH is spent on basic and clinical research; 26% is spent on prevention research, including vaccine research (12%). The remainder is spent on training and information dissemination.[10]

In the early years of the epidemic, increases in HIV/AIDS research funding were larger in size as the research enterprise ramped up to confront a new, emerging infectious disease. More recently, however, increases in NIH spending on HIV/AIDS research have lagged slightly behind the overall increases in the NIH budget. For example, between FY 1999 and FY 2000, spending on HIV/AIDS research increased 11% compared with a 14% increase in the overall NIH budget.[4,11]

What Is the Role of Clinical Trials?

A major component of clinical research is the process of testing and evaluating the safety and effectiveness of potential treatments. Such trials are funded by NIH, FDA, pharmaceutical companies, and others. They are conducted in a variety of settings including universities, clinics, and individual physicians' offices. While the primary aim of clinical trials is to determine which treatments work for which people, these trials are also a source of free or low-cost care for patients who are enrolled in them. In fact, in some cases, patients are paid for their participation. Generally speaking, before being approved by the FDA for sale in the U.S., medications must go through three stages of clinical trials12:

- Phase I trials seek to determine the safe dosage levels for a treatment being tested. Such trials usually have 10 to 20 patients enrolled.

- Phase II trials seek to determine the safety and effectiveness of the treatment with as many as several hundred patients enrolled.

- Phase III trials seek to determine the long-term benefits of the treatment with as many as several thousand patients enrolled.

NIH sponsors a series of extramural AIDS clinical trials networks including the Adult AIDS Clinical Trials Group, the Pediatric AIDS Clinical Trials Group, the Strategic Program for Innovative Research on AIDS, and the Terry Beirn Community Programs for Clinical Research on AIDS, which is based in primary care settings.

What Role Do Community-Based Groups and People with HIV/AIDS Play in HIV/AIDS Research?

People with HIV/AIDS and the community-based organizations that serve them have played an essential role in research. Community-based trial groups provided some of the early tests of AIDS drugs. AIDS activism has led to dramatic changes in public and private responses to AIDS, including speeding up the drug review and approval process at the Food and Drug Administration, increasing participation of women and minorities in clinical trials, and greater accountability among research institutions. People with HIV now are incorporated into the research and drug development process and provide valuable input into the design of clinical studies, the implementation of research programs, and the setting of research priorities.

How Are Women and Minority Americans Involved in HIV/AIDS Research?

Because women and minority Americans represent a significant portion of people living with HIV/AIDS, new AIDS cases, and new HIV infections, their involvement in HIV/AIDS research is critical. Yet, in the earlier years of the epidemic, women and minorities often were left out of many research trials and protocols, resulting in a lack of clinical data about the impact of HIV and HIV-related treatments on these populations.

The NIH Revitalization Act (P.L.103-43) required NIH and other research agencies to expand the involvement of women and minority Americans in all research. In 1994, NIH implemented Guidelines requiring applicants for NIH grants to address "the appropriate inclusion of women and minorities in clinical research."[13] The amount of NIH AIDS research funds spent on research focused on minority Americans has increased from $266 million in FY 1996 to $323 million in FY 1999.

According to the NIH, 63% of enrollees in NIH-sponsored AIDS clinical trials, underway in December 1997, were minority Americans.[13] NIH has increased its focus on women and HIV through efforts that include the Women's Interagency HIV Study, which investigates the nature and rate of disease progression in women, and the Women and Infants Transmission Study, which evaluates factors associated with perinatal (mother to fetus) HIV transmission.

According to NIH, women represented 34% of participants in NIH-sponsored clinical trials enrolled in December 1997,[13] but criticism about the inclusion of minorities and women in clinical trials still remains.[14]

What Has HIV/AIDS Research Produced?

After nearly 18 years of effort, the nation's investment in HIV/AIDS research has resulted in numerous advances including.[15,16,17,18]

- The identification of HIV, the viral agent causing AIDS;

- The development of a test to detect the presence of antibodies to HIV in blood and other tissues;

- A doubling of the average survival time for a person living with HIV/AIDS;

- The development of drugs to treat HIV infection that reduce the impact of the virus on the human body;

- Advances in the treatment and prevention of several HIV-related diseases and infections including Pneumocystis pneumonia, CMV retinitis, and toxoplasmosis;

- The identification of barriers to access to care for people with HIV and disparities in access and outcomes for some populations;

- A dramatic reduction in the number of new HIV infections in the U.S. due to successful community and individual level prevention interventions; and

- The discovery that the use of antiretroviral drugs can dramatically reduce the risk of transmission of HIV from a pregnant woman to a fetus.

Still, there is no cure for HIV, and the potential for the development of an effective vaccine is many years away.

How Has HIV/AIDS Research Helped in Other Areas?

Beyond its direct impact on the treatment and prevention of AIDS-related conditions, HIV/AIDS research has also led to major advances in other areas of science and medicine. HIV/AIDS research is helping to unravel the mysteries surrounding many other infectious, malignant, neurologic, autoimmune and metabolic diseases. Most importantly, HIV research has significantly enhanced our understanding of the immune system and the ways in which our bodies fight against disease and infection.

HIV/AIDS research has provided an entirely new paradigm for drug design and development to treat viral infections. For example, the recent development of the new flu drug, Relenza directly benefited from AIDS research. The drug known as 3TC, developed to treat AIDS, is now the most effective therapy for chronic hepatitis B infection. Drugs developed to prevent and treat AIDS-related opportunistic infections also provide benefit to patients undergoing cancer chemotherapy or receiving anti-transplant rejection therapy. AIDS is also providing new understanding of the relationship between viruses and cancer.[15,16] Additionally, HIV/AIDS research has contributed to:

- Accelerated research into viruses in general and retroviruses in particular;

- Provided insight into treatment with protease inhibitors of other conditions including bone loss and heart muscle damage;

- Enhanced understanding of the spread of infectious agents through the blood/brain barrier (which has implications for research on Alzheimer's disease, dementia, encephalitis, and meningitis);

- Improved treatment and prevention of infections among people with advanced breast cancer, organ transplants, or autoimmune conditions; and

- Improved diagnostic tests to detect cancer cells and tuberculosis.

What Are Current Challenges for HIV/AIDS Research?

There are several important challenges for HIV/AIDS research over the next decade that form the basis for current and future research priorities, both for the federal research effort and for those working in the private sector and in the community. These include[1]:

- *The global epidemic.* With more than 90% of new infections occurring in developing countries where therapeutic interventions are unaffordable and hard to deliver, HIV/AIDS research efforts are addressing the need to develop treatments that can be implemented in these countries and are accessible to their populations.

- *Health disparities in the U.S. and the impact of HIV on minorities, women, and young people.* Despite recent positive trends, HIV remains a leading cause of death among minority Americans, and HIV increasingly impacts minorities, women, and young people. Research challenges include: increasing the number of minority researchers conducting behavioral and clinical research; educating minority physicians about HIV treatment approaches; including women and minorities in clinical research in proportion to their increasing representation in the epidemic; developing and evaluating prevention interventions designed to reduce HIV risk behaviors and transmission in communities disproportionately impacted by HIV; and reducing barriers to prevention and treatment.

- *Improved therapies.* Researchers are focusing on the development of new, simpler, less toxic, and less expensive drugs to address the issues of side effects and complicated regimens.

- *Long-term clinical effectiveness research.* Clinical studies are needed to identify strategies for the long-term use of HIV antiretroviral therapy and answer questions such as when to begin therapy, how to manage side effects, how to improve adherence to HIV therapy and avoid the development of drug resistance, and how to treat patients for whom therapy is failing.

- *Prevention research.* Without a cure for HIV, prevention efforts continue to be the most cost-effective way to address the epidemic. Prevention priorities include management of sexually transmitted diseases; perinatal prevention, including enhancing understanding of breast-feeding risk; and the development of topical microbicides (microbicides, a synthetic or natural substance that can kill or neutralize HIV during sexual intercourse, offer a promising new prevention intervention).[19,20] In addition, understanding how to assist people in changing behaviors that place them at risk for HIV infection is a critical priority. This includes addressing the issue of complacency.[21]

- *Vaccines.* The NIH and many private and community organizations continue to make developing a vaccine against HIV a priority. Several AIDS vaccine trials are now underway.

- *The link between public and private investments and research.* The relationship between government-sponsored research, private industry research and research conducted by academic institutions is key to how scientific knowledge is produced and applied in the U.S., within and beyond the field of HIV research. Pharmaceutical companies, for example, frequently utilize the knowledge gained from NIH-supported HIV research to help them develop new drugs and other products. This has sometimes led to criticism of the high price of HIV-related drugs in the U.S. and around the world, and questions have been raised about whether drug makers should discount those prices to reflect the public investment and, more generally, how to make drugs and other new interventions more affordable to all people with HIV.

- *Translating research into practice.* To be effective, research efforts must continue to identify ways to translate knowledge into programs and practices. For example, although national guidelines exist for HIV/AIDS-related drug treatment and prophylaxis, challenges remain to putting these guidelines into practice throughout different clinical settings and among different providers and payers in the U.S.

Conclusion

As a new infectious disease that emerged at a time when many believed that the threat of infectious disease in the U.S. had largely been eliminated, HIV presented considerable challenges to scientific research. Overall, HIV/AIDS research has resulted in tremendous advances, including a dramatic reduction in AIDS-related mortality and the discovery of increasingly effective treatments for HIV disease and its related conditions. Despite these advances, however, the research community will be challenged with the need to continue to develop interventions to address an epidemic that increasingly affects racial and ethnic minorities, women, and young people throughout the U.S. and around the world.

Roles and Responsibilities within the NIH Institutes

The National Institute of Allergy and Infectious Diseases (NIAID) has the lead responsibility within the NIH for the discovery and development of interventions to treat or prevent HIV infection.

The National Cancer Institute (NCI) focuses its research on AIDS-related malignancies (about 30% of people with AIDS develop some form of malignancy). NCI houses the HIV Drug Resistance Program, the HIV and Malignancies Branch, and the NIH Vaccine Research Center, a joint project with NIAID.

The National Institute on Drug Abuse (NIDA) focuses on developing strategies to reduce drug related behaviors that are linked to the transmission of HIV.

The National Institute of Mental Health (NIMH) focuses on the impact of HIV on the central nervous system (CNS), mechanisms to motivate behavior change, behavioral prevention strategies in at-risk populations and therapeutics for CNS complications of HIV.

The National Center for Research Resources (NCRR) provides critical research technologies and shared resources across all NIH Institutes and Centers.

The National Heart, Lung and Blood Institute (NHLBI) supports research on the pulmonary, hematologic, and cardiac complications of HIV infection and research designed to maximize the safety and adequacy of the nation's blood supply.

The National Institute of Child Health and Human Development (NICHD) supports research focused on maternal, pediatric, and adolescent HIV infection and AIDS.

End Notes

1. Nathanson, N., M.D., Director, Office of AIDS Research, Testimony to Congress, 2000.

2. Joint United Nations Programme on HIV/AIDS, AIDS Epidemic Update: December 1999.

3. Centers for Disease Control and Prevention, HIV/AIDS Surveillance Report;11(No.1), 1999.

4. Department of Health and Human Services, Fiscal Year 2001 Justification of Estimates for Appropriations Committees (http://www.nih.gov/od/oar/public/pubs/oar2001cj.pdf).

5. National Institutes of Health, National Institute of Allergy and Infectious Diseases, HIV and Other Lentiviruses, (http://www.niaid.nih.gov/publications/hivaids/8.htm).

6. Centers for Disease Control and Prevention, CDC Update. A Glance at the HIV Epidemic, 2000.

7. Pharmaceutical Research and Manufacturers Association, Progress against AIDS Promises to Continue with 102 New Medicines in Development, 1999.

8. Association of American Medical Colleges, Maximizing the Investment Principles to Guide the Federal-Academic Partnership in Biomedical and Health Sciences Research, 1999 (http://www.aamc.org/research).

9. Kaiser Family Foundation, Federal HIV/AIDS Spending: A Budget Chartbook, 1999.

10. National Institutes of Health, Office of AIDS Research, Budget Authority by Activity.

11. Congressional Research Service, AIDS: Funding for Federal Government Programs: FY 1981-FY 2000, CRS Report to Congress, 1999.

12. National Institutes of Health, National Institute of Allergy and Infectious Diseases, Clinical Trials Research, 1999 (http://www.niaid.nih.gov/daids/therapeutics/geninfo/clintrials.htm).

13. National Institutes of Health, Fact Sheet on AIDS Research and Minority Populations, 1999.

14. Pear, R., "Research Neglects Women, Studies Find," *New York Times*, April 30, 2000.

15. National Institutes of Health, Overview of NIH HIV/AIDS Research Priorities, 1999.

16. AIDS Action, http://www.aidsaction.org/policy/research.html.

17. Center for AIDS Prevention Studies, Does HIV Prevention Work?, 1998 (http://www.caps.ucsf.edu).

18. Center for AIDS Prevention Studies, How is Science Used in HIV Prevention?, 1999 (http://www.caps.ucsf.edu).

19. American Foundation for AIDS Research, Microbicides: A New Weapon Against HIV, 2000 (http://www.amfar.org/media/Micro.pdf).

20. National Institutes of Health, National Institute of Allergy and Infectious Diseases, NIAID Topical Microbicide Research:

Developing New Tools to Protect Women from HIV/AIDS and other STDs, 2000 (http://www.niaid.nih.gov/factsheets/topmicro.htm).

21. Centers for Disease Control and Prevention, Combating Complacency in HIV Prevention, 1999 (http://www.cdc.gov/hiv/pubs/facts/combat.htm).

Chapter 61

Comprehensive International Program of Research on AIDS (CIPRA)

According to the latest figures released by the Joint United Nations Programme on HIV/AIDS (UNAIDS), approximately 40 million people worldwide are now living with AIDS. Ninety five percent of all people infected with HIV live in developing countries. Most of the 3 million deaths from HIV/AIDS-related illnesses in 2001 occurred in these countries, making AIDS the fourth leading cause of death worldwide and the leading cause of death in Africa. Children are not spared: in 2001, more than 800,000 were newly infected throughout the world.[1]

In response to these realities, the National Institute of Allergy and Infectious Diseases (NIAID) has developed a multifaceted global HIV/AIDS research agenda. The agenda builds upon the Institute's long-standing commitment to international infectious disease research by assisting those countries hardest hit by the AIDS scourge to expand their basic and clinical research capacities, enhance partnerships for public health, and foster education of scientists and clinicians.

The Comprehensive International Program of Research on AIDS (CIPRA), which recently awarded its first group of grants, is a part of NIAID's HIV/AIDS global research agenda. The first five grants provide up to $50,000 for up to two years. As research capacity grows in grantee countries, investigators can choose to apply for other types of CIPRA grants. The new grants will help scientists plan research

National Institute of Allergy and Infectious Diseases (NIAID), December 2001; available online at http://www.niaid.nih.gov/factsheets/cipra.htm.

programs, establish collaborations, build administrative infrastructure, and assemble applications for larger CIPRA grants. "We view these first grants as a bright beginning in what we expect will be a long-term and very exciting program," says Rod Hoff, Ph.D., an official in NIAID's Division of AIDS.

CIPRA grants are given only to institutions and investigators located in countries with an annual per capita income of less than $5,000. The infrastructure for research, training, and data collection is often deficient in these countries and CIPRA seeks to provide the infrastructure support needed to help grantees become full partners with their colleagues in the United States and other developed countries.

Awards have been made to institutions in Trinidad, Peru, China, Zambia and the Russian Federation.

Trinidad and Tobago

HIV/AIDS Prevention and Treatment in Trinidad and Tobago. About 500,000 Caribbeans currently live with HIV/AIDS, and the disease has killed 8,000 people in the region, according to the Caribbean Task Force on HIV/AIDS. The average prevalence of HIV infection is 2 percent, making the region second only to sub-Saharan Africa.[2] Most new infections in Trinidad and Tobago occur in heterosexuals 15 to 24 years old, resulting in a dramatic HIV increase in young women and children less than 15 years old.

This CIPRA grant will fund development of a program responsive to the particular needs of the epidemic in Trinidad and Tobago. Potentially, the program could serve as a model for other Caribbean countries with similar epidemiological and socioeconomic features. It will include assessment for site development and infrastructure needs, as well as plans for increasing the clinical and laboratory capacity needed to perform prevention and treatment intervention research, leading eventually to clinical trials.

Peru

HIV Pathogenesis, Prevention, and Treatment in the Andes. The aim of the project is to develop a regional capacity for HIV prevention and vaccine research in the Peruvian Andes. The investigators plan to submit a subsequent grant application that will consider a wide range of topics. These will include the interaction of other sexually transmitted diseases and HIV; resistance to anti-HIV drugs; effectiveness of preventive behavioral interventions for men who have sex with men; transmission from high to lower-risk populations; assessment of multi-drug resistant tuberculosis in HIV-infected people; evaluation of rapid diagnostic tests for HIV infection; and prevention of mother-to-child transmission of HIV.

China

CIPRA-China Planning and Organization. China's health ministry estimates that about 600,000 Chinese were living with HIV/AIDS in 2000. Given the recently observed rises in reported HIV infections and infection rates in many sub-populations in several parts of the country, the total number of people living with HIV/AIDS in China could well exceed one million by the end of 2001.[3] A consortium of Chinese research organizations, led by the National Center for AIDS Prevention and Control of the Chinese Academy of Preventive Medicine, will use this CIPRA grant to develop an agenda of integrated epidemiological, clinical and laboratory research; support the training of promising AIDS researchers; and develop a strong administrative and research infrastructure at the local, provincial, and national levels.

Zambia

Planning for Randomized Controlled Trials of ART in Lusaka, Zambia. Zambia has one of the highest rates of HIV seroprevalence in Africa. Due to recent government and drug company initiatives to reduce costs, it is expected that antiretroviral drugs will soon be more available to people needing them. However, minimal data are available on the best use of combination antiretroviral therapy (ART) in Zambia. The goal of this grant is to begin development of infrastructure and facilities for a research program on suitable ART for Zambia. In general, African countries have not previously developed systematic approaches to identifying simple and practical HIV treatment regimes. The grant represents the first effort in Zambia to undertake this task.

Russian Federation

HIV/AIDS and Opportunistic Infections in Intravenous Drug Users. Eastern Europe, and the Russian Federation in particular, are experiencing the fastest growing infection rate in the world. In St. Petersburg, Russia (which had an HIV infection incidence of 114 cases per 100,000 people in 2000), the spread of HIV/AIDS occurs primarily through intravenous drug use. The primary focus of this project will be epidemiological research and development of a prevention program, with a secondary focus on treating HIV/AIDS in intravenous drug users who have viral hepatitis and opportunistic infections.

References

1.   UNAIDS. AIDS Epidemic Update. Dec. 2001.

2.   UNAIDS. AIDS Epidemic Update. Dec. 2001.

3.   UNAIDS. AIDS Epidemic Update. Dec. 2001.

Chapter 62

The Thailand
Phase III Vaccine Study

The development of an effective HIV vaccine is a public health priority throughout the world. Because no one knows for sure which vaccine, or type of vaccine, will be most effective, multiple vaccines are being explored simultaneously. This particular trial is being conducted to address the urgent need for an HIV vaccine in Thailand and other developing nations. Because of the severe and escalating toll of HIV in Thailand, Thai government and public health officials have developed the Thai National Plan for HIV Vaccine Research. Through this plan, Thai officials are coordinating their efforts to help find an effective vaccine to slow the HIV epidemic in their country.

The VaxGen Phase III trial is part of that plan. VaxGen, Inc., a biomedical research company located in San Francisco, California, developed the candidate vaccine to be evaluated, AIDSVAX, and will fund most aspects of the study. VaxGen worked closely with Thai officials to ensure that AIDSVAX was designed to work against the subtypes of HIV most common in Thailand (i.e., subtypes B and E).

The Bangkok Metropolitan Administration (BMA) is leading the 3-year collaborative research trial. BMA is conducting the trial in conjunction with VaxGen, the Mahidol University Faculty of Tropical Medicine in Bangkok, and the HIV/AIDS Collaboration (a long-standing research collaborative between the Thai Ministry of Public Health and the CDC).

"Questions and Answers on the Thailand Phase III Vaccine Study and CDC's Collaboration," National Center for HIV, STD and TB Prevention, Centers for Disease Control and Prevention (CDC), February 1999; available online at http://www.cdc.gov/hiv/pubs/facts/vaccineqa.htm.

What is the trial designed to do?

The Phase III trial is designed to determine if AIDSVAX is effective in protecting against HIV infection and disease. While Phase I and II trials have already demonstrated that the vaccine is safe for use and is capable of inducing antibodies against HIV infection, it is not known if the level and type of antibodies produced will prevent HIV infection. This trial will answer that question. Large-scale human testing (called a Phase III trial) is the last and most important step in the evaluation process before a vaccine is considered for licensing.

How is the trial designed?

The trial is being conducted among uninfected injection drug users (IDUs) attending 17 drug treatment clinics in Bangkok. The design is a randomized, double-blind, placebo-controlled trial in which half of the 2,500 volunteers receive the AIDSVAX vaccine being evaluated and the other half receive placebo injections that do not include the vaccine. Neither the researchers nor the participants know which participants are in each half of the trial. To guard against any of the participants relaxing their preventive behaviors, all volunteers receive extensive counseling on how to protect themselves against HIV infection, as well as explicit warnings that it is unknown whether or not this vaccine will protect them from infection.

Why is this particular vaccine being evaluated?

Thai officials chose to work with VaxGen to evaluate this vaccine because it has proven safe and effective in stimulating an immune response against HIV subtypes E and B, the subtypes most common in Thailand. If AIDSVAX proves to have a protective effect, it would therefore be effective against the subtypes causing the local Thai epidemic. AIDSVAX is also the first vaccine to receive approval for large-scale human testing (Phase III trials).

How does this vaccine work?

AIDSVAX uses a genetically engineered protein (gp120) from the surface of the human immunodeficiency virus. When injected into the body, it stimulates production of antibodies to attack any future invading HIV. Researchers hope the antibodies will prevent the virus from binding to, and infecting, healthy T-cells. AIDSVAX is a bivalent vaccine, meaning that it uses gp120 proteins from the surface of two different strains of HIV. The formulation of AIDSVAX being tested in Thailand uses HIV subtypes E and B, the subtypes most common in Thailand.

Why do only some of the participants receive the vaccine? Do the other participants get any benefit from the trial?

A placebo-controlled design (where some of the participants receive the vaccine being tested and some receive no vaccine) is currently the only scientifically sound way to determine if a vaccine works. In order to determine how effective the vaccine is, researchers will compare the rate of HIV infection in participants who receive the vaccine to the rate among those that receive the placebo injection. If people in the vaccine group have lower rates of infection than people with similar risk behaviors in the group that receives the placebo injection, then researchers will know the vaccine works. If the rates of infection are the same in both groups, researchers will know the vaccine does not work.

Everyone in the trial, regardless of the vaccine's effectiveness, is expected to benefit from participation in the trial. First, all IDUs participating in the trial are automatically enrolled in drug treatment and maintenance programs at the Thai clinics to help them stop using drugs and reduce their risk for HIV infection. Second, all volunteers receive the best available counseling on how to reduce their risk for HIV infection through behavior change. Individualized counseling sessions are based on CDC guidelines for the type of risk-reduction counseling that is most effective. Finally, all volunteers are encouraged to participate in group education sessions that focus on building peer support for reducing HIV risk.

In the Thailand AIDSVAX trial, one in two participants will receive the trial vaccine (the other will receive a placebo), yet in the U.S. AIDSVAX trial, two out of three participants will receive the trial vaccine (the other will receive a placebo). Why the difference?

The primary reason for the difference in vaccine to placebo ratio in the two studies is to account for the wider genetic diversity (range of HIV strains) in the United States, compared to Thailand. In the U.S., the prevalent subtype B has been present since the mid-to-late 1970s and has over two decades to genetically diverge. By comparison, the

Thai epidemic did not begin until 1988, and the subtype E viruses predominant there are not as diverse.

Many researchers believe genetic diversity may have an effect on vaccine protection, and that an HIV vaccine that is protective against some strains may not be effective against others. It is therefore important to ensure that each study will produce enough data to reliably analyze the vaccine's protective effect against the range of strains present in that nation. To statistically account for the wider genetic diversity in the U.S., it was necessary to include a greater proportion of vaccinated individuals in the U.S. study.

How do you expect to determine if the vaccine prevents infection, if you are counseling everyone to protect themselves from exposure?

Health officials have an obligation to ensure that all participants benefit from proven prevention methods as we search for new ones. And while risk-reduction counseling has proven effective in reducing IDUs' risk for HIV infection, it has not proven effective in totally eliminating HIV risk. If behavior change programs were 100% effective, we would not need an HIV vaccine. Regardless of the best efforts at HIV prevention counseling, some individuals will continue to take risks. By comparing the rates of infection among those at risk in both groups, researchers will be able to determine if the vaccine helps protect these individuals from infection.

Do the participants know that some do not receive any vaccine?

Yes. Because of possible language and educational barriers, Thai health officials have worked with CDC, local clinic staff, and IDUs themselves to design an extensive process to ensure that volunteers understand what their participation in the trial means, exactly what they receive and do not receive as part of the trial, and that trial participation does not protect them from infection. Potentially eligible volunteers participate in an education session on the nature of the study (which includes a video) and then are given the opportunity to ask questions. Following this session, they complete a comprehension test, followed by discussion of the correct answers. After taking materials home to discuss the study with their family and peers, potential participants are asked to return to complete a second comprehension test. Those who are unable to pass the comprehension test are not enrolled. Those who do pass then undergo the informed consent process before being enrolled. All counseling sessions and materials are in the native language and have been locally evaluated for reading level and comprehension.

If participants become infected during the course of the trial, are they provided medical care?

Yes, the BMA has committed to providing medical care to any participants who become infected according to the Bangkok Metropolitan Administration Guidelines for Clinical Care of HIV-Infected Patients (27 May 1998). These guidelines state that HIV-infected persons will receive prophylaxis for tuberculosis and *Pneumocystis carinii* pneumonia (PCP), and that two antiretroviral drugs—AZT and ddI, ddC, or 3TC—will be administered to HIV-infected individuals when their CD4 counts drop below 500 or if the person develops an HIV-related disease. As part of the trial, participants are provided CD4 and viral load monitoring. CDC is working with BMA to ensure that local standards of care are implemented and that the Thai Ministry of Public Health and local physicians continue to review the standards as clinical management evolves.

Why not provide participants who become infected the same treatments available in the United States?

Thai government and health officials feel very strongly that treatment should follow the protocols they have established for their country. The triple drug therapies currently being used in the United States are not considered feasible for use in Thailand, not only because of cost constraints, but also because of issues related to the complexity of the regimen, the necessary follow-up and monitoring of patients, and tolerance to the therapies. Additionally, providing therapies not routinely available in Thailand to trial participants would be considered an unfair inducement to join the trial.

Why has there been skepticism about the potential effectiveness of AIDSVAX?

The AIDSVAX vaccine was developed over a period of a decade. The first version of the vaccine was based on only one strain of HIV. Because of the increasing genetic diversity of HIV across the globe, many believed it was important to add additional strains. VaxGen has since improved the vaccine, which is now based on these two strains of HIV.

For use in Thailand for example, it was necessary to add an HIV strain from the subtype E virus, which is predominant in Thailand. The vaccine used in Thailand is composed of both subtype B (MN strain) and subtype E (A244 strain) antigens. For other areas of the world where the HIV subtypes may differ, the vaccine would have to be manipulated based on the strains common in those particular areas.

Additionally, no one knows for sure what type of immune response in vaccine recipients will be needed to prevent HIV infection. Some researchers believe that antibodies alone will be effective, but others believe that both antibodies and specialized immune cells (called killer T-cells) will be required to protect against infection. The VaxGen vaccine induces only an antibody response, while other vaccines under development combine this approach with a killer T-cell response. This and other studies ultimately will be required to determine whether either approach works.

Has this vaccine been studied in the United States? Why conduct the study in Thailand?

VaxGen is conducting a similar trial in the United States, but with a version of AIDSVAX designed to protect against the HIV strains common in North America. That study, which began in June 1998, will involve 5,000 volunteers at high risk for sexual HIV infection in 30-40 cities.

Thai health officials have decided to evaluate the AIDSVAX formula designed to work in Asia and the Pacific Rim as part of their efforts to find a vaccine that will be effective in their country. They are evaluating the vaccine among IDUs because HIV is now spreading rapidly among that population in Thailand. Among IDUs in Bangkok, 6% become infected each year, despite methadone treatment, education and counseling on HIV prevention, and easy access to sterile needles. A vaccine is urgently needed to slow this epidemic.

What is CDC's role in the trial?

For nearly a decade, CDC has worked closely with Thai public health officials to design and evaluate prevention efforts to help stop the Thai HIV epidemic. In 1990, CDC established a permanent field station in Thailand and a collaborative research program with the Thai Ministry of Public Health—the HIV/AIDS Collaboration. Through this long-standing collaboration, CDC has worked closely with Thailand to address its evolving prevention needs.

Over the past several years, CDC has applied its experience in studying disease transmission and prevention to help the Thai government prepare to implement vaccine studies. Since 1995, this collaboration has involved a range of activities, including measuring the level of new (or incident) HIV infections in Thailand, determining the genetic characterization of incident HIV infections, identifying risk factors for infection, identifying a group of individuals who were willing to participate and could be followed over time to evaluate risk behaviors and infection, and working with the community to build the understanding and support necessary to implement vaccine studies.

In addition, in collaboration with the BMA, Faculty of Tropical Medicine of Mahidol University, and VaxGen, CDC has provided technical assistance in the development of the protocol, data forms, questionnaires, study procedures, and informational materials.

As the VaxGen study proceeds, CDC will continue to provide technical consultation as needed, laboratory testing and processing, and assistance in the analysis of study results. More importantly, perhaps, CDC will provide scientific support in the design and implementation of effective risk-reduction counseling for study volunteers and in the monitoring of behavioral risk factors. It is critical that participants in the study not abandon proven prevention methods (i.e., safer drug-related and sexual behaviors) as we search for new ones.

What ethical reviews were done (in the U.S. and Thailand) before beginning this trial?

To ensure an ethically sound study, all plans for the study, as well as consent procedures and educational materials, have been carefully reviewed and approved by multiple committees in Thailand, the United States, and internationally.

In Thailand, the trial has received an ethics review and approval from the Bangkok Metropolitan Administration, the Faculty of Tropical Medicine of Mahidol University, the Ethical and Scientific Review Committees of the Thailand Ministry of Public Health (MOPH), and the Thailand Food and Drug Administration. The Thailand MOPH also requested independent review and approval from UNAIDS. The UNAIDS review was conducted by the UNAIDS Vaccine Advisory Committee and a number of outside international experts on vaccine trials.

In the United States, the trial has received an ethics review and approval from the U.S. Food and Drug Administration and will soon receive additional approvals based on ethics reviews by the CDC Institutional Review Board (including representation by NIH) and the

449

NIH Office for the Protection of Research Risks. Additionally, study plans have been presented to the Ethics Subcommittee of the CDC External Advisory Group.

Is CDC involved in other vaccine trials?

Currently, the only other Phase III trial underway is the VaxGen study in the United States. CDC is planning to assist VaxGen with its U.S. study as well, but has not yet begun those efforts. CDC's role in that trial will be similar, and the agency will work to evaluate the impact of the trial on both participant and community attitudes and behaviors. Additionally, CDC will provide expertise in HIV surveillance in order to assess HIV subtypes and resistance. This information will be critical, not only for the communities currently involved, but also for the future evaluation and implementation of vaccine strategies.

How does CDC's role complement that of NIH in HIV vaccine development?

CDC and NIH bring unique expertise and experience to the search for an HIV vaccine. In general, NIH has led the nation's basic research efforts to develop vaccines that may prevent HIV infection. This involves extensive cellular and laboratory research on the mechanisms of infection and the development of strategies to interfere with those mechanisms. NIH also is responsible for coordinating the simultaneous evaluation of multiple vaccine candidates.

To complement NIH's expertise, CDC has a long history in the field of vaccine evaluation, including evaluation of the measles vaccine, the hepatitis B vaccine, and the vaccine for *Haemophilus influenzae* type B disease. As the nation's lead prevention agency, CDC will be responsible for developing policies and procedures for effectively using an HIV vaccine, once a safe and effective vaccine is available. CDC has extensive experience in HIV prevention research and in working with states and communities to design and evaluate HIV prevention strategies. Until now, CDC's vaccine efforts have related primarily to working with communities and individuals to help researchers better understand attitudes and behaviors related to vaccines, including what factors influence people's willingness to participate in vaccine studies and use a vaccine and how vaccine studies may influence risk behaviors. Now, as large-scale evaluations of HIV vaccine candidates begin, CDC will play an increasingly important role in the design and evaluation of these studies and their impact on HIV transmission and related attitudes and behaviors.

Chapter 63

HIV/AIDS Clinical Trials

An Introduction to Clinical Trials

Choosing to participate in a clinical trial is an important personal decision. The following frequently asked questions provide detailed information about clinical trials. In addition, it is often helpful to talk to a physician, family members, or friends about deciding to join a trial. After identifying some trial options, the next step is to contact the study research staff and ask questions about specific trials.

What is a clinical trial?

A clinical trial is a research study to answer specific questions about vaccines, new therapies or new ways of using known treatments. Clinical trials (also called medical research and research studies) are used to determine whether new drugs or treatments are both safe and effective. Carefully conducted clinical trials are the fastest and safest way to find treatments that work in people.

All text in this chapter is from Centers for Disease Control and Prevention (CDC), 2002. Under the heading "An Introduction to Clinical Trials," available online at http://www.clinicaltrials.gov/ct/gui/info/whatis; under the heading "Combination Therapy with IL-2 Plus Antiretroviral Drugs to Treat HIV Infection," available online at http://www.clinicaltrials.gov/ct/gui/show/NCT00004737; under the heading "Nutrition Intervention in AIDS Wasting," available online at http://clinicaltrials.gov/ct/gui/show/NCT00006167; and under the heading "Screening Protocol for HIV Vaccine Studies," available online at http://www.clincialtrials.gov/ct/gui/show/NCT00031304.

Why participate in a clinical trial?

Participants in clinical trials can play a more active role in their own health care, gain access to new research treatments before they are widely available, and help others by contributing to medical research.

Where do the ideas for trials come from?

Ideas for clinical trials usually come from researchers. After researchers test new therapies or procedures in the laboratory and in animal studies, the treatments with the most promising laboratory results are moved into clinical trials. During a trial, more and more information is gained about a new treatment, its risks and how well it may or may not work.

Who sponsors clinical trials?

Clinical trials are sponsored or funded by a variety of organizations or individuals such as physicians, medical institutions, foundations, voluntary groups, and pharmaceutical companies, in addition to federal agencies such as the National Institutes of Health (NIH), the Department of Defense (DOD), and the Department of Veteran's Affairs (VA). Trials can take place in a variety of locations, such as hospitals, universities, doctors' offices, or community clinics.

What is a protocol?

A protocol is a study plan on which all clinical trials are based. The plan is carefully designed to safeguard the health of the participants as well as answer specific research questions. A protocol describes what types of people may participate in the trial; the schedule of tests, procedures, medications, and dosages; and the length of the study. While in a clinical trial, participants following a protocol are seen regularly by the research staff to monitor their health and to determine the safety and effectiveness of their treatment.

What is a placebo?

A placebo is an inactive pill, liquid, or powder that has no treatment value. In clinical trials, experimental treatments are often compared with placebos to assess the treatment's effectiveness. In some studies, the participants in the control group will receive a placebo instead of an active drug or treatment.

What is a control or control group?

A control is the standard by which experimental observations are evaluated. In many clinical trials, one group of patients will be given an experimental drug or treatment, while the control group is given either a standard treatment for the illness or a placebo.

What are the different types of clinical trials?

Treatment trials test new treatments, new combinations of drugs, or new approaches to surgery or radiation therapy.

Prevention trials look for better ways to prevent disease in people who have never had the disease or to prevent a disease from returning. These approaches may include medicines, vitamins, vaccines, minerals, or lifestyle changes.

Screening trials test the best way to detect certain diseases or health conditions.

Quality of Life trials (or Supportive Care trials) explore ways to improve comfort and the quality of life for individuals with a chronic illness.

What are the phases of clinical trials?

Clinical trials are conducted in phases. The trials at each phase have a different purpose and help scientists answer different questions:

- In Phase I trials, researchers test a new drug or treatment in a small group of people (20-80) for the first time to evaluate its safety, determine a safe dosage range, and identify side effects.

- In Phase II trials, the study drug or treatment is given to a larger group of people (100-300) to see if it is effective and to further evaluate its safety.

- In Phase III trials, the study drug or treatment is given to large groups of people (1,000-3,000) to confirm its effectiveness, monitor side effects, compare it to commonly used treatments, and collect information that will allow the drug or treatment to be used safely.

- In Phase IV trials, post marketing studies delineate additional information including the drug's risks, benefits, and optimal use.

What is an expanded access protocol?

Most human use of investigational new drugs takes place in controlled clinical trials conducted to assess safety and efficacy of new drugs. Data from the trials can serve as the basis for the drug marketing application. Sometimes, patients do not qualify for these carefully-controlled trials because of other health problems, age, or other factors. For patients who may benefit from the drug use but don't qualify for the trials, FDA regulations enable manufacturers of investigational new drugs to provide for expanded access use of the drug. For example, a treatment IND (Investigational New Drug application) or treatment protocol is a relatively unrestricted study. The primary intent of a treatment IND/protocol is to provide for access to the new drug for people with a life-threatening or serious disease for which there is no good alternative treatment. A secondary purpose for a treatment IND/protocol is to generate additional information about the drug, especially its safety. Expanded access protocols can be undertaken only if clinical investigators are actively studying the new treatment in well-controlled studies, or all studies have been completed. There must be evidence that the drug may be an effective treatment in patients like those to be treated under the protocol. The drug cannot expose patients to unreasonable risks given the severity of the disease to be treated.

Some investigational drugs are available from pharmaceutical manufacturers through expanded access programs listed in Clinical Trials.gov. Expanded access protocols are generally managed by the manufacturer, with the investigational treatment administered by researchers or doctors in office-based practice. If you or a loved one are interested in treatment with an investigational drug under an expanded access protocol listed in ClinicalTrials.gov, review the protocol eligibility criteria and location information and inquire at the Contact Information number.

Participation in Clinical Trials

For those considering participation in a clinical trial, the following frequently asked questions are important in understanding the role of the participant and the unique process of clinical trials.

Who can participate in a clinical trial?

All clinical trials have guidelines about who can participate. Using inclusion/exclusion criteria is an important principle of medical research that helps to produce reliable results. The factors that allow someone to participate in a clinical trial are called inclusion criteria and those that disallow someone from participating are called exclusion criteria. These criteria are based on such factors as age, gender, the type and stage of a disease, previous treatment history, and other medical conditions. Before joining a clinical trial, a participant must qualify for the study. Some research studies seek participants with illnesses or conditions to be studied in the clinical trial, while others need healthy participants. It is important to note that inclusion and exclusion criteria are not used to reject people personally. Instead, the criteria are used to identify appropriate participants and keep them safe. The criteria help ensure that researchers will be able to answer the questions they plan to study.

What happens during a clinical trial?

The clinical trial process depends on the kind of trial being conducted The clinical trial team includes doctors and nurses as well as social workers and other health care professionals. They check the health of the participant at the beginning of the trial, give specific instructions for participating in the trial, monitor the participant carefully during the trial, and stay in touch after the trial is completed.

Some clinical trials involve more tests and doctor visits than the participant would normally have for an illness or condition. For all types of trials, the participant works with a research team. Clinical trial participation is most successful when the protocol is carefully followed and there is frequent contact with the research staff.

What is informed consent?

Informed consent is the process of learning the key facts about a clinical trial before deciding whether or not to participate. It is also a continuing process throughout the study to provide information for participants. To help someone decide whether or not to participate, the doctors and nurses involved in the trial explain the details of the study. If the participant's native language is not English, translation assistance can be provided. Then the research team provides an informed consent document that includes details about the study, such as its purpose, duration, required procedures, and key contacts. Risks and potential benefits are explained in the informed consent document. The participant then decides whether or not to sign the document.

Informed consent is not a contract, and the participant may withdraw from the trial at any time.

What kind of preparation should a potential participant make for the meeting with the research coordinator or doctor?

- Plan ahead and write down possible questions to ask.
- Ask a friend or relative to come along for support and to hear the responses to the questions.
- Bring a tape recorder to record the discussion to replay later.

What should people consider before participating in a trial?

People should know as much as possible about the clinical trial and feel comfortable asking the members of the health care team questions about it, the care expected while in a trial, and the cost of the trial. The following questions might be helpful for the participant to discuss with the health care team. Some of the answers to these questions are found in the informed consent document.

- What is the purpose of the study?
- Who is going to be in the study?
- Why do researchers believe the new treatment being tested may be effective? Has it been tested before?
- What kinds of tests and treatments are involved?
- How do the possible risks, side effects, and benefits in the study compare with my current treatment?
- How might this trial affect my daily life?
- How long will the trial last?
- Will hospitalization be required?
- Who will pay for the treatment?
- Will I be reimbursed for other expenses?
- What type of long-term follow up care is part of this study?
- How will I know that the treatment is working? Will results of the trials be provided to me?
- Who will be in charge of my care?

Does a participant continue to work with a primary health care provider while in a trial?

Yes. Most clinical trials provide short-term treatments related to a designated illness or condition, but do not provide extended or complete primary health care. In addition, by having the health care provider work with the research team, the participant can ensure that other medications or treatments will not conflict with the protocol.

What are side effects and adverse reactions?

Side effects are any undesired actions or effects of drug or treatment. Negative or adverse effects may include headache, nausea, hair loss, skin irritation, or other physical problems. Experimental treatments must be evaluated for both immediate and long-term side effects.

What are the benefits and risks of participating in a clinical trial?

Benefits: Clinical trials that are well-designed and well-executed are the best treatment approach for eligible participants to:

- Play an active role in their own health care.
- Gain access to new research treatments before they are widely available.
- Obtain expert medical care at leading health care facilities during the trial.
- Help others by contributing to medical research.

Risks: There are risks to clinical trials.

- There may be unpleasant, serious or even life-threatening side effects to treatment.
- The treatment may not be effective for the participant.
- The protocol may require more of their time and attention than would a non-protocol treatment, including trips to the study site, more treatments, hospital stays or complex dosage requirements.

How is the safety of the participant protected?

The ethical and legal codes that govern medical practice also apply to clinical trials. In addition, most clinical research is federally regulated with built in safeguards to protect the participants. The trial follows a carefully controlled protocol, a study plan which details what researchers will do in the study. As a clinical trial progresses, researchers report the results of the trial at scientific meetings, to medical journals, and to various government agencies. Individual participants' names will remain secret and will not be mentioned in these reports.

Every clinical trial in the U.S. must be approved and monitored by an Institutional Review Board (IRB) to make sure the risks are as low as possible and are worth any potential benefits. An IRB is an independent committee of physicians, statisticians, community advocates, and others that ensures that a clinical trial is ethical and the rights of study participants are protected. All institutions that conduct or support biomedical research involving people must, by federal regulation, have an IRB that initially approves and periodically reviews the research.

Can a participant leave a clinical trial after it has begun?

Yes. A participant can leave a clinical trial, at any time. When withdrawing from the trial, the participant should let the research team know about it, and the reasons for leaving the study.

Combination Therapy with IL-2 Plus Antiretroviral Drugs to Treat HIV Infection

This study will test whether the drug Interleukin-2 (IL-2), given together with antiretroviral drugs, can reduce the number of serious infections or prolong survival in people with HIV infection. IL-2 is a protein naturally produced by white blood cells called lymphocytes, which are important cells of the immune system. Lymphocytes from patients with HIV do not produce IL-2 normally and the total numbers of lymphocytes gradually decline with progressive disease. Administration of IL-2 has been shown capable of increasing the number of lymphocytes in treated patients above that usually reached through use of antiretroviral drugs alone.

Patients with HIV infection 18 years and older who have no symptoms of significant HIV illness and no history of opportunistic infections may be eligible for this 6-year study. Candidates will be screened with a medical history and physical examination, including blood tests and urinalysis. Those enrolled in the study will be randomly assigned to one of two treatment groups, as follows:

- Group 1 will receive antiretroviral therapy alone. Patients in this group will be evaluated every 4 months with a physical examination and blood tests.

- Group 2 will receive antiretroviral therapy plus IL-2. In addition to antiretroviral drugs, patients will receive IL-2 injections under the skin twice a day, 5 days a week (one treatment cycle). The 5-day cycle will be repeated every 8 weeks for 3 cycles. Subsequent cycles will be scheduled based on the treatment response. Outpatients will be taught how to self-administer injections.

  Group 2 patients will be evaluated with a physical examination and blood tests every month for the first 6 months of treatment. Subsequent visits will be scheduled on an individual basis, but will be no less often than once every 4 months. Patients may need to be monitored daily during the 5 days of each injection cycle. Blood tests will also be done on day 5 of the first cycle and 1 month after the first cycle to evaluate drug side effects for possible dosage adjustments.

Further Study Details

The purpose of this study is to compare the effects of subcutaneous recombinant interleukin-2 (SC rIL-2) and no SC rIL-2 on disease progression and death over a 5-year follow-up period in patients with HIV-1 infection and absolute CD4+ cell counts of greater than or equal to 300/mm who are taking combination antiretroviral therapy.

Eligibility: Inclusion Criteria

- Documentation of HIV-1 infection by any licensed ELISA test and confirmed by a second method (e.g. Western Blot); or any one of the following at any time: detectable HIV p24 antigen, quantifiable plasma HIV RNA, or detectable proviral DNA.

- Absolute CD4(+) cell count of greater than or equal to 300/mm(3) within 45 days prior to randomization. (For patients who are status post-splenectomy, also a CD4(+) cell percentage greater than 20 percent).

- No evidence of active clinical disease for at least one year, in the judgment of the clinician, for any AIDS-defining illness or any of the following conditions: extrapulmonary *Pneumocystis carinii* disease; multi-dermatomal herpes zoster (greater than or equal to 10 lesions in a non-contiguous site); American trypanosomiasis (Chagas disease) of the CNS; *Penicillium marneffei* disease; visceral leishmaniasis; non-Hodgkin's lymphoma of any cell-type; Hodgkin's lymphoma; bartonellosis; microsporidiosis (greater than 1 month's duration); nocardiosis; invasive aspergillosis; or Rhodococcus equi disease.

- Age greater than or equal to 18 years.

- Laboratory values (within 45 days prior to randomization): AST or ALT less than or equal to 5 times the upper limit of normal (ULN); Total or direct bilirubin less than or equal to 2 times ULN (Patients with hyperbilirubinemia due to Gilbert's syndrome or indinavir therapy may have a serum bilirubin up to 5 times ULN); Creatinine less than or equal to 2.0 mg/dL (177 micro mol/L); Platelet count greater than or equal to 50,000/mm(3); On or initiating combination antiretroviral therapy at the time of randomization. Antiretroviral therapy can include agents (approved and investigational) administered through routine care or through participation in clinical trials or expanded access programs.

- Signed informed consent form.

Exclusion Criteria

- Prior rIL-2 therapy.

- Concurrent malignancy requiring cytotoxic chemotherapy.

- Use of systemic corticosteroids, immunosuppressants, or cytotoxic agents within 45 days prior to study randomization.

- Any CNS abnormality that requires ongoing treatment with antiseizure medication.

- Current or historical autoimmune/inflammatory diseases including: Inflammatory bowel disease (Crohn's disease, ulcerative colitis); Psoriasis; Optic neuritis; or any autoimmune/inflammatory diseases with potentially life-threatening complications.

- Pregnancy. (For women of childbearing potential, a negative pregnancy test, serum or urine, is required within 14 days prior to randomization).

- Breastfeeding.

Nutrition Intervention in AIDS Wasting

There are no guidelines for appropriate nutritional management of weight loss or wasting in HIV infection. Some treatments may increase weight, but without improving muscle mass or quality of life. In this clinical trial AIDS patients with wasting are randomized to one of three nutritional strategies and studied over a 12-week period: 1) optimal oral nutrition with counseling and protein and calorie supplementation, and a placebo pill; 2) optimal oral nutrition with the oral androgen, oxandrolone at 20 mg daily; and 3) optimal oral nutrition with progressive resistance training (PRT). In all participants, dietary intervention is maximized by weekly personalized counseling to address individual issues and concerns. Two primary outcomes are assessed: thigh muscle mass and quality of life. Our findings can be used to develop guidelines for standards of nutritional care among AIDS patient with the wasting syndrome.

Eligibility

Ages eligible for study are 18 years and above. Both genders are eligible for this study.

Inclusion Criteria

- Loss of 10% of usual body weight, or loss of 5% of usual body weight within the previous 6 months, or BMI 20kg/m². If the candidate is taking a protease inhibitor, he/she must have not regained weight since initiating the medication over a period of at least 4 weeks prior to screening.
- Documented HIV-positive
- Able to eat
- English-speaking
- Compliance with medical regimens
- For heterosexually active women: willingness to use an effective means of birth control
- Patient and physician not planning to start new treatments for HIV infection or weight loss during the 12 weeks of study.

Exclusion Criteria

- Vomiting 1 time/day or diarrhea 4 times/day on average in the previous week

- Fever 101° F within the previous week
- Receiving induction treatment for one of the following (new diagnosis or recurrence within 4 weeks):

    Pneumocystis carinii pneumonia

    Cryptococcal meningitis

    Cytomegalovirus retinitis or pneumonitis

    Toxoplasmosis

    Mycobacterium avium complex

    Visceral Kaposi's Sarcoma

    Lymphoma Pulmonary tuberculosis

- Received corticosteroids, estrogens, progesterones, androgens, oral anticoagulants, or growth hormone within the previous three months
- History of life-threatening reaction to oxandrolone or testosterone
- Currently pregnant
- History of congestive heart failure, myocardial infarction, angina/coronary artery disease, uncontrolled hypertension, cerebrovascular accident, hepatic failure, bleeding disorder, diabetes, nephrotic syndrome, cancer of the breast or prostate, or hypercalcemia
- Milk product allergy
- Current use of injected drugs
- Participation in an exercise program or strength training within the previous 4 weeks
- Any medical condition which renders the participant physically incapable of performing strength exercises
- Serum total testosterone level at least 300ng/ml, unless patient and primary physician prepared to begin testosterone injections concurrent with study enrollment (men only).

Screening Protocol for HIV Vaccine Studies

Healthy volunteers will be screened under this protocol for possible participation in a study testing a vaccine against HIV, the virus that causes AIDS. Healthy adults 18 to 60 years of age may be eligible for this study. Participants must be in good general health with no history of significant medical problems or abnormal laboratory test results. Pregnant or breast-feeding women and people infected with HIV will not be enrolled. Participants enrolled in this protocol will undergo the following tests and procedures within 8 weeks before the start of the experimental vaccine study:

- Medical history, including history of sexual activity and drug use.

- Physical examination.

- Pregnancy test for women of childbearing age.

- Blood and urine tests to evaluate possible medical problems such as liver and kidney function; to evaluate immune function; and to test for HIV, hepatitis and syphilis.

Individuals who are identified through this screening protocol as possible candidates for an HIV vaccine trial will be provided additional information about study options.

Further Study Details

The purpose of this study is to screen subjects to determine if they are suitable candidates for Phase I HIV vaccine trials. All work will be conducted at the National Institutes of Health. Healthy, HIV-negative subjects will be recruited and screened. The results of this study will be used to determine if the subject meets all of the eligibility requirements for participation in Phase I HIV trials of preventative vaccines or therapeutic vaccines. Educational materials on vaccines will be reviewed with and provided to subjects before enrollment into the study.

Eligibility

Both genders are eligible for this study.

Inclusion Criteria

Eligibility determination for the HIV trial will be dependent on results of laboratory tests and answers to the self-administered and/ or interview questions performed at this study.

- Age: 18-60 years of age.

- Good general health without clinically significant medical history, physical examination findings, or clinically significant abnormal laboratory results. A clinically significant condition or process includes the following:

  A condition that is chronic or recurring and is life threatening.

  A process that would affect the immune response, such as an autoimmune disease or HIV infection.

  A process that would require medication that affects the immune response.

  A condition for which repeated injections or blood draws may pose additional risk to the participant.

  A condition that requires active medical intervention or monitoring to avert grave danger to the participant's health or well-being.

  A condition or process in which signs or symptoms could be confused with reactions to vaccine.

- Willingness to follow-up for planned duration of the study (6 months or longer).

- Able and willing to give informed consent.

- Agree to have blood stored for future tests.

Exclusion Criteria

- Known to be HIV-1 positive (seropositive).

- Women who are known to be pregnant and/or breast feeding.

Chapter 64

Taking Part in Research Studies: What Questions You Should Ask

A research study is a way for finding answers to difficult scientific or health questions. For example, scientists may want to understand more about how AIDS is spread by asking people about their activities in a survey. Another example is when doctors might do a research study to find out whether a new medicine helps people improve their eyesight.

Following is a list of important questions you should ask of anyone who wants you or members of your family or community to be part of a research study.

Who put this study together?

- Who is running or in charge of this study?

- Whose idea was this study?

- How were people like me part of putting it together?

- Who are the researchers? Are they doctors or scientists? Who do they work for?

- Have they done studies like this before?

National Center for HIV, STD and TB Prevention, Centers for Disease Control and Prevention (CDC), updated August 13, 1998; available online at http://www.cdc.gov/hiv/pubs/brochure/unc3bro.htm. Despite the older date of this document, the information will be helpful to those considering taking part in a research study.

- Is the government part of this study? Who else is a part of this study?

- Who is paying for this study?

- Who will make money from the results of this study?

How can people like me share their ideas as you do this study?

- How will the study be explained in my community?

- Who of people like me will look at this study before it starts?

- Who of people like me are you talking to as you do this study? A Community Advisory Board?

- Who from the study can I go to with ideas, questions, or complaints?

- How will people like me find out about how the study is going?

Who is going to be in this study?

- What kinds of people are you looking for? Why?

- Are you trying to get minorities in this study?

- Are you including people less than 18 years old?

- How are you finding people for this study?

- Is transportation and/or daycare provided for people in this study?

- Do I need to sign to participate?

- Will you answer all of my questions before I sign the consent form?

- Can I quit the study after signing the consent form?

- If I quit the study, will anything happen to me?

What will I get out of this study?

- What are the benefits?

- Is payment involved? How will I be paid?

- Will I get free health care or other services if I participate? For how long?

- Will I get general health care and/or psychological care if I participate? For how long?

How will I be protected from harm?

- Do I stand a chance of being harmed in this study? In the future?
- Does the study protect me from all types of harm?
- If I get harmed, who will take care of me? Who is responsible?
- If I get harmed in any way, will I get all needed treatment?
- Who pays for treatment?

How will my privacy be protected?

- Who is going to see the information I give?
- Will my name be used with the information?
- What happens to the information I gave if I quit the study?
- Is there a written guarantee of privacy?

What do I have to do in this study?

- When did you start this study? How long will it last?
- How much of this study have you already done?
- Have there been any problems so far?
- Will I get treated the same as everyone else?
- What kinds of different treatments are offered in this study?
- Is there a real and a fake treatment?

What will be left behind after the study is over?

- What will happen to the information people give? How will it be kept?
- What are you going to do with the results of the study?
- How will the public learn about the results?
- Will results be in places where the public can see them?
- Are you going to send me a copy of the results? When?
- What other studies are you planning to do here?

Part Seven

HIV/AIDS
Statistical Information

Chapter 65

HIV/AIDS Statistics: An Overview

HIV/AIDS Worldwide

As of the end of 2001, an estimated 40 million people worldwide—37.2 million adults and 2.7 million children younger than 15 years—were living with HIV/AIDS. More than 70 percent of these people (28.1 million) live in Sub-Saharan Africa; another 15 percent (6.1 million) live in South and Southeast Asia.[1]

Worldwide, approximately one in every 100 adults aged 15 to 49 is HIV-infected. In Sub-Saharan Africa, about 8.4 percent of all adults in this age group are HIV-infected. In 16 African countries, the prevalence of HIV infection among adults aged 15 to 49 exceeds 10 percent.[1]

Approximately 48 percent of adults living with HIV/AIDS worldwide are women.[1]

An estimated 5 million new HIV infections occurred worldwide during 2001; that is, about 14,000 infections each day. More than 95 percent of these new infections occurred in developing countries.[1]

In 2001, approximately 6,000 young people aged 15 to 24 became infected with HIV every day—that is, about five every minute.[1]

In 2001 alone, HIV/AIDS-associated illnesses caused the deaths of approximately 3 million people worldwide, including an estimated 580,000 children younger than 15 years.[1]

"HIV/AIDS Statistics," National Institute of Allergy and Infectious Diseases (NIAID), February 2002; available online at http://www.niaid.nih.gov/factsheets/aidsstat.htm.

Worldwide, more than 80 percent of all adult HIV infections have resulted from heterosexual intercourse.[1]

HIV/AIDS in the United States

The Centers for Disease Control and Prevention (CDC) estimate that 850,000 to 950,000 U.S. residents are living with HIV infection, one-quarter of whom are unaware of their infection.[2]

Approximately 40,000 new HIV infections occur each year in the United States, about 70 percent among men and 30 percent among women. Of these newly infected people, half are younger than 25 years of age.[3,4]

Of new infections among men in the United States, CDC estimates that approximately 60 percent of men were infected through homosexual sex, 25 percent through injection drug use, and 15 percent through heterosexual sex. Of newly infected men, approximately 50 percent are black, 30 percent are white, 20 percent are Hispanic, and a small percentage are members of other racial/ethnic groups.[4]

Of new infections among women in the United States, CDC estimates that approximately 75 percent of women were infected through heterosexual sex and 25 percent through injection drug use. Of newly infected women, approximately 64 percent are black, 18 percent are white, 18 percent are Hispanic, and a small percentage are members of other racial/ethnic groups.[4]

In the United States, 793,026 cases of AIDS had been reported to the CDC through June 30, 2001.[5]

The estimated number of new adult/adolescent AIDS cases diagnosed in the United States was 49,407 in 1997, 42,508 in 1998, 40,671 in 1999, and 40,106 in 2000.[5]

The estimated number of new pediatric AIDS cases (cases among individuals younger than age 13) in the United States fell from 949 in 1992 to 105 in 2000.[5]

The rate of adult/adolescent AIDS cases reported in the United States in 2000 (per 100,000 population) was 74.2 among blacks, 30.4 among Hispanics, 12.7 among American Indians/Alaska Natives, 7.9 among whites, and 4.3 among Asians/Pacific Islanders.[6]

From 1985 to 2000, the proportion of adult/adolescent AIDS cases in the United States reported in women increased from 7 percent to 25 percent.[6]

As of the end of 2000, an estimated 338,978 people in the United States were living with AIDS.[5]

As of June 30, 2001, 457,667 deaths among people with AIDS had been reported to the CDC.[5] AIDS is now the fifth leading cause of death in the United States among people aged 25 to 44, and is the leading cause of death for black men in this age group. Among black women in this age group, HIV ranks third.[7]

The estimated annual number of AIDS-related deaths in the United States fell approximately 70 percent from 1995 to 1999, from 51,117 deaths in 1995 to 15,245 deaths in 2000.[5]

Of the estimated 15,245 AIDS-related deaths in the United States in 1999, approximately 50 percent were among blacks, 30 percent among whites, 18 percent among Hispanics, and less than 1 percent among Asians/Pacific Islanders and American Indians/Alaska Natives.[5]

References

1. UNAIDS. Report on the Global HIV/AIDS Epidemic: December 2001.

2. Fleming, P.L. et al. HIV Prevalence in the United States, 2000. 9th Conference on Retroviruses and Opportunistic Infections, Seattle, Wash., Feb. 24-28, 2002. Abstract 11.

3. Centers for Disease Control and Prevention (CDC). HIV and AIDS—United States, 1981-2001. *MMWR* 2001;50:430-434.

4. Centers for Disease Control and Prevention (CDC). HIV Prevention Strategic Plan through 2005. January 2001.

5. Centers for Disease Control and Prevention (CDC). HIV/AIDS Surveillance Report 2001;13(no.1):1-41.

6. Centers for Disease Control and Prevention (CDC). HIV/AIDS Surveillance Report 2000;12(no.2):1-44.

7. Hoyert, D.L. et al. Deaths: Final data for 1999. National Vital Statistics Reports; vol. 49, no.

8. Hyattsville, Maryland: National Center for Health Statistics, 2001.

Chapter 66

Surveillance of Health Care Workers with HIV/AIDS

Of the adults reported with AIDS in the United States through June 30, 2001, 23,473 had been employed in health care. These cases represented 5.1 percent of the 461,495 AIDS cases reported to CDC for whom occupational information was known (information on employment in the health care setting was missing for 322,537 reported AIDS cases).

The type of job is known for 22,000 (94%) of the 23,473 reported health care workers with AIDS. The specific occupations are as follows: 1,746 physicians, 117 surgeons, 5,105 nurses, 482 dental workers, 453 paramedics, 3,046 technicians, 1,042 therapists, and 5,222 health aides. The remainder are maintenance workers, administrative staff, etc. Overall, 73% of the health care workers with AIDS, including 1,374 physicians, 87 surgeons, 3,791 nurses, 378 dental workers, and 315 paramedics, are reported to have died.

CDC is aware of 57 health care workers in the United States who have been documented as having seroconverted to HIV following occupational exposures. Twenty-six have developed AIDS. These individuals who seroconverted include 19 laboratory workers (16 of whom were clinical laboratory workers), 24 nurses, 6 physicians, 2 surgical technicians, 1 dialysis technician, 1 respiratory therapist, 1 health aide, 1 embalmer/morgue technician, and 2 housekeeper/maintenance

National Center for HIV, STD and TB Prevention, Centers for Disease Control and Prevention (CDC), updated February 2002; available online at http://www.cdc.gov/hiv/pubs/facts/hcwsurv.htm.

worker. The exposures were as follows: 48 had percutaneous (puncture/cut injury) exposure, 5 had mucocutaneous (mucous membrane and/or skin) exposure, 2 had both percutaneous and mucocutaneous exposure, and 2 had an unknown route of exposure. Forty-nine health care workers were exposed to HIV-infected blood, 3 to concentrated virus in a laboratory, 1 to visibly bloody fluid, and 4 to an unspecified fluid.

CDC is also aware of 137 other cases of HIV infection or AIDS among health care workers who have not reported other risk factors for HIV infection and who report a history of occupational exposure to blood, body fluids, or HIV-infected laboratory material, but for whom seroconversion after exposure was not documented. The number of these workers who acquired their infection through occupational exposures is unknown.

For information about prevention of occupational transmission, see the CDC fact sheet titled "Preventing Occupational HIV Transmission to Healthcare Personnel," September 2001.

Chapter 67

HIV/AIDS among African Americans

In the United States, the impact of HIV and AIDS in the African American community has been devastating. Through December 2000, CDC had received reports of 774,467 AIDS cases—of those, 292,522 cases occurred among African Americans. Representing only an estimated 12% of the total U.S. population, African Americans make up almost 38% of all AIDS cases reported in this country. Of persons infected with HIV, it is estimated that almost 129,000 African Americans were living with AIDS at the end of 1999.

In 2000, more African Americans were reported with AIDS than any other racial/ethnic group.

- 19,890 cases were reported among African Americans, representing nearly half (47%) of the 42,156 AIDS cases reported that year.

- Almost two-thirds (63%) of all women reported with AIDS were African American.

- African American children also represented almost two-thirds (65%) of all reported pediatric AIDS cases.

- The 2000 rate of reported AIDS cases among African Americans was 58.1 per 100,000 population, more than 2 times the rate for Hispanics and 8 times the rate for whites.

National Center for HIV, STD and TB Prevention, Centers for Disease Control and Prevention (CDC), updated March 11, 2002; available online at http://www.cdc.gov/hiv/pubs/facts/afam.htm.

Data on HIV and AIDS diagnoses in 25 states with integrated reporting systems show the increased impact of the epidemic on the African American community in the last few years. In these states, during the period from January 1996 through June 1999, African Americans represented a high proportion (50%) of all AIDS diagnoses, but an even greater proportion (57%) of all HIV diagnoses. And among young people (ages 13 to 24), 65% of the HIV diagnoses were among African Americans.

Prevention Efforts Must Focus on High-Risk Behaviors

Adult/Adolescent Men. Among African American men reported with AIDS, men who have sex with men (MSM) represent the largest proportion (37%) of reported cases since the epidemic began. The second most common exposure category for African American men is injection drug use (34%), and heterosexual exposure accounts for 8% of cumulative cases.

Adult/Adolescent Women. Among African American women reported with AIDS, injection drug use has accounted for 41% of all AIDS case reports since the epidemic began, with 38% due to heterosexual contact.

Interrelated Prevention Challenges in African American Communities

Looking at select seroprevalence studies among high-risk populations gives an even clearer picture of why the epidemic continues to spread in communities of color. The data suggest that three interrelated issues play a role—the continued health disparities between economic classes, the challenges related to controlling substance abuse, and the intersection of substance abuse with the epidemic of HIV and other sexually transmitted diseases (STDs).

- *Substance abuse* is fueling the sexual spread of HIV in the United States, especially in minority communities with high rates of STDs. Studies of HIV prevalence among patients in drug treatment centers and STD clinics find the rates of HIV infection among African Americans to be significantly higher than those among whites. Sharing needles and trading sex for drugs are two ways that substance abuse can lead to HIV and other STD transmission, putting sex partners and children of drug users at risk as well. Comprehensive programs for drug users must provide the information, skills, and support necessary to reduce both injection-related and sexual risks. At the same time, HIV prevention and treatment, substance abuse prevention, and sexually transmitted disease treatment and prevention services must be better integrated to take advantage of the multiple opportunities for intervention.

- *Prevention efforts must be improved* and sustained for young gay men. In a sample of young men who have sex with men (ages 15-22) in seven urban areas, researchers found that, overall, 7% were infected with HIV (range, 2%-12%). A significantly higher percentage of African American MSM (14%) than white MSM (3%) were infected.

It is clear that the public sector alone cannot successfully combat HIV and AIDS in the African American community. Overcoming the current barriers to HIV prevention and treatment requires that local leaders acknowledge the severity of the continuing epidemic among African Americans and play an even greater role in combating HIV/AIDS in their own communities. Additionally, HIV prevention strategies known to be effective (both behavioral and biomedical) must be available and accessible for all populations at risk.

Chapter 68

HIV/AIDS among Hispanic Americans

The United States has a large and growing Hispanic population that is heavily affected by the HIV/AIDS epidemic. In 2000, Hispanics represented 13% of the U.S. population (including residents of Puerto Rico), but accounted for 19% of the total number of new U.S. AIDS cases reported that year (8,173 of 42,156 cases). The AIDS incidence rate per 100,000 population (the number of new cases of a disease that occur during a specific time period) among Hispanics in 2000 was 22.5, more than 3 times the rate for whites (6.6), but lower than the rate for African Americans (58.1).

Hispanics in the United States include a diverse mixture of ethnic groups and cultures. HIV exposure risks for U.S.-born Hispanics and Hispanics born in other countries vary greatly, indicating a need for specifically targeted prevention efforts.

Historical Trends in AIDS Cases among Hispanics in the U.S.

Between 1993 and 1999, the number of persons living with AIDS increased, as a result of the 1993 expanded AIDS case definition and, more recently, improved survival among those who have benefited from the new combination drug therapies. During that period, the

"HIV/AIDS among Hispanics in the United States," National Center for HIV, STD and TB Prevention, Centers for Disease Control and Prevention (CDC), updated March 11, 2002; available online at http://www.cdc.gov/hiv/pubs/facts/Hispanic.htm.

characteristics of persons living with AIDS were changing, reflecting an expansion of the epidemic, particularly in minority populations. In 1993, 18% of those estimated to be living with AIDS were Hispanic, while in 1999, 20% were Hispanic. In comparison, non-Hispanic whites represented 46% of people estimated to be living with AIDS in 1993, but only 38% in 1999.

Cumulatively, males account for the largest proportion (81%) of AIDS cases reported among Hispanics in the United States, although the proportion of cases among females is rising. Females represent 19% of cumulative AIDS cases among Hispanics, but account for 23% of cases reported in 2000 alone. Sixty percent of Hispanics reported with AIDS in 2000 were born in the U.S.; of those, 42% were born in Puerto Rico.

From the beginning of the epidemic through December 2000, 114,019 Hispanic men have been reported with AIDS in the United States. Of these cases, men who have sex with men (MSM) represent 42%, injection drug users (IDUs) account for 35%, and 6% of cases were due to heterosexual contact. About 7% of cases were among Hispanic men who both had sex with men and injected drugs. Among men born in Puerto Rico, however, injection drug use accounts for a significantly higher proportion of cases than male-male sex.

For adult and adolescent Hispanic women, heterosexual contact accounts for the largest proportion (47%) of cumulative AIDS cases, most of which are linked to sex with an injection drug user. Injection drug use accounts for an additional 40% of AIDS cases among U.S. Hispanic women.

Building Better Prevention Programs for Hispanics

While race and ethnicity alone are not risk factors for HIV infection, underlying social and economic conditions (such as language or cultural diversity, higher rates of poverty and substance abuse, or limited access to or use of health care) may increase the risk for infection in some Hispanic American communities.

Transmission related to substance abuse continues to be a significant problem among Hispanics living in the United States, especially among those of Puerto Rican origin. Studies of patients in drug treatment centers find HIV prevalence among Hispanics to be substantially higher in some regions of the country, particularly the Northeast and Midwest. Comprehensive programs for drug users must provide the information, skills, and support necessary to reduce both injection-related and sexual risks. In addition, HIV prevention and treatment, substance abuse prevention, and sexually transmitted disease treatment and prevention services must be better integrated to take advantage of the multiple opportunities for intervention.

Prevention messages must be tailored to the affected communities. Hispanic populations need interventions that (1) are consistent with their values and beliefs and (2) include skills-building activities to facilitate changes in sexual behavior. Further, because the HIV/AIDS epidemic among Hispanics living in the U.S. reflects to a large extent the exposure modes and cultural modes of the individuals' birthplaces, an understanding of these behaviors and differences is important in targeting prevention efforts. For example, some high-risk behaviors associated with drug abuse (such as use of shooting galleries) may be more predominant among Puerto Rico-born Hispanics than among other Hispanics. Therefore, for these populations, prevention strategies should emphasize (1) preventing and treating substance abuse and (2) decreasing needle-sharing and the use of shooting galleries. For Hispanics born in Mexico, Cuba, and Central and South America, CDC data indicate that male-male sex is the primary mode of HIV transmission. Messages targeted to these populations must be based on an understanding of their cultural attitudes toward homosexuality and bisexuality, which may be different from those of other populations at high risk for infection.

To improve prevention programs in Hispanic communities across the United States, in addition to addressing underlying social and economic conditions, we must apply the lessons we have already learned about the design of culturally appropriate HIV prevention efforts for each Hispanic population.

Chapter 69

HIV/AIDS among U.S. Women

Between 1992 and 1999, the number of persons living with AIDS increased, as a result of the 1993 expanded AIDS case definition and, more recently, improved survival among those who have benefited from the new combination drug therapies. During that 7-year period, a growing proportion of persons living with AIDS were women, reflecting the ongoing shift in populations affected by the epidemic. In 1992, women accounted for 14% of adults/adolescents living with AIDS— by 1999, the proportion had grown to 20%.

Since 1985, the proportion of all AIDS cases reported among adult and adolescent women has more than tripled, from 7% in 1985 to 25% in 1999. The epidemic has increased most dramatically among women of color. African American and Hispanic women together represent less than one-fourth of all U.S. women, yet they account for more than three-fourths (78%) of AIDS cases reported to date among women in our country. In 2000 alone, African American and Hispanic women represented an even greater proportion (80%) of cases reported in women.

While HIV/AIDS-related deaths among women continued to decrease in 1999, largely as a result of recent advances in HIV treatment, HIV/AIDS was the 5th leading cause of death for U.S. women aged 25-44. Among African American women in this same age group, HIV/AIDS was the third leading cause of death in 1999.

"HIV/AIDS among U.S. Women: Minority and Young Women at Continuing Risk," National Center for HIV, STD and TB Prevention, Centers for Disease Control and Prevention (CDC), updated March 11, 2002; available online at http://www.cdc.gov/hiv/pubs/facts/women.htm.

Heterosexual Contact Now Is Greatest Risk for Women

Sex with drug users plays large role. In 2000, 38% of women reported with AIDS were infected through heterosexual exposure to HIV; injection drug use accounted for 25% of cases. In addition to the direct risks associated with drug injection (sharing needles), drug use also is fueling the heterosexual spread of the epidemic. A significant proportion of women infected heterosexually were infected through sex with an injection drug user. Reducing the toll of the epidemic among women will require efforts to combat substance abuse, in addition to reducing HIV risk behaviors.

Many HIV/AIDS cases among women in the United States are initially reported without risk information, suggesting that women may be unaware of their partners' risk factors or that the health care system is not documenting their risk. Historically, more than two-thirds of AIDS cases among women initially reported without identified risk were later reclassified as heterosexual transmission, and just over one-fourth were attributed to injection drug use.

Prevention Needs of Women

Pay attention to prevention for women. The AIDS epidemic is far from over. Scientists believe that cases of HIV infection reported among 13- to 24-year-olds are indicative of overall trends in HIV incidence (the number of new infections in a given time period, usually a year) because this age group has more recently initiated high-risk behaviors—and females made up nearly half (47%) of HIV cases in this age group reported from the 34 areas with confidential HIV reporting for adults and adolescents in 2000. Further, for all years combined, young African American and Hispanic women account for three-fourths of HIV infections reported among females between the ages of 13 and 24 in these areas.

Implement programs that have been proven effective in changing risky behaviors among women and sustaining those changes over time, maintaining a focus on both the uninfected and infected populations of women.

Increase emphasis on prevention and treatment services for young women and women of color. Knowledge about preventive behaviors and awareness of the need to practice them is critical for each and every generation of young women—prevention programs should be comprehensive and should include participation by parents as well as the educational system. Community-based programs must reach out-of-school youth in settings such as youth detention centers and shelters for runaways.

Address the intersection of drug use and sexual HIV transmission. Women are at risk of acquiring HIV sexually from a partner who injects drugs and from sharing needles themselves. Additionally, women who use noninjection drugs (e.g., crack cocaine, methamphetamines) are at greater risk of acquiring HIV sexually, especially if they trade sex for drugs or money.

Develop and widely disseminate effective female-controlled prevention methods. More options are urgently needed for women who are unwilling or unable to negotiate condom use with a male partner. CDC is collaborating with scientists around the world to evaluate the prevention effectiveness of the female condom and to research and develop topical microbicides that can kill HIV and the pathogens that cause STDs.

Better integrate prevention and treatment services for women across the board, including the prevention and treatment of other STDs and substance abuse and access to antiretroviral therapy.

Chapter 70

HIV Prevalence among America's Youth

In the United States, HIV-related death has the greatest impact on young and middle-aged adults, particularly racial and ethnic minorities. In 1999, HIV was the fifth leading cause of death for Americans between the ages of 25 and 44. Among African American men in this age group, HIV infection has been the leading cause of death since 1991. In 1999, among black women 25-44 years old, HIV infection was the third leading cause of death. Many of these young adults likely were infected in their teens and twenties. It has been estimated that at least half of all new HIV infections in the United States are among people under 25, and the majority of young people are infected sexually (Rosenberg PS, Biggar RJ, Goedert JJ. Declining age at HIV infection in the United States [letter]. *New Engl J Med* 1994;330:789-90).

In 2000, 1,688 young people (ages 13 to 24) were reported with AIDS, bringing the cumulative total to 31,293 cases of AIDS in this age group. Among young men aged 13- to 24-years, 49% of all AIDS cases reported in 2000 were among men who have sex with men (MSM); 10% were among injection drug users (IDUs); and 9% were among young men infected heterosexually. In 2000, among young women the same age, 45% of all AIDS cases reported were acquired heterosexually and 11% were acquired through injection drug use. Among both males and females in this age group, the proportion of

"Young People at Risk: HIV/AIDS among America's Youth," National Center for HIV, STD and TB Prevention, Centers for Disease Control and Prevention (CDC), updated March 11, 2002; available online at http://www.cdc.gov/hiv/pubs/facts/youth.htm.

cases with exposure risk not reported or identified (26% for males and 43% for females) will decrease and the proportion of cases attributed to sexual contact and injection drug use will increase as follow-up investigations are completed and cases are reclassified into these categories.

Surveillance data analyzed from 25 states with integrated HIV and AIDS reporting systems for the period between January 1996 and June 1999 indicate that young people (aged 13 to 24) accounted for a much greater proportion of HIV (13%) than AIDS cases (3%). These data also show that even though AIDS incidence (the number of new cases diagnosed during a given time period, usually a year) is declining, there has not been a comparable decline in the number of newly diagnosed HIV cases among youth.

Scientists believe that cases of HIV infection diagnosed among 13- to 24-year-olds are indicative of overall trends in HIV incidence (the number of new infections in a given time period, usually a year) because this age group has more recently initiated high-risk behaviors. Females made up nearly half (47%) of HIV cases in this age group reported from the 34 areas with confidential HIV reporting for adults and adolescents in 2000—and in young people between the ages of 13 and 19, a much greater proportion of HIV infections was reported among females (61%) than among males (39%). Cumulatively, young African Americans are most heavily affected, accounting for 56% of all HIV cases ever reported among 13- to 24-year-olds in these 34 areas.

Improving HIV Prevention for Young People

CDC research has shown that early, clear communications between parents and young people about sex is an important step in helping adolescents adopt and maintain protective sexual behaviors. In addition, a wide range of activities must be implemented in communities to reduce the toll HIV infection and AIDS takes on young Americans.

School-based programs are critical for reaching youth before behaviors are established. Because risk behaviors do not exist independently, topics such as HIV, STDs, unintended pregnancy, tobacco, nutrition, and physical activity should be integrated and ongoing for all students in kindergarten through high school. The specific scope and content of these school health programs should be locally determined and consistent with parental and community values. Research has clearly shown that the most effective programs are comprehensive ones that include a focus on delaying sexual behavior and provide information on how sexually active young people can protect themselves. Evidence of prevention success can be seen in trends from the Youth Risk Behavior Survey conducted over an 8-year period, which show both a decline in sexual risk behaviors and an increase in condom use among sexually active youth. The percentage of sexually experienced high school students decreased from 54.1% in 1991 to 49.9% in 1999, while condom use among sexually active students increased from 46.2% to 58.0%. These findings represent a reversal in the trend toward increased sexual risk among teens that began in the 1970s and point to the success of comprehensive prevention efforts to both delay first intercourse among teens and increase condom use among young people who are sexually active.

Efforts to reach out-of-school youth are made by community-based programs. Addressing the needs of adolescents who are most vulnerable to HIV infection, such as homeless or runaway youth, juvenile offenders, or school drop-outs, is critically important. For example, a 1993 serosurveillance survey of females in four juvenile detention centers found that between 1% and 5% were HIV infected (median 2.8%).

Prevention efforts for young gay and bisexual men must be sustained. Targeted, sustained prevention efforts are urgently needed for young MSM as they come of age and initiate high-risk sexual behavior. Ongoing studies show that both HIV prevalence and risk behaviors remain high among young MSM. In a sample of young MSM ages 15-22 in seven urban areas, researchers found that, overall, 7% were infected with HIV, with higher prevalence among young African American (14%) and Hispanic (7%) men than among young white men (3%).

We must address sexual and drug-related risk. Many students report using alcohol or drugs when they have sex, and 1 in 50 high school students reports having injected an illegal drug. Surveillance data from the 34 states with integrated HIV and AIDS reporting systems suggest that drug injection led to at least 6% of HIV diagnoses reported among those aged 13-24 in 2000, with an additional 50% attributed to sexual transmission (both heterosexual and MSM).

STD treatment must play a role in prevention programs for young people. An estimated 12 million cases of STDs other than HIV are diagnosed annually in the United States, and about two-thirds of those are among people under the age of 25. Research has shown that biological factors make people who are infected with an STD more likely to become infected with HIV if exposed sexually; and HIV-infected people with STDs also are more likely to transmit HIV to their sex partners. Expanding STD treatment is critical to reducing the consequences of these diseases and helping to reduce risks of transmitting HIV among youth.

Evaluation of factors influencing risk behavior must be ongoing. Both broad-based surveys of the extent of risk behaviors among young people and focused studies of the factors contributing to risk and behavioral intent among specific groups of adolescents must be conducted and analyzed.

For young people, it is critical to prevent patterns of risky behaviors before they start. HIV prevention efforts must be sustained and designed to reach each new generation of Americans.

Part Eight

Additional Help
and Information

Chapter 71

Glossary of AIDS-Related Terms

Acquired Immunity: See Passive Immunity.

Acquired Immune Deficiency Syndrome (AIDS): The most severe manifestation of infection with the human immunodeficiency virus (HIV). The Centers for Disease Control and Prevention (CDC) lists numerous opportunistic infections and cancers that, in the presence of HIV infection, constitute an AIDS diagnosis. In 1993, CDC expanded the criteria for an AIDS diagnosis in adults and adolescents to include CD4+ T-cell count at or below 200 cells per microliter in the presence of HIV infection. In persons (age 5 and older) with normally functioning immune systems, CD4+ T-cell counts usually range from 500-1,500 cells per microliter. Persons living with AIDS often have infections of the lungs, brain, eyes, and other organs, and frequently suffer debilitating weight loss, diarrhea, and a type of cancer called Kaposi's Sarcoma. See HIV Disease; Opportunistic Infections; AIDS Wasting Syndrome.

AACTG: See Adult AIDS Clinical Trials Group.

ACTIS: See AIDS Clinical Trials Information Service.

Active Immunity: Protection from a disease as a result of previous exposure to the disease-causing infectious agent or antigen. The protection

---

"Glossary of HIV/AIDS-Related Terms, 4th Edition," HIV/AIDS Treatment Information Service (ATIS; now AIDSinfo), Department of Health and Human Service (DHHS), 2002.

can be a result of having had the disease or having received a vaccine to prevent getting the disease.

Acupuncture: A Chinese medical treatment involving the insertion of very fine sterile needles into the body at specific points according to a mapping of energy pathways. Historically, acupuncture is one component of an overall program of Chinese medicine that includes theory, practice, diagnosis, physiology, and the use of herbal preparations. Acupuncture is used to control pain and to treat other conditions such as allergies or addiction withdrawal. See Alternative Medicine.

Acute HIV Infection: The period of rapid viral replication immediately following exposure to HIV. An estimated 80 to 90 percent of individuals with primary HIV infection develop an acute syndrome characterized by flu-like symptoms of fever, malaise, lymphadenopathy, pharyngitis, headache, myalgia, and sometimes rash. Following primary infection, seroconversion and a broad HIV-1 specific immune response occur, usually within an average of 3 weeks after transmission of HIV. It was previously thought that HIV was relatively dormant during this phase. However, it is now known that during the time of primary infection, high levels of plasma HIV RNA can be documented.

Acute HIV Infection and Early Diseases Research Program (AIEDRP): A program funded by the National Institute of Allergy and Infectious Diseases (NIAID) focusing on innovative ways to study how HIV-1 causes disease in adults. Scientists will use interventions, such as highly active antiretroviral therapy (HAART) given in the acute and early phases of infection, to increase their understanding of the mechanisms and course of HIV disease. Information about this program can be found at http://aiedrp.fhcrc.org.

ADAP: See AIDS Drugs Assistance Programs.

Adenopathy: Any disease involving or causing enlargement of glandular tissues, especially one involving the lymph nodes.

Adherence: The extent to which the patient continues the agreed-upon mode of treatment or intervention as prescribed.

Adjuvant: An ingredient added to a prescription or solution that facilitates or modifies the action of the principal ingredient. May be used in HIV therapies or for HIV vaccines.

Administration: (Route of Administration.) How a drug or therapy is introduced into the body. Systemic administration means that the drug goes throughout the body (usually carried in the bloodstream), and includes oral (by mouth), intravenous (injection into the vein, IV), intramuscular (injection into a muscle, IM), intrathecal (injection into the spinal canal), subcutaneous (injection beneath the skin, SQ), and rectal administrations. Local administration means that the drug is applied or introduced into the specific area affected by the disease, such as application directly onto the affected skin surface (topical administration). The effects of most therapies depend upon the ability of the drug to reach the affected area; thus the route of administration and consequent distribution of a drug in the body are important determinants of its effectiveness.

Adult AIDS Clinical Trials Group (AACTG): The largest HIV clinical trial organization in the world. It plays a major role in setting standards of care for HIV infection and opportunistic diseases related to HIV/AIDS in the United States and the developed world. The AACTG has been pivotal in providing the data necessary for the approval of therapeutic agents, as well as the treatment and prevention strategies, for many opportunistic infections and malignancies. The AACTG is composed of, and directed by, leading clinical scientists in HIV/AIDS therapeutic research and funded through the National Institute of Allergy and Infectious Diseases. Internet address: http://aactg.s-3.com.

Adverse Reaction: (Adverse Event.) An unwanted effect caused by the administration of drugs. Onset may be sudden or develop over time. See Side Effects.

Aerosolized: A form of administration in which a drug, such as pentamidine, is turned into a fine spray or mist by a nebulizer and inhaled.

AETC: See AIDS Education and Training Centers.

Affected Community: Persons living with HIV and AIDS and other related individuals, including their families, friends, and advocates whose lives are directly influenced by HIV infection and its physical, psychological, and sociological ramifications.

Agammaglobulinemia: A nearly total absence of immunoglobulins resulting in the loss of ability to produce immune antibodies. See Antibodies.

Agency for Healthcare Research and Quality (AHRQ): Provides evidence-based information on health care outcomes, quality, cost, use, and access. Information from AHRQ's research helps people make more informed decisions and improve the quality of health care services. AHRQ was formerly known as the Agency for Health Care Policy and Research. Internet address: http://www.ahrq.gov.

AHRQ: See Agency for Healthcare Research and Quality.

AIDS: See Acquired Immunodeficiency Syndrome.

AIDS Clinical Trials Information Service (ACTIS): Provides quick and easy access to information on federally and privately funded clinical trials that evaluate experimental drugs and other therapies for adults and children at all stages of HIV infection. ACTIS is co-sponsored by the Food and Drug Administration, the National Institute of Allergy and Infectious Diseases, the Centers for Disease Control and Prevention, and the National Library of Medicine (see entries for these organizations). Internet address: http://www.actis.org.

AIDS Dementia Complex (ADC): (HIV-associated dementia or HAD.) A degenerative neurological condition attributed to HIV infection, characterized by a group of clinical presentations including loss of coordination, mood swings, loss of inhibitions, and widespread cognitive dysfunction. It is the most common central nervous system complication of HIV infection. Characteristically, it manifests itself after the patient develops major opportunistic infections or AIDS-related cancers. However, patients can also have this syndrome before these major systemic complications occur. The cause of ADC has not been determined exactly, but it may result from HIV infection of cells or inflammatory reactions to such infections.

AIDSDrugs: An online database service of the National Library of Medicine with information about drugs undergoing testing against HIV infection, AIDS, AIDS-related complex, and related opportunistic diseases. Internet address: http://www.actis.org.

AIDS Drug Assistance Programs (ADAP): State-based programs funded in part by Title II of the Ryan White C.A.R.E. Act that provide therapeutics (including devices necessary to administer pharmaceuticals) to treat HIV disease or prevent the serious deterioration of health, including treatment of opportunistic infections. ADAP formularies and eligibility criteria are determined state-by-state with a focus on serving low-income individuals who have limited or no coverage from private insurance or Medicaid.

AIDS Education and Training Centers (AETC): The Health Resources and Services Administration (HRSA) supports the National AIDS Education and Training Centers (AETCs) Program. This is a network of 15 regional centers that conduct targeted, multidiscipli-nary HIV education and training programs for health care providers. The mission of these centers is to increase the number of health care providers who are effectively educated and motivated to counsel, diag-nose, treat, and manage individuals with HIV infection and to assist in the prevention of high risk behaviors which may lead to infection. Internet address: http://www.aids-ed.org.

AIDSLINE: An online database service of the National Library of Medicine with citations and abstracts covering the published scien-tific and medical literature on AIDS and related topics. Internet ad-dress: http://gateway.nlm.nih.gov.

AIDS-Related Cancers: Several cancers are more common or more aggressive in persons living with HIV. These malignancies include certain types of immune system cancers known as lymphomas, Kaposi's Sarcoma, and anogenital cancers that primarily affect the anus and the cervix. HIV, or the immune suppression it induces, ap-pears to play a role in the development of these cancers.

AIDS-Related Complex (ARC): (Early Symptomatic HIV Infection) 1. A group of common complications found in early stage HIV infection. They include progressive generalized lymphadenopathy (PGL), recur-rent fever, unexplained weight loss, swollen lymph nodes, diarrhea, herpes, hairy leukoplakia, fungus infection of the mouth and throat and/or the presence of HIV antibodies. 2. Symptoms that appear to be related to infection by HIV. They include an unexplained, chronic deficiency of white blood cells (leukopenia) or a poorly functioning lymphatic system with swelling of the lymph nodes (lymphadenopa-thy) lasting for more than 3 months without the opportunistic infec-tions required for a diagnosis of AIDS. See AIDS Wasting Syndrome.

AIDS Research Advisory Committee (ARAC): A board that ad-vises and makes recommendations to the Director, National Institute of Allergy and Infectious Diseases, on all aspects of HIV-related re-search, vaccine development, pathogenesis, and epidemiology.

AIDS Service Organization (ASO): A health association, support agency, or other service actively involved in the prevention and treat-ment of AIDS.

AIDSTrials: An online database service of the National Library of Medicine with information about clinical trials of agents (e.g., drugs) under evaluation against HIV infection, AIDS, and related opportu-nistic diseases. Internet address: http://www.actis.org.

AIDS Wasting Syndrome: The involuntary weight loss of 10 percent of baseline body weight plus either chronic diarrhea (two loose stools per day for more than 30 days) or chronic weakness and documented fever (for 30 days or more, intermittent or constant) in the absence of a concurrent illness or condition other than HIV infection that would explain the findings.

Alkaline Phosphatase: An enzyme normally present in certain cells within the liver, bone, kidney, intestine, and placenta. When the cells are destroyed in those tissues, more of the enzyme leaks into the blood, and levels rise in proportion to the severity of the condition. Measurement of this enzyme is used as an indication of the health of the liver.

Alopecia: Loss of hair that frequently occurs in patients undergoing chemotherapy for cancer or suffering from other diseases, such as AIDS, where cell-killing, or cytotoxic, drugs are used.

Alpha Interferon (Interferon alpha): A protein—one of three major classes of interferons—that the body produces in response to infections. In persons who are HIV positive, elevated interferon levels are regarded as an indication of disease progression. See Interferon.

Alternative Medicine: A broad category of treatment systems (e.g., chiropractic, herbal medicine, acupuncture, homeopathy, naturopathy, and spiritual devotions) or culturally based healing traditions such as Chinese, Ayurvedic, and Christian Science. Alternative medicines share the common characteristic of non acceptance by the biomedical (i.e., mainstream Western) establishment. Alternative medicine is also referred to as complementary medicine. The designation alternative medicine is not equivalent to holistic medicine, a narrower term. For more information, contact the National Center for Complementary and Alternative Medicine Clearinghouse (NCCAM). Internet address: http://nccam.nih.gov.

Alveolar: Pertaining to the alveoli sacs, the site of gas exchange in the lungs.

Amebiasis: An inflammation of the intestines caused by infestation with *Entamoeba histolytica* (a type of ameba) and characterized by frequent, loose stools flecked with blood and mucus.

Amino Acids: Any of a class of nitrogen-containing acids. Some 22 amino acids are commonly found in animals and humans. Chains of amino acids synthesized by living systems are called polypeptides (up to about 50 amino acids) and proteins (more than 50 amino acids). See Peptide; Proteins.

Anaphylactic Shock: A life-threatening allergic reaction character-ized by a swelling of body tissues (including the throat) and a sudden decline in blood pressure. Symptoms include difficulty breathing, vio-lent coughing, and chest constriction.

Anemia: A lower than normal number of red blood cells.

Anergy: 1. The loss or weakening of the body's immunity to an irri-tating agent, or antigen. Patients may be so immunologically sup-pressed that they are unable to produce a reaction to an antigen. For example, such patients will usually not test positive for tuberculosis (TB) on a tuberculin skin test (or Mantoux test). The lack of a reac-tion indicates anergy. 2. Researchers in cell culture have shown that CD4+ T-cells can be turned off by a signal from HIV that leaves them unable to respond to further immune system stimulation.

Angiogenesis: The process of forming new blood vessels. Angiogen-esis is essential for the growth of tumors, especially Kaposi's Sarcoma.

Angiomatosis: A condition characterized by the formation of a tumor that is composed chiefly of blood or lymphatic vessels. See Kaposi's Sarcoma.

Anorexia: The lack or loss of appetite that leads to significant de-cline in weight.

Antenatal: Occurring before birth.

Antibiotic: A natural or synthetic substance that inhibits the growth of micro-organisms such as bacteria or fungi. Some antibiotics are used to treat infectious diseases.

Antibodies: Molecules in the blood or other body fluids that tag, de-stroy, or neutralize bacteria, viruses, or other harmful toxins (antigens). They are members of a class of proteins known as immunoglobulins, which are produced and secreted by B lymphocytes in response to stimulation by antigens. An antibody is specific to an antigen.

Antibody-Dependent Cell-Mediated Cytotoxicity (ADCC): An immune response in which antibodies bind to target cells, identify-ing them for attack by the immune system.

Antibody-Mediated Immunity: Also called humoral immunity. Immunity that results from the activity of antibodies in blood and lymphoid tissue.

Antifungal: A substance that kills or inhibits the growth of a fun-gus.

Antigen: Any substance that stimulates the immune system to produce antibodies (proteins that fight antigens). Antigens are often foreign substances such as bacteria or viruses that invade the body.

Antigen Presentation: The event of providing fragments of foreign proteins, including viruses and bacteria, to the helper T-cells. The presentation occurs through the display of the fragments of foreign proteins on the surface of the antigen-presenting cells (APC).

Antigen-Presenting Cell (APC): The cell type that collects foreign material (e.g., antigen) and digests it into pieces that can be recognized by the immune system. The APC presents the antigen to the helper T-cells, the CD4+ T-cells; this results in the initiation of expansion of an immune response targeted against the foreign material. APCs are B cells, macrophages, or dendritic cells.

Antineoplastic: A substance that prevents the development, growth, or proliferation of malignant (tumor) cells.

Antiprotozoal: A substance that kills or inhibits the multiplication of single-celled micro-organisms called protozoa.

Antiretroviral Drugs: Substances used to kill or inhibit the multiplication of retroviruses such as HIV.

Antisense Drugs: An antisense, nucleic acid-related compound is the mirror image of the genetic sequence that it is supposed to inactivate. It is a synthetic segment of DNA or RNA that locks onto a strand of natural DNA or RNA with a complementary sequence of nucleotides. By binding to either the target DNA or RNA, the antisense drug prohibits the normal functioning and expression of the gene. This prevents the building of new virus particles or the infection of new host cells.

Antitoxins: Antibodies that recognize and inactivate toxins produced by certain bacteria, plants, or animals.

Antiviral: A substance or process that destroys a virus or suppresses its replication (i.e., reproduction).

Aphasia: Loss of ability to speak or understand speech.

Aphthous Ulcer: A painful oral or esophageal sore of unknown cause that has a deep eroded base. Aphthous ulcers are common in persons living with HIV.

Apoptosis: "Cellular suicide," also known as programmed cell death. HIV may induce apoptosis in both infected and uninfected immune system cells. Normally when CD4+ T-cells mature in the thymus gland, a small proportion of these cells is unable to distinguish self from nonself. Because these cells would otherwise attack the body's own tissues, they receive a biochemical signal from other cells that results in apoptosis. See Tumor Necrosis Factor.

Approved Drugs: In the U.S., the Food and Drug Administration (FDA) must approve a substance as a drug before it can be marketed. The approval process involves several steps, including preclinical laboratory and animal studies, clinical trials for safety and efficacy, filing of a New Drug Application (NDA) by the manufacturer of the drug, FDA review of the application, and FDA approval/rejection of application.

ARC: See AIDS-Related Complex.

ARM: One group of participants in a comparative clinical trial, all of whom receive the same treatment. The other arm(s) receive(s) a different treatment regimen.

ART: Antiretroviral therapy.

Arthralgia: A pain in a joint.

ASO: See AIDS Service Organization.

Aspergillosis: A fungal infection—resulting from the fungus Aspergillus—of the lungs that can spread through the blood to other organs. Symptoms include fever, chills, difficulty in breathing, and coughing up blood. If the infection reaches the brain, it may cause dementia.

Assembly and Budding: Names for a portion of the processes by which new HIV is formed in infected host cells. Viral core proteins, enzymes, and RNA (ribonucleic acid) gather just inside the cell's membrane, while the viral envelope proteins aggregate within the membrane. An immature viral particle is formed and then pinches off from the cell, acquiring an envelope and the cellular and HIV proteins from the cell membrane. The immature viral particle then undergoes processing by an HIV enzyme called protease to become an infectious virus.

Asymptomatic: Without symptoms. Usually used in the HIV/AIDS literature to describe a person who has a positive reaction to one of several tests for HIV antibodies but who shows no clinical symptoms of the disease.

Ataxia: Lack of muscular coordination.

Attenuated: Weakened or decreased. For example, an attenuated virus can no longer produce disease but might be used to produce a vaccine.

Autoantibody: 1. An antibody that is active against some of the tissues of the organism that produced it. 2. An antibody directed against the body's own tissue.

Autoimmunization: The induction of an immune response to a body's own cells (tissue).

Autoinoculation: Inoculation of a microorganism obtained by contact with a lesion on one's own body, producing a secondary infection.

Autologous: Pertaining to the same organism or one of its parts; originating within an organism itself. For instance, donating your own blood for your future surgery is known as an autologous transfusion.

Avascular Necrosis (AVN): Also referred to as osteonecrosis. A disease resulting from temporary or permanent loss of blood supply to the bone. It is a possible late complication that may be associated with Highly Active Antiretroviral Therapy (HAART). The most common site is the femoral head. Many patients have other risk factors including alcohol abuse, hyperlipidemia, corticosteroid use, and hypercoagulability (increased clotting ability of the blood).

AVN: See Avascular Necrosis.

Bactericidal: (Bacteriocidal) Capable of killing bacteria.

Bacteriostatic: Capable of inhibiting reproduction of bacteria.

Bacterium: A microscopic organism composed of a single cell. Many bacteria can cause disease in humans.

Baculovirus: A virus of insects used in the production of some HIV vaccines. See Vaccine.

Baseline: 1. Information gathered at the beginning of a study from which variations found in the study are measured. 2. A known value or quantity with which an unknown is compared when measured or assessed. 3. The initial time point in a clinical trial, just before a volunteer starts to receive the experimental treatment undergoing testing. At this reference point, measurable values such as CD4 count are recorded. Safety and efficacy of a drug are often determined by monitoring changes from the baseline values.

Basophil: A type of white blood cell, also called a granular leukocyte, filled with granules of toxic chemicals that can digest micro-organisms. Basophils, as well as other types of white blood cells, are responsible for the symptoms of allergy.

B Cell Lymphoma: See Lymphoma.

B Cells: See B Lymphocytes.

BDNA Test: (bDNA): See Branched DNA Assay.

Beta 2 Microglobulin: Protein tightly bound to the surface of many nucleated cells, articularly those of the immune system. Elevated microglobulin levels occur in a variety of diseases. While elevated microglobulin is not specific to HIV, there is a correlation between this marker and the progression of HIV disease.

Bilirubin: A red pigment occurring in liver bile, blood, and urine. Its measurement can be used as an indication of the health of the liver. Bilirubin is the product of the breakdown of hemoglobin in red blood cells. It is removed from the blood and processed by the liver, which secretes it into the digestive tract. An elevated level of bilirubin in blood serum is an indication of liver disease or drug-induced liver impairment.

Binding Antibody: As related to HIV infection: An antibody that attaches to some part of HIV. Binding antibodies may or may not adversely affect the virus.

Bioavailability: The extent to which an oral medication is absorbed in the digestive tract and reaches the bloodstream, thereby permitting access to the site of action.

Biological Response Modifiers (BRMs): Substances, either natural or synthesized, that boost, direct, or restore normal immune defenses. BRMs include interferons, interleukins, thymus, hormones, and monoclonal antibodies.

Biopsy: Surgical removal of a piece of tissue from a living subject for microscopic examination to make a diagnosis (e.g., to determine whether abnormal cells such as cancer cells are present).

Biotechnology: 1. Use of living organisms or their products to make or modify a substance. These include recombinant DNA techniques (genetic engineering). 2. Industrial application of the results of biological research, particularly in fields such as recombinant DNA or gene splicing, which permits the production of synthetic hormones or enzymes by combining genetic material from different species.

Blinded Study: A clinical trial in which participants are unaware as to whether they are in the experimental or control arm of the study. See Double Blind Study.

BLIPS: The transient detection of a viral load level after a period of time when viral load was undetectable. It is usually defined as a viral load of 50 to 500 copies/mL after viral load <50 copies/mL on at least two consecutive occasions.

Blood-Brain Barrier: A selective barrier (obstacle) between circulating blood and brain tissues that prevents damaging substances from reaching the brain. Certain compounds readily cross the blood/brain barrier; others are completely blocked.

B Lymphocytes (B Cells): One of the two major classes of lymphocytes, B lymphocytes are blood cells of the immune system, derived from the bone marrow and spleen; they are involved in the production of antibodies. During infections, these cells are transformed into plasma cells that produce large quantities of antibody directed at specific pathogens. When antibodies bind to foreign proteins, such as those that occur naturally on the surfaces of bacteria, they mark the foreign cells for consumption by other cells of the immune system. This transformation occurs through interactions with various types of T-cells and other components of the immune system. In persons living with AIDS, the functional ability of both the B and the T lymphocytes is damaged, with the T lymphocytes being the principal site of infection by HIV.

Body Fat Redistribution Syndrome (BFR): See Fat Redistribution.

Body Fluids: Any fluid in the human body, such as blood, urine, saliva (spit), sputum, tears, semen, mother's milk, or vaginal secretions. Only blood, semen, mother's milk, and vaginal secretions have been linked directly to the transmission of HIV.

Bone Marrow: Soft tissue located in the cavities of the bones where blood cells such as erythrocytes, leukocytes, and platelets are formed.

Bone Marrow Suppression: A side effect of many anticancer and antiviral drugs, including AZT. Leads to a decrease in white blood cells, red blood cells, and platelets. Such reductions in turn result in anemia, bacterial infections, and spontaneous or excess bleeding.

Booster: A second or later dose of a vaccine given to increase the immune response to the original dose.

Branched DNA Assay: (bDNA test) A test developed by Bayer (formerly Chiron Corporation) for measuring the amount of HIV (as well as other viruses) in blood plasma. Test results are calibrated in numbers of virus particle equivalents per milliliter of plasma. The bDNA test is similar in results but not in technique to the Polymerase Chain Reaction (PCR) test. bDNA testing is currently being used to evaluate the effectiveness of drug treatment regimens and to gauge HIV disease progression. Newer versions, or generations, of these assays are being developed; they will be able to detect smaller numbers of copies of HIV in a blood sample. See Viral Burden.

Breakthrough Infection: An infection caused by the infectious agent the substance is designed to protect against. As it pertains to a vaccine trial, the infection may be caused by exposure to the infectious agent before the vaccine has taken effect, or before all doses of the vaccine have been given.

Bronchoscopy: Visual examination of the bronchial passages of the lungs through the tube of an endoscope (usually a curved flexible tube containing fibers that carry light down the tube and project an enlarged image up the tube to the viewer) that is inserted into the upper lungs. Can be used for extraction of material from the lungs. See Endoscopy.

Budding: See Assembly and Budding.

Buffalo Hump: See Lipodystrophy.

Burkitt's Lymphoma: A B-cell type lymphoma.

Cachexia: General ill health and malnutrition, marked by weakness and emaciation, usually associated with serious disease. See AIDS Wasting Syndrome.

Candida: Yeast-like fungi commonly found in the normal flora of the mouth, skin, intestinal tract, and vagina, which can become clinically infectious in immune-compromised persons. See Candidiasis, Fungus, Thrush.

Candidiasis: An infection with a yeast-like fungus of the Candida family, generally Candida albicans. Candidiasis of the esophagus, trachea, bronchi, or lungs is an indicator disease for AIDS. Oral or recurrent vaginal candida infection is an early sign of immune system deterioration. See Opportunistic Infections; Thrush; Vaginal Candidiasis.

Carcinogen: Any cancer-producing substance.

CAT Scan: See C-T Scan.

CBC: See Complete Blood Count.

CBCT: See Community-Based Clinical Trial.

CBO: See Community-Based Organization.

CCR5: Cell surface molecule, which is needed along with the primary receptor, the CD4 molecule, in order to fuse with the membranes of the immune system cells. Researchers have found that the strains of HIV most often transmitted from person to person require the CCR5 molecule and CD4 molecule in order for HIV to enter the cell. In addition to its role in fusion, CKR5 is a receptor for certain immune-signaling molecules called chemokines that are known to suppress HIV infection of cells. See Chemokines; CXCR4.

CDC: See Centers for Disease Control and Prevention.

CD4 (T4) or CD4+ Cells: 1. A type of T-cell involved in protecting against viral, fungal, and protozoal infections. These cells normally orchestrate the immune response, signaling other cells in the immune system to perform their special functions. Also known as T helper cells. 2. HIV's preferred targets are cells that have a docking molecule called cluster designation 4 (CD4) on their surfaces. Cells with this molecule are known as CD4-positive (or CD4+) cells. Destruction of CD4+ lymphocytes is the major cause of the immunodeficiency observed in AIDS, and decreasing CD4+ lymphocyte levels appear to be the best indicator for developing opportunistic infections. Although CD4 counts fall, the total T-cell level remains fairly constant through the course of HIV disease, due to a concomitant increase in the CD8+ cells. The ratio of CD4+ to CD8+ cells is therefore an important measure of disease progression. See CD8 (T8) Cells; Immunodeficiency.

CD8 (T8) Cells: White blood cells with the CD8 protein on their surface. These white blood cells kill some cancer cells and cells infected by intracellular pathogens (some bacteria, viruses, and mycoplasma). Also called cytotoxic T-cells, T8 cells, cytotoxic T lymphocytes.

CDC National AIDS Hotline (CDC-NAH): Provides education, information, and referrals for persons living with HIV, their families and friends, health professionals, and the general public on HIV/AIDS issues, including risk factors, transmission, prevention, and testing. The Hotline number is 1-800-342-AIDS (1-800-342-2437). Internet Address: http://www.ashastd.org/nah/index.html.

CDC National Prevention Information Network (CDC-NPIN): The National Prevention Information Network (NPIN) is a national reference, referral and distribution service for information on HIV/AIDS, STDs, and TB, sponsored by the Centers for Disease Control and Prevention (CDC). All of the NPIN's services are designed to facilitate sharing of information and resources among people working in HIV, STD, and TB prevention, treatment, and support services. NPIN staff serves a diverse network of people who work in international, national, state, and local settings. Internet address: http://www.cdcnpin.org/.

Cell Lines: Specific cell types artificially maintained in the laboratory (i.e., in vitro) for scientific purposes.

Cell-Mediated Immunity (CMI): This branch of the immune system exists primarily to deal with viruses, which are more insidious than bacteria because they invade the host (e.g., human) cells, where they can hide from the antibody-making cells of the immune system. With this system, the reaction to foreign material is performed by specific defense cells, such as killer T-cells, macrophages, and other white blood cells rather than by antibodies.

Cellular Immunity: See Cell-Mediated Immunity.

Centers for Disease Control and Prevention (CDC): The U.S. Department of Health and Human Services agency with the mission to promote health and quality of life by preventing and controlling disease, injury, and disability. CDC operates 11 Centers including the National Center for HIV, STD, and TB Prevention. CDC assesses the status and characteristics of the HIV epidemic and conducts epidemiologic, laboratory, and surveillance investigations. Internet address: http://www.cdc.gov.

Central Nervous System (CNS): The central nervous system is composed of the brain, spinal cord, and meninges (protective membranes surrounding them).

Central Nervous System (CNS) Damage: (By HIV infection.) Although monocytes and macrophages can be infected by HIV, they appear to be relatively resistant to killing. However, these cells travel throughout the body and carry HIV to various organs, especially the lungs and the brain. Persons living with HIV often experience abnormalities in the central nervous system. Investigators have hypothesized that an accumulation of HIV in brain and nerve cells or the inappropriate release of cytokines or toxic byproducts of these cells may be to blame for the neurological manifestations of HIV disease.

Centers for Medicare and Medicaid Services (CMS): A federal agency within the U.S. Department of Health and Human Services.

CMS runs the Medicare and Medicaid programs, two national health care programs that benefit about 75 million Americans. And with the Health Resources and Services Administration, CMS runs the State Children's Health Insurance Program (SCHIP), a program that is expected to cover many of the approximately 10 million uninsured children in the United States. CMS also regulates all laboratory testing (except research) performed on humans in the United States. (Formerly the Health Care Financing Administration (HCFA)). Internet address: http://cms.hhs.gov.

Cerebral: Pertaining to the cerebrum, the main portion of the brain.

Cerebrospinal Fluid (CSF): Fluid that bathes the brain and the spinal cord. A sample of this fluid is often removed from the body for diagnostic purposes by a lumbar puncture (spinal tap). See Lumbar Puncture.

Cervical Cancer: A malignant neoplasm of the uterine cervix. See Cervical Dysplasia; Cervix; Pap Smear.

Cervical Dysplasia: Abnormality in the size, shape, and organization of adult cells of the cervix. It is often a precursor lesion for cervical cancer. Studies indicate an increase in prevalence of cervical dysplasia among women living with HIV. Additional studies have documented that a higher prevalence is associated with greater immune suppression. HIV infection also may adversely affect the clinical course and treatment of cervical dysplasia and cancer.

Cervical Intraepithelial Neoplasia (CIN1, CIN2, CIN3): Dysplasia of the cervix epithelium, often premalignant (i.e., precancerous). Considerable evidence implicates human papilloma virus (HPV) in the development of CIN. Immunosuppression may also play an important role in facilitating infection or persistence of HPV in the genital tract and progression of HPV-induced neoplasia. See Condyloma; Neoplasm.

Cervix: The lower terminus of the uterus that juts into the lower vagina and contains a narrow canal connecting the upper and lower parts of a woman's reproductive tract.

Challenge: In vaccine experiments, the deliberate exposure of an immunized animal to the infectious agent.

Chancroid: A highly contagious sexually transmitted disease caused by the *Haemophilus ducreyi bacterium* with symptoms appearing 3 to 5 days after exposure. It appears as a tender papule that becomes pustular and then ulcerative.

Chemokines: Also called beta chemokines. Studies of the relationship between HIV and these immune system chemicals have shown the complex exchanges that take place when HIV and white blood cells meet. Chemokines are intracellular messenger molecules secreted by CD8+ cells whose major function is to attract immune cells to sites of infection. Recent research has shown that HIV-1 needs access to chemokine receptors on the cell surface to infect the cell. Several chemokines—called RANTES, MIP-1A, and MIP-1B—interfere with HIV replication by occupying these receptors. Findings suggest that one mechanism these molecules use to suppress HIV infectivity is to block the process of fusion used by the virus to enter cells.

Chemoprophylaxis: The use of a drug or chemical to prevent a disease.

Chemotherapy: In general, it is the use of medications to treat any disease. It is more commonly used to described medications to treat cancer. The treatment, mostly of cancer, uses a series of cytotoxic drugs that attack cancerous cells. This treatment commonly has adverse side effects that may include the temporary loss of the body's natural immunity to infections, loss of hair, digestive upset, and a general feeling of illness. Although unpleasant, the adverse effects of treatment are tolerated considering the life-threatening nature of the cancers.

Chlamydia: A sexually transmitted disease (STD) caused by Chlamydia trachomatis that infects the genital tract. The infection is frequently asymptomatic (i.e., shows no symptoms), but if left untreated, it can cause sterility in women.

Chronic Idiopathic Demyelinating Polyneuropathy (CIPD): Chronic, spontaneous loss or destruction of myelin. Myelin is a soft, white, somewhat fatty material that forms a thick sheath around the core of myelinated nerve fiber. Patients show progressive, usually symmetric weakness in the upper and lower extremities. Patients with clinical progression of the syndrome after 4 to 6 weeks by definition have CIPD. Treatment in most centers consists of giving IV-immune globulin for 4 to 5 days or plasmapheresis (5 to 6 exchanges over 2 weeks).

CIPD: See Chronic Idiopathic Demyelinating Polyneuropathy.

Circumoral Paresthesia: An abnormal sensation, such as burning or prickling around the mouth, often in the absence of an external stimulus. See Paresthesia.

Clade: Also called a subtype. A clade is a group of related HIV isolates classified according to their degree of genetic similarity (such as the percentage of identity within their envelope genes). There are currently three groups of HIV-1 isolates: M, N, and O. Isolate M (major strains) consists of at least ten clades, A through J. Group O (outer strains) may consist of a similar number of clades. French researchers reported the discovery of a new HIV-1 isolate that cannot be categorized in either group M or O. The new isolate was found in a Cameroonian woman with AIDS. They suggested that this new isolate be classified as group N (for new or for non-M-non-O). See Isolate.

Clinical: Pertaining to or founded on observation and treatment of patients, as distinguished from theoretical or basic science.

Clinical Alert: The National Institutes of Health, in conjunction with the editors of several biomedical journals, publish these bulletins on urgent cases in which timely and broad dissemination of results of clinical trials could prevent morbidity (sickness) and mortality (death). The Clinical Alert does not become a barrier to subsequent publication of the full research paper. Clinical Alerts are widely distributed electronically through the National Library of Medicine and through standard mailings. Internet Address: http://www.nlm.nih.gov/databases/alerts/clinical_alerts.html.

Clinical Endpoint: See Endpoint.

Clinical Latency: The period of time a virus or bacteria or other organism is living or developing in the body without causing symptoms. The period of time in which a person with HIV infection does not exhibit any evidence of disease or sickness. Even early in the disease, HIV is active within lymphoid organs where large amounts of virus become trapped in the follicular dendritic cells (FDC) network. Surrounding tissues are areas rich in CD4+ T-cells. These cells increasingly become infected, and viral particles accumulate both in infected cells and as free virus.

Clinical Practice Guidelines: Systematically developed statements by panels of expert practitioners to assist clinicians and patients in making decisions about appropriate health care for specific clinical circumstances. Internet Address: (National Guideline Clearinghouse) http://www.guideline.gov.

Clinical Trial: A scientifically designed and executed investigation of the effects of an intervention (drug, vaccine, biologic or behavioral) administered to human subjects. The goal is to define the safety, clinical efficacy, and pharmacological effects (including toxicity, side effects, incompatibilities, or interactions) of the drug. The U.S. government, through the FDA, requires strict testing of all new drugs and vaccines prior to their approval for use as therapeutic agents. See Phase I, II, III, and IV Trials.

ClinicalTrials.Gov: A service of the National Institutes of Health through its National Library of Medicine that provides a comprehensive database of clinical trials for all serious and life threatening diseases, including HIV/AIDS. The website is designed to provide patients, family members and members of the public with current information about clinical research studies and other trial information. Internet address: http://clinicaltrials.gov.

Clone: 1. A group of genetically identical cells or organisms descended from a common ancestor. 2. To produce genetically identical copies. 3. A genetically identical replication of a living cell that is valuable for the investigation and reproduction of test cultures.

CMS: See Centers for Medicare and Medicaid Services.

CMV: See Cytomegalovirus.

CMV Retinitis: See Cytomegalovirus Retinitis.

CNS: See Central Nervous System.

Coccidioidomycosis: An infectious fungal disease caused by the inhalation of spores of *Coccidioides immitis*, which are carried on windblown dust particles. The disease is endemic in hot, dry regions of the Southwestern United States and Central and South America. It is considered an AIDS-defining opportunistic infection in persons with HIV infection. Also called desert fever, San Joaquin Valley fever, or Valley fever. See Fungus; Opportunistic Infections.

Codon: A sequence of three nucleotides of messenger RNA that specifies addition of a particular amino acid to, or termination of, a polypeptide chain during protein synthesis. See Ribonucleic Acid.

Cofactors: 1. Substances, micro-organisms, or characteristics of individuals that may influence the progression of a disease or the likelihood of becoming ill. 2. A substance, such as a metallic ion or coenzyme, that must be associated with an enzyme for the enzyme to function. 3. A situation or activity that may increase a person's susceptibility to AIDS. Examples of cofactors are other infections, drug and alcohol use, poor nutrition, genetic factors, and stress. In HIV immunology, the concept of cofactors is being expanded and new cofactors have been identified. A recent example is the discovery of the interaction of CXCR4 (fusin) and CD4 to facilitate entry of HIV into cells.

Cognitive Impairment: Loss of the ability to process, learn, and remember information.

Cohort: In epidemiology, a group of individuals with some characteristics in common.

Colitis: Inflammation of the colon.

Combination Therapy: Two or more drugs or treatments used together to achieve optimum results against HIV infection and/or AIDS. Combination drug therapy has proven more effective in decreasing viral load than monotherapy (single-drug therapy). An example of combination therapy would be the use of two nucleoside analog drugs plus either a protease inhibitor or a non-nucleoside reverse transcription inhibitor. See Synergism.

Community-Based Clinical Trial (CBCT): A clinical trial conducted primarily through primary-care physicians rather than academic research facilities.

Community-Based Organization (CBO): A service organization that provides social services at the local level.

Community Planning: Community planning groups are responsible for developing comprehensive HIV prevention plans that are directly responsive to the epidemics in their jurisdictions. The goal of HIV Prevention Community Planning is to improve the effectiveness of HIV prevention programs. Together in partnership, representatives of affected populations, epidemiologists, behavioral scientists, HIV/AIDS prevention service providers, health department staff, and others analyze the course of the epidemic in their jurisdiction, determine their priority intervention needs, and identify interventions to meet those needs. CDC supports implementation of an effective planning process.

Community Programs for Clinical Research on Aids (CPCRA): The CPCRA, founded in 1989, and called the Terry Beirn Community Programs for Clinical Research on AIDS since 1992, is a network of research units composed of community based health care providers who offer their patients the opportunity to participate in research where they get their health care. The 15 CPCRA units comprise a variety of clinical settings, including private physicians' practices, university, and veterans' hospital clinics; drug treatment centers; and freestanding community clinics. Patients at these clinics are eligible for participation in CPCRA studies. The CPCRA, funded by the National Institute of Allergy and Infectious Diseases (NIAID), is targeted to serve populations underrepresented in previous clinical trials efforts. The research focus and scientific agenda of the CPCRA is identifying and improving treatment options in the day-to-day clinical care of people with HIV. Internet address: http://www.cpcra.org.

Compassionate Use: A method of providing experimental therapeutics prior to final FDA approval for use in humans. This procedure is used with very sick individuals who have no other treatment options. Often, case-by-case approval must be obtained from the FDA.

Complement: A group of proteins in normal blood serum and plasma that, in combination with antibodies, causes the destruction of antigens, particularly bacteria and foreign blood cells.

Complement Cascade: A precise sequence of events, usually triggered by an antigen-antibody complex, in which each component of the complement system is activated in turn. See Antibodies; Antigen.

Complementary and Alternative Therapy: Broad range of healing philosophies, approaches, and therapies that Western (conventional) medicine does not commonly use to promote well being or treat health conditions. Examples include acupuncture, herbs, etc. For more information contact the NCCAM. Internet address: http://www.nccam.nih.gov. See Alternative Medicine.

Complete Blood Count (CBC): A frequently ordered blood test that provides the white count, red blood cell count, red cell indices, hematocrit, and hemoglobulin in a microliter of whole blood.

Computed Tomography Scan: See C-T Scan.

Concomitant Drugs: Drugs that are taken together. Certain concomitant medications may have adverse interactions.

Condyloma: A wart-like skin growth usually on the external genitalia or perianal area.

Condyloma Acuminatum: A wart in the genital and perianal area. Although the lesions are usually few in number, they may aggregate to form large cauliflower-like masses. Caused by the human papilloma virus (HPV), it is infectious and autoinoculable (i.e., capable of being transmitted by inoculation from one part of the body to another). Also called genital warts, venereal warts, or verruca acuminata.

Contagious: In the context of HIV, has come to be more popularly known as any infectious disease capable of being transmitted by casual contact from person to another. Casual contact can be defined as normal day-to-day contact among people at home, school, work, or in the community. A contagious pathogen (e.g., chicken pox) can be transmitted by casual contact. An infectious pathogen, on the other hand, is transmitted by direct or intimate contact (e.g., sex). HIV is infectious, not contagious.

Contraindication: A specific circumstance when the use of certain treatments could be harmful.

Controlled Trials: Control is a standard against which experimental observations may be evaluated. In clinical trials, one group of patients is given an experimental drug, while another group (i.e., the control group) is given either a standard treatment for the disease or a placebo.

Co-Receptors: A group of proteins that have been found to block the entry of HIV into immune cells.

Core: The protein capsule surrounding a virus' DNA or RNA. In HIV, p55, the precursor molecule to the core, is broken down into the smaller protein molecules of p24, p17, p7, and p6. HIV's core is primarily composed of p24.

Core Protein: See Core.

Correlates of Immunity/Correlates of Protection: The immune responses that protect an individual from a certain disease. The precise identities of the correlates of immunity in HIV are unknown.

CPCRA: See Community Programs for Clinical Research on AIDS.

Creatinine: A protein found in muscles and blood, and excreted by the kidneys in the urine. The level of creatinine in the blood or urine provides a measure of kidney function.

Cross-Resistance: The phenomenon in which a microbe that has acquired resistance to one drug through direct exposure, also turns out to have resistance to one or more other drugs to which it has not been exposed. Cross-resistance arises because the biological mechanism of resistance to several drugs is the same and arises through the identical genetic mutations.

Cryotherapy: The use of liquid nitrogen to freeze and destroy a lesion or growth, sometimes used to induce scar formation and healing to prevent further spread of a condition.

Cryptococcal Meningitis: A life-threatening infection of the membranes surrounding the brain and the spinal cord caused by the fungus

Cryptococcus neoformans. Symptoms include headache, dizziness, stiff neck, and if untreated, coma and death. See Cryptococcus neoformans; Cryptococcosis.

Cryptococcus Neoformans: A fungus found in soil contaminated by bird droppings. Most people have been exposed to this organism, which does not usually cause disease in healthy people. In persons with impaired immune systems this organism can cause disease.

Cryptococcosis: An infectious disease due to the fungus Cryptococcus neoformans, which is acquired via the respiratory tract. It can spread from the lungs to the central nervous system (especially the membranes surrounding the brain), the skin, the skeletal system, and the urinary tract. It is considered an AIDS defining opportunistic infection in persons infected with HIV. See Cryptococcal Meningitis.

Cryptosporidiosis: A diarrheal disease caused by the protozoa Cryptosporidium which grows in the intestines. Symptoms include abdominal cramps and severe chronic diarrhea. It is considered an AIDS defining opportunistic infection in persons with HIV infection. Cryptosporidiosis usually occurs late in the course of HIV disease as immunological deterioration progresses. See Cryptosporidium.

Cryptosporidium: The protozoan (parasite *Cryptosporidium parvum*) which causes cryptosporidiosis. The parasite is found in the intestines of animals and may be transmitted to humans by direct contact with an infected animal, by eating contaminated food, or by drinking contaminated water. The parasite grows in the intestines and in people with HIV disease causes cryptosporidiosis. See Cryptosporidiosis.

CSF: See Cerebrospinal Fluid.

C-T Scan (Computed Tomography Scan): Radiography (using x-rays). An x-ray in which a three-dimensional image of a body structure is constructed by computer from a series of cross-sectional images made along an axis. Also called CAT scan. See Magnetic Resonance Imaging (MRI).

CTL: See Cytotoxic T Lymphocyte.

Cutaneous: Of, pertaining to, or affecting the skin.

CXCR4: A cell molecule that acts as a cofactor or co-receptor for the entry of HIV into immune system cells. Early in the epidemic, CD4 molecules were found to be the primary receptor for HIV on immune system cells. Recent data indicate that a second molecule, CXCR4, is also required for fusion and entry of certain strains of HIV into cells.

New studies indicate a multistage interplay between HIV and two receptors on white blood cells. After binding to the receptor CD4, the virus fuses with a second receptor, CXCR4, which normally binds to chemokines. This double clasp may then signal the receptors to move the virus into the cell. Also called fusin.

Cytokines: A protein produced by white blood cells, that acts as a messenger between cells. Cytokines can stimulate or inhibit the growth and activity of various immune cells. Cytokines are essential for a coordinated immune response and can also be used as immunologic adjuvants. HIV replication is regulated by a delicate balance among the body's own cytokines. By altering that balance one can influence the replication of the virus in the test tube and potentially even in the body. See also Interleukins; Tumor Necrosis Factor.

Cytomegalovirus (CMV): A common herpes virus that is a common cause of opportunistic diseases in persons with AIDS and other persons with immune suppression. Most adults in the U.S. have been infected by CMV; however the virus does not cause disease in healthy people. Because the virus remains in the body for life, it can cause disease if the immune system becomes severely damaged or suppressed by drugs. While CMV can infect most organs of the body, persons with AIDS are most susceptible to CMV retinitis (disease of the eye) and colitis (disease of the colon). See Cytomegalovirus Retinitis.

Cytomegalovirus (CMV) Retinitis: An eye disease common among persons who are living with HIV. Without treatment, persons with CMV retinitis can lose their vision. CMV infection can affect both eyes and is the most common cause of blindness among persons with AIDS. See Cytomegalovirus.

Cytopenia: Deficiency in the cellular elements of the blood.

Cytotoxic: An agent or process that is toxic or destructive to cells.

Cytotoxic T Lymphocyte (CTL): A lymphocyte that is able to kill foreign cells marked for destruction by the cellular immune system. CTLs can destroy cancer cells and cells infected with viruses, fungi, or certain bacteria. CTLs are also known as killer T-cells; they carry the CD8 marker. CTLs kill virus-infected cells, whereas antibodies generally target free-floating viruses in the blood. See also CD8 (T8) Cells.

Data Safety And Monitoring Board (DSMB): An independent committee, composed of community representatives and clinical research experts, that reviews data while a clinical trial is in progress to ensure that participants are not exposed to undue risk. A DSMB may recommend that a trial be stopped if there are safety concerns or if the trial objectives have been achieved.

DAIDS: See Division of Acquired Immunodeficiency Syndrome.

Deletion: Elimination of a gene (i.e., from a chromosome) either in nature or in the laboratory.

Dementia: Chronic intellectual impairment (i.e., loss of mental capacity) with organic origins that affects a person's ability to function in a social or occupational setting. See AIDS Dementia Complex.

Demyelination: Destruction, removal, or loss of the myelin sheath of a nerve or nerves.

Dendrite: Any of the usual branching protoplasmic processes that conduct impulses toward the body of a nerve cell.

Dendritic Cells: Patrolling immune system cells that may begin the HIV disease process by carrying the virus from the site of the infection to the lymph nodes, where other immune cells become infected. Dendritic cells travel through the body and bind to foreign invaders—such as HIV—especially in external tissues, such as the skin and the membranes of the gut, lungs, and reproductive tract. They then ferry the foreign substance to the lymph nodes to stimulate T-cells and initiate an immune response. In laboratory experiments, the dendritic cells that carry HIV also bind to CD4+ T-cells, thereby allowing HIV to infect the CD4+ T-cells. CD4+ T-cells are the primary immune system cells targeted by HIV and depleted during HIV infection.

Deoxyribonucleic Acid (DNA): The molecular chain found in genes within the nucleus of each cell, which carries the genetic information that enables cells to reproduce. DNA is the principal constituent of chromosomes, the structures that transmit hereditary characteristics.

Department Of Health And Human Services (DHHS or HHS): The U.S. government's principal agency for protecting the health of all Americans and providing essential human services, especially for those who are least able to help themselves. DHHS includes more than 300 programs, covering a wide spectrum of activities. The Department's programs are administered by operating divisions, including as the Centers for Disease Control and Prevention, the Food and Drug Administration, and the National Institutes of Health. DHHS works closely with state and local governments, and many DHHS-funded services are provided at the local level by state or county agencies, or through private-sector grantees. Internet address: http://www.hhs.gov.

Desensitization: Gradually increasing the dose of a medicine in order to overcome severe reactions. Desensitization procedures have become popular when administering certain medications including some antiretroviral medicines and antibiotics.

DHHS: See Department of Health and Human Services.

Diabetes Mellitus (DM): A disorder of carbohydrate metabolism characterized by elevated blood glucose (blood sugar) levels and glucose in the urine resulting from inadequate production or use of insulin. Insulin is the hormone that allows glucose to leave the bloodstream and enter body cells, where it is used for energy generation or stored for future use. Diabetes mellitus can also lead to long-term complications that include the development of neuropathy (swelling and wasting of the nerves), retinopathy (nonswelling eye disorder), nephropathy (swelling or breakdown disorder of the kidneys), generalized degenerative changes in large and small blood vessels, and increased susceptibility to infections. See Hyperglycemia.

Diagnosis: The determination of the presence of a specific disease or infection, usually accomplished by evaluating clinical symptoms and laboratory tests.

Diarrhea: Uncontrolled, loose, and frequent bowel movements caused by diet, infection, medication, and irritation or inflammation of the intestine. Severe or prolonged diarrhea can lead to weight loss and malnutrition. The excessive loss of fluid that may occur with AIDS-related diarrhea can be life threatening. There are many possible causes of diarrhea in persons who have AIDS. The most common infectious organisms causing AIDS-related diarrhea include cytomegalovirus (CMV), the parasites *Cryptosporidium, Microsporidia*, and *Giardia lamblia*, and the bacteria *Mycobacterium avium* and *Mycobacterium intracellulare*. Other bacteria and parasites that cause diarrheal symptoms in otherwise healthy people may cause more severe, prolonged, or recurrent diarrhea in persons with HIV or AIDS. See *Cryptosporidium; Giardiasis; Microsporidiosis; Mycobacterium avium complex (MAC)*.

Diplopia: Double vision.

Disseminated: Spread of a disease throughout the body.

Division of Acquired Immunodeficiency Syndrome (DAIDS): A division of NIAID, it was formed in 1986 to address the national research needs created by the advent and spread of the HIV/AIDS epidemic; to increase basic knowledge of the pathogenesis, natural history, and transmission of HIV disease; and to support research to promote HIV detection, treatment, and prevention. Internet address: http://www. niaid.nih.gov/daids.

DNA: See Deoxyribonucleic Acid.

Domain: A region of a gene or gene product. See Gene.

Dose-Ranging Study: A clinical trial in which two or more doses of an agent (such as a drug) are tested against each other to determine which dose works best and is least harmful.

Dose-Response Relationship: The relationship between the dose of some agent (such as a drug), or the extent of exposure, and a physiological response. A dose-response effect means that as the dose increases, so does the effect.

Double-Blind Study: A clinical trial design in which neither the participating individuals nor the study staff know which patients are receiving the experimental drug and which are receiving a placebo (or another therapy). Double-blind trials are thought to produce objective results, since the expectations of the doctor and the patient about the experimental drug do not affect the outcome. See Blinded Study.

Drug-Drug Interaction: A modification of the effect of a drug when administered with another drug. The effect may be an increase or a decrease in the action of either substance, or it may be an adverse effect that is not normally associated with either drug.

Drug Resistance: The ability of some disease-causing microorganisms, such as bacteria, viruses, and mycoplasma, to adapt themselves, to grow, and to multiply even in the presence of drugs that usually kill them. See Cross-Resistance.

DSMB: See Data Safety and Monitoring Board.

Dysplasia: Any abnormal development of tissues or organs. In pathology, alteration in size, shape, and organization of adult cells.

Dyspnea: Difficult or labored breathing.

Efficacy: (Of a drug or treatment) The maximum ability of a drug or treatment to produce a result regardless of dosage. A drug passes efficacy trials if it is effective at the dose tested and against the illness for which it is prescribed. In the procedure mandated by the FDA, Phase II clinical trials gauge efficacy, and Phase III trials confirm it.

ELISA: (Enzyme-Linked Immunosorbent Assay) A type of enzyme immunoassay (EIA) to determine the presence of antibodies to HIV in the blood or oral fluids. Repeatedly reactive (i.e., two or more) ELISA test results should be validated with an independent supplemental test of high specificity. In the U.S. the validation test used most often is the Western Blot test.

Empirical: Based on experimental data, not on a theory.

Encephalitis: A brain inflammation of viral or other microbial origin. Symptoms include headaches, neck pain, fever, nausea, vomiting, and nervous system problems. Several types of opportunistic infections can cause encephalitis.

Endemic: Pertaining to diseases associated with particular locales or population groups.

Endogenous: Relating to or produced by the body.

Endoscopy: Viewing the inside of a body cavity (e.g., colon) with an endoscope, a device using flexible fiber optics.

Endotoxin: A toxin present inside a bacterial cell.

Endpoint: A category of data used to compare the outcome in different arms of a clinical trial. Common endpoints are severe toxicity, disease progression, or death.

End-Stage Disease: Final period or phase in the course of a disease leading to a person's death.

Enteric: Pertaining to the intestines.

Enteritis: Inflammation of the intestine.

ENV: (env) The env gene gives rise to the two major viral glycoproteins (gp120 and gp41) that are associated with the membrane envelope surrounding each HIV-1 virion.

Entry Inhibitors: Compounds designed to disrupt the interactions between the HIV virus and the cell surface. These compounds can block or prevent binding to human cell surface receptions (CD4, CCR5, and CXCR4, for instance), or prevent fusion of the HIV virus to the cell. No drugs that employ these mechanisms have been approved by the FDA. Some compounds are in clinical trials.

Envelope: The outer coat, or envelope, of HIV is composed of two layers of fat-like molecules called lipids taken from the membranes of human cells. Embedded in the envelope are numerous cellular proteins, as well as mushroom-shaped HIV proteins that protrude from the surface. Each mushroom is thought to consist of a cap made of four glycoprotein molecules (called gp120) and a stem consisting of four gp41 molecules embedded in the envelope. The virus uses these proteins to attach to and infect cells.

Enzyme: A cellular protein whose shape allows it to hold together several other molecules in close proximity to each other. In this way, enzymes are able to induce chemical reactions in other substances with little expenditure of energy and without being changed themselves. Basically, an enzyme acts as a catalyst.

Eosinophil: A type of white blood cell, called granulocyte, that can digest micro-organisms. The granules can be stained by the acid dye eosin for microscopic examination.

Eosinophilic Folliculitis: An inflammatory reaction around hair follicles, characterized by very itchy papules (small elevations or bumps on the skin) that may grow together to form plaques. It involves invasion of the follicles by eosinophils. This disorder almost always occurs in HIV-infected persons with CD4+T-cell counts below 200, so it is an important cutaneous marker of a specific stage of HIV disease.

Epidemic: A disease that spreads rapidly through a demographic segment of the human population, such as everyone in a given geographic area; a military base, or similar population unit; or everyone of a certain age or sex, such as the children or women of a region. Epidemic diseases can be spread from person to person or from a contaminated source such as food or water.

Epidemiologic Surveillance: The ongoing and systematic collection, analysis, and interpretation of data about a disease or health condition. As part of a surveillance system to monitor the HIV epidemic in the U.S., the Centers for Disease Control and Prevention (CDC) in collaboration with state and local health departments, other federal agencies, blood collection agencies, and medical research institutions, conducts standardized HIV seroprevalence surveys in designated subgroups of the U.S. population. Collecting blood samples for the purpose of surveillance is called serosurveillance.

Epidemiology: The branch of medical science that deals with the study of incidence and distribution and control of a disease in a population.

Epithelium: The covering of the internal and external organs of the body. Also the lining of vessels, body cavities, glands, and organs. It consists of cells bound together by connective material and varies in the number of layers and the kinds of cells.

Epitope: A unique shape or marker carried on an antigen's surface that triggers a corresponding antibody response. See Antibodies; Antigen.

Epstein-Barr Virus (EBV): A herpes-like virus that causes one of the two kinds of mononucleosis (the other is caused by CMV). It infects the nose and throat and is contagious. EBV lies dormant in the lymph glands and has been associated with Burkitt's lymphoma and hairy leukoplakia.

Erythema: Redness or inflammation of the skin or mucous membranes.

Erythema Multiforme: A type of hypersensitivity reaction (rash) that occurs in response to medications, infections, or illness. The exact cause is unknown. Approximately 90% of erythema multiforme cases are associated with herpes simplex or mycoplasma infections. The disorder occurs primarily in children and young adults. A severe form of this condition is called Stevens-Johnson Syndrome.

Erythrocytes: Red blood cells whose major function is to carry oxygen to cells.

Etiology: The study or theory of the factors that cause disease.

Exclusion/Inclusion Criteria: The medical or social standards determining whether a person may or may not be allowed to enter a clinical trial. For example, some trials may not include persons with chronic liver disease, or may exclude persons with certain drug allergies; others may exclude men or women or only include persons with a lowered T-cell count.

Exogenous: Developed or originating outside the body.

Exotoxin: A toxic substance, made by bacteria released outside the bacterial cell.

Expanded Access: Refers to any of the FDA procedures, such as compassionate use, parallel track, and treatment IND, that distribute experimental drugs to patients who are failing on currently available treatments for their condition and also are unable to participate in ongoing clinical trials.

Experimental Drug: A drug that is not FDA licensed for use in humans, or as a treatment for a particular condition. See Off-Label Use.

Expression System: In HIV vaccine production, cells into which an HIV gene has been inserted to produce desired HIV proteins.

Fat Redistribution: Also called body fat redistribution syndrome (BFR). Changes in body fat distribution, sometimes referred to as lipodystrophy syndrome or fat redistribution syndrome, have been observed in patients taking protease inhibitors. Changes may include visceral fat accumulation (protease paunch), dorsocervical fat accumulation (buffalo hump), extremity wasting with venous prominence, facial thinning, breast enlargement, and lipomatosis.

FDA: See Food and Drug Administration.

FDC: See Follicular Dendritic Cells.

Floaters: Drifting dark spots within the field of vision. Floaters can be caused by infection with Cytomegalovirus (CMV) retinitis, but also can appear in persons as a normal part of the aging process.

Follicle: A small anatomical sac, cavity, or deep narrow mouthed depression (e.g., a hair follicle).

Follicular Dendritic Cells (FDCs): Cells found in the germinal centers of lymphoid organs. FDCs have thread-like tentacles that form a web-like network to trap invaders and present them to other cells of the immune system for destruction. See Lymphoid Organs.

Food And Drug Administration (FDA): The U.S. Department of Health and Human Services agency responsible for ensuring the safety and effectiveness of all drugs, biologics, vaccines, and medical devices, including those used in the diagnosis, treatment, and prevention of HIV infection, AIDS, and AIDS-related opportunistic infections. The FDA also works with the blood banking industry to safeguard the nation's blood supply. Internet address: http://www.fda.gov.

Functional Antibody: An antibody that binds to an antigen and has an effect. For example, neutralizing antibodies inactivate HIV or prevent it from infecting other cells.

Fungus: One of a group of primitive, nonvascular organisms including mushrooms, yeasts, rusts, and molds.

Fusin: See CXCR4.

Fusion Inhibitor: A class of antiretroviral agents that binds to the gp41 envelope protein and blocks the structural changes necessary for the virus to fuse with the host CD4 cell. When the virus cannot penetrate the host cell membrane and infect the cell, HIV replication within that host cell is prevented.

Fusion Mechanism: Fusion is an integral step in the process whereby HIV enters cells. Researchers have found that in addition to the primary receptor, the CD4 molecule, other cofactors, such as CCR5 and CXCR4 are needed in order for HIV to fuse with the membranes of the immune system cells.

GAG: (gag) A gene of HIV that codes for the core protein p55. p55 is the precursor of HIV proteins p17, p24, p7, and p6. These form HIV's capsid, the inner protein shell surrounding HIV's strand of RNA.

Gamma Globulin: One of the proteins in blood serum that contains antibodies. Passive immunizing agents obtained from pooled human plasma. See Globulins; Immunoglobulin G.

Gamma Interferon: A T-cell-derived stimulating substance that suppresses virus reproduction, stimulates other T-cells, and activates macrophage cells.

Ganglion: A mass of nervous tissue, composed principally of nerve-cell bodies, usually lying outside the central nervous system.

GART: Genotypic Antiretroviral Resistance Test. See Genotypic Assay.

Gastrointestinal (GI): Relating to the stomach and intestines.

Gene: 1. A unit of DNA that carries information for the biosynthesis of a specific product in the cell. 2. Ultimate unit by which inheritable characteristics are transmitted to succeeding generations in all living organisms. Genes are contained by, and arranged along the length of, the chromosome. Alteration of either gene number or arrangement can result in mutation (a change in the inheritable traits).

Gene Therapy: Any of a number of experimental treatments in which cell genes are altered. Some gene therapies attempt to provoke new immune activity; some try to render cells resistant to infection; some involve the development of enzymes that destroy viral or cancerous genetic material within cells.

Genetic Engineering: The technique by which genetic material from one organism is inserted into a foreign cell in order to mass-produce the protein encoded by the inserted genes. This relatively new technique manipulates the DNA (genetic material) of cells. For example, in this technique, the genes, which are actually portions of molecules of DNA, are removed from the donor organism (insect, plant, mammal, or other organism) and spliced into the genetic material of a virus; the virus is then allowed to infect recipient bacteria. In this way the bacteria become recipients of both viral and foreign genetic material.

Genital Ulcer Disease: Ulcerative lesions on the genitals usually caused by a sexually transmitted disease such as herpes, syphilis, or chancroid. The presence of genital ulcers may increase the risk of transmitting HIV.

Genital Warts: See Condyloma.

Genitourinary Tract: The organs concerned with the production and excretion of urine and those concerned with reproduction. Also called genitourinary system, urogenital system, or urogenital tract.

Genome: The complete set of genes in the chromosomes of each cell of a particular organism.

Genotypic Assay: A test that determines if HIV has become resistant to the antiviral drug(s) the patient is currently taking. The test analyzes a sample of the virus from the patient's blood to identify any mutations in the virus that are associated with resistance to specific drugs. Also known as GART (Genotypic Antiretroviral Resistance Assay).

Germinal Centers: One of a series of follicles or cavities around the periphery of lymph nodes. Germinal centers are the site of antibody production and are populated mostly by B cells but include a few T-cells and macrophages. As HIV infection progresses, the germinal centers gradually decay.

Giardiasis: A common protozoal infection of the small intestine, spread via contaminated food and water and direct person-to-person contact.

Globulins: Simple proteins found in the blood serum, which contain various molecules central to the immune system function. See Immunoglobulin.

Glycoprotein: A conjugated protein in which the nonprotein group is a carbohydrate (i.e., a sugar molecule). Also called glucoprotein.

Gonorrhea: An infection caused by *Neisseria gonorrhoeae*. Although gonorrhea is considered primarily a sexually transmitted disease it can also be transmitted to newborns during the birth process.

GP41: (gp41) Glycoprotein 41, a protein embedded in the outer envelope of HIV. Plays a key role in HIV's infection of CD4+ T-cells by facilitating the fusion of the viral and the cell membranes. See GP120.

GP120: (gp120) Glycoprotein 120, a protein that protrudes from the surface of HIV and binds to CD4+ T-cells. In a two-step process that allows HIV to breach the membrane of T-cells, gp120-CD4 complex refolds to reveal a second structure that binds to CCR5, one of several chemokine co-receptors used by the virus to gain entry into T-cells.

GP160: (gp160) Glycoprotein 160, a precursor of HIV envelope proteins gp41 and gp120.

Granulocyte: A type of white blood cell filled with granules of compounds that digest micro-organisms. Granulocytes are part of the innate immune system and have broad-based activity.

Granulocyte-Colony Stimulating Factor (G-CSF): A cytokine that stimulates the growth of granulocytes, a type of white blood cell. G-CSF alleviates the neutropenia that is a side effect of certain drugs.

Granulocyte Macrophage-Colony Stimulating Factor (GM-CSF): A cytokine that stimulates the growth of granulocytes and macrophages. Like the granulocyte colony-stimulating factor GM-CSF, it alleviates neutropenia but is less specific and has more side effects than G-CSF.

Granulocytopenia: A lack or low level of granulocytes in the blood. Often used interchangeably with neutropenia.

HAART: See Highly Active Antiretroviral Therapy.

Hairy Leukoplakia: See Oral Hairy Leukoplakia.

Half-Life: The time required for half the amount of a drug to be eliminated from the body.

HAM/TSP: See HTLV-I-associated myelopathy/tropical spastic paraparesis.

HCFA: Health Care Financing Administration. Now known as The Centers for Medicare and Medicaid Services (CMS).

HCSUS: See HIV Cost and Services Utilization Study.

Health Resources and Services Administration (HRSA): A U.S. Department of Health and Human Services agency that directs national health programs which improve the health of the Nation by assuring quality health care to underserved, vulnerable, and special-need populations and by promoting appropriate health professions workforce capacity and practice, particularly in primary care and public health. Among other functions, HRSA administers the Ryan White CARE Act Titles I, II, III(b), IV, SPNS, and AETCs to provide treatment and services for those affected by HIV/AIDS. HRSA administers programs to demonstrate how communities can organize their health care resources to develop an integrated, comprehensive, culturally competent system to care for those with AIDS and HIV infection. HRSA also administers education and training programs for health care providers and community service workers who care for persons living with HIV or AIDS. Internet address: http://www.hrsa.dhhs.gov.

HELLP Syndrome: A rare but potentially life-threatening syndrome that includes hemolysis, elevated liver enzymes, and low platelets that can occur during the third trimester of pregnancy Mitochondrial fatty acid oxidation can occur in pregnant women. Some speculate that the presence of this condition may enhance susceptibility to the syndrome. Receiving nucleoside analog drugs may also increase susceptibility.

Helper/Suppressor Ratio (of T-cells): T-cells are lymphocytes (white blood cells) that are formed in the thymus and are part of the immune system. They have been found to be abnormal in persons with AIDS. The normal ratio of helper T-cells (also known as CD4+ T-cells) to suppressor T-cells (also known as CD8+ T-cells) is approximately 2:1. This ratio becomes inverted in persons with AIDS but also may be abnormal for a host of other temporary reasons.

Helper T-cells: Lymphocytes bearing the CD4 marker that are responsible for many immune system functions, including turning antibody production on and off.

Hematocrit: A laboratory measurement that determines the percentage of packed red blood cells in a given volume of blood. In women, red blood cells are normally 37 to 47 percent of their blood, and in men, red blood cells are normally 40 to 54 percent of their blood.

Hematotoxic: Poisonous to the blood or bone marrow.

Hemoglobin: The component of red blood cells that carries oxygen.

Hemolysis: The rupture of red blood cells.

Hemophilia: An inherited disease that affects mostly males and prevents normal blood clotting. It is treated by lifelong injections of a synthetic version of the clotting factor lacking in persons with the disease. The new recombinant clotting factor is extracted from normal blood and if not heat treated can carry HIV.

Hepatic: Pertaining to the liver.

Hepatic Steatosis: Fatty liver caused by liver toxins such as carbon tetrachloride, and other factors such as alcohol, medications (steroids, minocycline), obesity, diabetes mellitus, cystic fibrosis, total lipodystrophy, and pregnancy.

Hepatitis: An inflammation of the liver. May be caused by bacterial or viral infection, parasitic infestation, alcohol, drugs, toxins, or transfusion of incompatible blood. Although many cases of hepatitis are not a serious threat to health, the disease can become chronic and can sometimes lead to liver failure and death. There are four major types of viral hepatitis: 1. hepatitis A, caused by infection with the hepatitis A virus, which is spread by fecal-oral contact; 2. hepatitis B, caused by infection with the hepatitis B virus (HBV), which is most commonly passed on to a partner during intercourse, especially during anal sex, as well as through sharing of drug needles; 3. non-A, non-B hepatitis, caused by the hepatitis C virus, which appears to be spread through sexual contact as well as through sharing of drug needles (another type of non-A, non-B hepatitis is caused by the hepatitis E virus, principally spread through contaminated water); 4. delta hepatitis, which occurs only in persons who are already infected with HBV and is caused by the HDV virus; most cases of delta hepatitis occur among people who are frequently exposed to blood and blood products, such as persons with hemophilia.

Hepatitis C/Co-Infection with HIV: Approximately 40% of patients infected with HIV are also infected with the hepatitis C virus (HCV), mainly because both viruses share the same routes of transmission. HCV is one of most important causes of chronic liver disease in the U.S. It has been demonstrated in clinical studies that HIV infection causes a more rapid progression of chronic hepatitis C to cirrhosis and liver failure in HIV-infected persons.

Hepatomegaly: Enlargement of the liver.

Herpes Viruses: A group of viruses that includes herpes simplex type 1 (HSV-1), herpes simplex type 2 (HSV-2), cytomegalovirus (CMV), Epstein-Barr virus (EBV), *varicella zoster* virus (VZV), human herpes virus type 6 (HHV-6), and HHV-8, a herpes virus associated with Kaposi's Sarcoma. See entries under names of some of the individual viruses.

Herpes Simplex Virus 1 (HSV-1): A virus that causes cold sores or fever blisters on the mouth or around the eyes, and can be transmitted to the genital region. Stress, trauma, other infections, or suppression of the immune system can reactivate the latent virus.

Herpes Simplex Virus 2 (HSV-2): A virus causing painful sores of the anus or genitals that may lie dormant in nerve tissue. It can be reactivated to produce symptoms. HSV-2 may be transmitted to a newborn child during birth from an infected mother, causing retardation and/or other serious complications. HSV-2 is a precursor of cervical cancer.

Herpes Varicella Zoster Virus (VZV): The varicella virus causes chicken pox in children and may reappear in adults as herpes zoster. Also called shingles, herpes zoster consists of very painful blisters on the skin that follow nerve pathways.

Highly Active Antiretroviral Therapy (HAART): The name given to treatment regimens recommended by leading HIV experts to aggressively suppress viral replication and progress of HIV disease. The usual HAART regimen combines three or more different drugs, such as two nucleoside reverse transcriptase inhibitors (NRTIs) and a protease inhibitor, two NRTIs and a non-nucleoside reverse transcriptase inhibitor (NNRTI), or other combinations. These treatment regimens have been shown to reduce the amount of virus so that it becomes undetectable in a patient's blood.

Histocompatibility Testing: A method of matching the self-antigens on the tissues of a transplant donor with those of a recipient. The closer the match, the better the chance that the transplant will not be rejected. See Human Leukocyte Antigens.

Histoplasmosis: A fungal infection, commonly of the lungs, caused by the fungus Histoplasma capsulatum. This fungus is commonly found in bird and/or bat droppings in the Ohio and Mississippi Valley region, the Caribbean Islands, and in Central and South America. It is spread by breathing in the spores of the fungus. Persons with severely damaged immune systems, such as those with AIDS, are vulnerable to a very serious disease known as progressive disseminated histoplasmosis. Nationwide, about 5% of persons with AIDS have histoplasmosis, but in geographic areas where the fungus is common, persons with AIDS are at high risk for disseminated histoplasmosis.

HIV-1: See Human Immunodeficiency Virus Type 1.

531

HIV-2: See Human Immunodeficiency Virus Type 2.

HIV-Associated Dementia: See AIDS Dementia Complex.

HIV Cost and Services Utilization Study (HCSUS): A study using a national sample representative of the adult U.S. population infected with HIV and receiving ongoing care that found significant variation in service utilization and receipt of medication. Women were more likely than men to use the emergency department and be hospitalized, and less likely to have received antiretroviral therapy including a protease inhibitor or non-nucleoside reverse transcriptase inhibitor by early 1998.

HIV Disease: During the initial infection with HIV, when the virus comes in contact with the mucosal surface and finds susceptible T-cells, the first site at which there is truly massive production of the virus is lymphoid tissue. This leads to a burst of massive viremia, with wide dissemination of the virus to lymphoid organs. The resulting immune response to suppress the virus is only partially successful and some virus escape. Eventually, this results in high viral turnover that leads to destruction of the immune system. HIV disease is, therefore, characterized by a gradual deterioration of immune functions. During the course of infection, crucial immune cells, called CD4+ T-cells, are disabled and killed, and their numbers progressively decline. See Acquired Immunodeficiency Syndrome; Human Immunodeficiency Virus Type 1.

HIV Prevention Trials Network (HPTN): A worldwide collaborative clinical trials network established by the National Institutes of Health to evaluate the safety and the efficacy of non-vaccine prevention interventions, alone or in combination, using HIV incidence as the primary endpoint. Internet address: http://www.hptn.org.

HIV-Related Tuberculosis: See Tuberculosis.

HIV Set Point: The rate of virus replication that stabilizes and remains at a particular level in each individual after the period of primary infection.

HIV Vaccine Trials Network (HVTN): Formed in 1999 by the Division of AIDS (DAIDS) of the National Institute of Allergy and Infectious Diseases. The HVTN mission is to develop and test prevention HIV vaccines through multi-center clinical trials in a global network of domestic and international sites. Internet address: http://www.hvtn.org.

HIV Viral Load: See Viral Load Test.

HLA: See Human Leukocyte Antigens.

Hodgkin's Disease: A progressive malignant cancer of the lymphatic system. Symptoms include lymphadenopathy, wasting, weakness, fever, itching, night sweats, and anemia. Treatment includes radiation and chemotherapy. See Lymphoma.

Holistic Medicine: Healing traditions that promote the protection and restoration of health through theories reputedly based on the body's natural ability to heal itself and through manipulation of various ways body components affect each other and are influenced by the external environment.

Homologous: With regards to immunology, tissue or serum derived from members of a single species.

Hormone: An active chemical substance formed in one part of the body and carried in the blood to other parts of the body where it stimulates or suppresses cell and tissue activity. See Pituitary Gland.

Host: A plant or animal harboring another organism.

Host Factors: The body's potent mechanisms for containing HIV, including immune system cells called CD8+ T-cells which may prove more effective than any antiretroviral drug in controlling HIV infection.

HPTN: See HIV Prevention Trials Network.

HPV: See Human Papilloma Virus.

HRSA: See Health Resources and Services Administration.

HTLV-I: See Human T-cell Lymphotropic Virus Type I.

HTLV-II: See Human T-cell Lymphotropic Virus Type II.

HTLV-I-Associated Myelopathy/Tropical Spastic Paraparesis (HAM/TSP): A chronic, degenerative neurological disease that causes the demyelination of the spinal cord. It is believed to be due to adult acquired infection with HTLV-I. The disease involves hyperreflexia, spasticity and weakness of the lower limbs, gait abnormality with bladder and sphincter involvement. Patients often present with complaints of incontinence or constipation and difficulty walking.

Human Growth Hormone (HGH): A peptide hormone secreted by the anterior pituitary gland in the brain. HGH enhances tissue growth by stimulating protein formation. A recombinant (genetically engineered) HGH, called Serostim, has been approved by FDA as a treatment for AIDS wasting syndrome.

Human Immunodeficiency Virus Type 1 (HIV-1): 1. The retrovirus isolated and recognized as the etiologic (i.e., causing or contributing to the cause of a disease) agent of AIDS. HIV-1 is classified as a lentivirus in a subgroup of retroviruses. 2. The genetic material of a retrovirus such as HIV is the RNA itself. HIV inserts its own RNA into the host cell's DNA, preventing the host cell from carrying out its natural functions and turning it into an HIV factory. See Lentivirus; Retrovirus.

Human Immunodeficiency Virus Type 2 (HIV-2): A virus closely related to HIV-1 that has also been found to cause AIDS. It was first isolated in West Africa. Although HIV-1 and HIV-2 are similar in their viral structure, modes of transmission, and resulting opportunistic infections, they have differed in their geographic patterns of infection.

Human Leukocyte Antigens (HLA): Marker molecules on cell surfaces that identify cells as self and prevent the immune system from attacking them.

Human Papilloma Virus (HPV): HPV is transmitted through sexual contact and is the virus that causes genital warts and plays a causative role in cervical dysplasia and cervical cancer. HPV affects more than 24 million Americans; CDC estimates that there are at least 500,000 new cases each year. In HIV-positive women, the prevalence and persistence of HPV infection increases with decreasing CD4 counts and increasing HIV RNA levels. There is no specific cure for an HPV infection. Interferon is used in the treatment of refractory or recurrent genital warts. Cryotherapy, laser treatment, or conventional surgery can remove the warts.

Human T-cell Lymphotropic Virus Type I (HTLVI): HTLV-I and HTLV-II, like all retroviruses, are single-stranded RNA viruses containing a genome that replicates through a DNA intermediary. This unique life cycle is made possible by the presence of a virally encoded enzyme, reverse transcriptase, which converts a single-stranded viral RNA into a double-stranded DNA provirus that can then be integrated into the host genome. HTLV-I has an affinity for T lymphocytes; it appears to be the causative agent of certain T-cell leukemias, T-cell lymphomas, and HTLV-I-associated myelopathy/tropical spastic paraparesis (HAM/TSP).

Human T-cell Lymphotropic Virus Type II (HTLVII): A virus closely related to HTLV-I, it shares 60% genomic homology (structural similarity) with HTLV-I. It is found predominantly in IV drug users and Native Americans, as well as Caribbean and South American Indian groups. HTLV-II has not been clearly been linked to any disease, but has been associated with several cases of myelopathy/tropical spastic paraparesis (HAM/TSP)-like neurological disease.

Humoral Immunity: The branch of the immune system that relies primarily on antibodies. See Cell-Mediated Immunity.

HVTN: See HIV Vaccine Trials Network.

Hydroxyurea: An inexpensive prescription drug used for the treatment of sickle-cell anemia and some forms of leukemia, which has been used investigationally for the treatment of HIV. Its potential safety and effectiveness for treatment of HIV have not been established, and clinicians should be aware of important safety precautions regarding its use. Hydroxyurea does not have direct antiretroviral activity; rather, it inhibits the cellular enzyme ribonucleotide reductase, resulting in reduced intracellular levels of deoxynucleoside triphosphates (dNTPs) that are necessary for DNA synthesis. For the most current information about the use of hydroxyurea in HIV treatment regimens, please see the "Guidelines for the Use of Antiretroviral Agents in HIV-Infected Adults and Adolescents," available at http://www.hivatis.org.

Hypergammaglobulinemia: Abnormally high levels of immunoglobulins in the blood. Common in persons with HIV.

Hyperglycemia: An abnormally high concentration of glucose in the circulating blood, seen especially in patients with diabetes mellitus. Hyperglycemia, new onset diabetes mellitus, diabetic ketoacidosis, and exacerbation of existing diabetes mellitus in patients receiving protease inhibitors have been reported.

Hyperlipidemia: An increase in the blood levels of triglycerides and cholesterol that can lead to cardiovascular disease and pancreatitis. As related to HIV: A side effect of HAART; all protease inhibitors have been shown to cause hyperlipidemia in clinical studies.

Hyperplasia: Abnormal increase in the elements composing a part (as tissue cells).

Hyperthermia: An unproven and dangerous experimental procedure that involves temporarily heating a patient's body core to temperatures of up to 108° F on the theory that this temperature kills free HIV and HIV-containing cells. One method for accomplishing this is by passing patients' blood through an external heater. This is called extra-corporeal whole body hyperthermia.

Hypogammaglobulinemia: Abnormally low levels of immunoglobulins. See Antibodies.

Hypogonadism: Deficiency in the secretory activity of the ovaries or testes. Prior studies have shown that 45% of patients with AIDS and 27% of HIV-infected patients without AIDS have subnormal testosterone levels. Replacement therapy is recommended for men with low or low-normal levels. Testosterone is an anabolic steroid that may restore nitrogen balance and lean body mass in patients with wasting.

Hypothesis: A supposition or assumption advanced as a basis for reasoning or argument, or as a guide to experimental investigation.

Hypoxia: Reduction of oxygen supply to tissues.

Idiopathic: Without a known cause.

Idiopathic Thrombocytopenia Purpura (ITP): See Immune Thrombocytopenic Purpura.

IHS: See Indian Health Service.

Immune Complex: Clusters formed when antigens and antibodies bind together.

Immune Deficiency: A breakdown or inability of certain parts of the immune system to function, thus making a person susceptible to certain diseases that they would not ordinarily develop.

Immune Response: The activity of the immune system against foreign substances.

Immune System: The body's complicated natural defense against disruption caused by invading foreign agents (e.g., microbes, viruses). There are two aspects of the immune system's response to disease: innate and acquired. The innate part of the response is mobilized very quickly in response to infection and does not depend on recognizing specific proteins or antigens foreign to an individual's normal tissue. It includes complements, macrophages, dendritic cells, and granulocytes. The acquired, or learned, immune response arises when dendritic cells and macrophages present pieces of antigen to lymphocytes, which are genetically programmed to recognize very specific amino acid sequences. The ultimate result is the creation of cloned populations of antibody-producing B cells and cytotoxic T lymphocytes primed to respond to a unique pathogen.

Immune Thrombocytopenic Purpura (ITP): Also called idiopathic immune thrombocytopenic purpura. A condition in which the body produces antibodies against the platelets in the blood, which are cells responsible for blood clotting. ITP is very common in persons infected with HIV.

Immunity: A natural or acquired resistance to a specific disease. Immunity may be partial or complete, long lasting, or temporary.

Immunization: To protect against an infectious disease by vaccination, usually with a weakened (attenuated) or killed form of the disease-causing microorganism. While people are usually immunized against an infectious disease by getting vaccinated, having a disease such as measles, mumps, or rubella one time usually prevents or immunizes a person from getting this disease again.

Immunocompetent: 1. Capable of developing an immune response. 2. Possessing a normal immune system.

Immunocompromised: Refers to an immune system in which the ability to resist or fight off infections and tumors is subnormal.

Immunodeficiency: Breakdown in immunocompetence, when certain parts of the immune system no longer function. This condition makes a person more susceptible to certain diseases.

Immunogen: A substance, also called an antigen, capable of provoking an immune response.

Immunogenicity: The ability of an antigen or vaccine to stimulate an immune response.

Immunoglobulin (Ig): Also called immune serum globulin. A class of proteins also known as antibodies made by the B cells of the immune system in response to a specific antigen. There are five classes of immunoglobulins: IgA, IgD, IgE, IgG, and IgM.

Immunoglobulin A (IgA): A class of antibodies often formed as a dimer (i.e., two antibody molecules attached to each other end to end), that is secreted into bodily fluids such as saliva. IgA protects the body's mucosal surfaces from infections.

Immunoglobulin D (IgD): A class of antibodies that is present in low concentration in serum The primary function of IgD appears to be as an antigen receptor on mature B cells.

Immunoglobulin E (IgE): A class of antibodies involved in anti-parasite immunity and in allergies.

Immunoglobulin G (IgG): A class of antibodies composed of two identical light and two identical heavy polypeptide chains. IgG acts on antigens by agglutinating (clumping cells together) them. In pregnancy, IgG crosses the placenta to the fetus and protects it against red cell antigens and white cell antigens. Also called gamma globulin.

Immunoglobulin M (IgM): A class of antibodies that is made by the body as the initial response to an antigen. If IgM is made in response to a vaccination, a booster shot will result in a switch from IgM to mostly immunoglobulin G.

Immunomodulator: Any substance that influences the immune system. See Interleukin-2; Immunostimulant; Immunosuppression.

Immunostimulant: Any agent or substance that triggers or enhances the body's defense; also called immunopotentiator.

Immunosuppression: A state of the body in which the immune system is damaged and does not perform its normal functions. Immunosuppression may be induced by drugs (e.g., in chemotherapy) or result from certain disease processes, such as HIV infection.

Immunotherapy: Treatment aimed at reconstituting an impaired immune system.

Immunotoxin: A plant or animal toxin (i.e., poison) that is attached to a monoclonal antibody and used to destroy a specific target cell.

Incidence: The number of new cases (e.g., of a disease) occurring in a given population over a certain period of time.

Inclusion/Exclusion Criteria: The medical or social standards determining whether a person may or may not be allowed to enter a clinical trial. For example, some trials may not allow persons with chronic liver disease or with certain drug allergies; others may exclude men or women, or only include persons with a lowered T-cell count.

Incubation Period: The time interval between the initial infection with a pathogen (e.g., HIV) and the appearance of the first symptom or sign of disease.

IND: See Investigational New Drug.

Indian Health Service (IHS): An agency within the U.S. Department of Health and Human Services responsible for providing federal health services to American Indians and Alaska Natives. The IHS currently provides health services to approximately 1.5 million American Indians and Alaska Natives who belong to more than 557 federally recognized tribes in 34 states. Internet address: http://www.ihs.gov.

Infection: The state or condition in which the body (or part of the body) is invaded by an infectious agent (e.g., a bacterium, fungus, or virus), which multiplies and produces an injurious effect (active infection). As related to HIV: Infection typically begins when HIV encounters a CD4+ cell. The HIV surface protein gp120 binds tightly to the CD4 molecule on the cell's surface. The membranes of the virus and the cell fuse, a process governed by gp41, another surface protein. The viral core, containing HIV's RNA, proteins, and enzymes, is released into the cell.

Infectious: An infection capable of being transmitted by direct or intimate contact (e.g., sex).

Informed Consent: The permission granted by a participant in a research study (including medical research) after receiving comprehensive information about the study. This is a statement of trust between the institution performing the research procedure and the person (e.g., a patient) on whom the research procedures are to be performed. This includes, for example, the type of protection available to people considering entering a drug trial. Before entering the trial, participants must sign a consent form that contains an explanation of: (a) why the research is being done, (b) what the researchers want to accomplish, (c) what will be done during the trial and for how long, (d) what the risks associated with the trial are, (e) what benefits can be expected from the trial, (f) what other treatments are available, and (g) the participant's right to leave the trial at any time. Informed consent also pertains to situations where certain tests need to be performed. See Clinical Trial.

Infusion: The process of administering therapeutic fluid, other than blood, to an individual by slowly injecting a dilute solution of the compound into a vein. Infusions are often used when the digestive system does not absorb appreciable quantities of a drug or when the drug is too toxic or the volume is too large to be given by quick injection.

Inoculation: The introduction of a substance (inoculum; e.g., a vaccine, serum, or virus) into the body to produce or to increase immunity to the disease or condition associated with the substance. See Vaccine.

Institutional Review Board (IRB): 1. A committee of physicians, statisticians, researchers, community advocates, and others that ensures that a clinical trial is ethical and that the rights of study participants are protected. All clinical trials in the U.S. must be approved by an IRB before they begin. 2. Every institution that conducts or supports biomedical or behavioral research involving human subjects must, by federal regulation, have an IRB that initially approves and periodically reviews the research so as to protect the rights of human subjects.

Integrase: A little-understood enzyme that plays a vital role in the HIV-infection process. Integrase inserts HIV's genes into a cell's normal DNA. It operates after reverse transcriptase has created a DNA version of the RNA form of HIV genes present in virus particles. Substances that inhibit integrase are being studied in HIV-infected patients.

Integrase Inhibitors: A class of experimental anti-HIV drugs that prevents the HIV integrase enzyme from inserting viral DNA into a host cell's normal DNA.

Integration: As related to HIV: The process by which the viral DNA migrates to the cell's nucleus, where it is spliced into the host's DNA with the help of viral integrase. Once incorporated, HIV DNA is called the provirus and is duplicated together with the cell's genes every time the cell divides. Recent reports suggest that HIV DNA can also integrate into the DNA of nondividing cells such as macrophages and brain and nerve cells.

Intensification: The addition of antiretroviral agents to an existing regimen, usually because of a failure to achieve the desired virologic response.

Intent to Treat: Analysis of clinical trial results that includes all data from patients in the groups to which they were randomized (i.e., assigned through random distribution) even if they never received the treatment.

Interaction: See Drug-Drug Interaction.

Interferon: One of a number of antiviral proteins that modulate the immune response. Interferon alpha is secreted by a virally infected cell and strengthens the defenses of nearby uninfected cells. A manufactured version of Interferon (trade names: Roferon, Intron A) is an FDA-approved treatment for Kaposi's Sarcoma, hepatitis B, and hepatitis C. Interferon gamma is synthesized by immune system cells (Natural Killer [NK] Cells and CD4 cells). It activates macrophages and helps orient the immune system to a mode that promotes cellular immunity (Th1 response).

Interleukins: One of a large group of glycoproteins that act as cytokines. The interleukins are secreted by and affect many different cells in the immune system. See Biotechnology; B Lymphocytes; Genetic Engineering; Killer T-cells; Natural Killer Cells (NK); Lymphocyte; T-cells.

Interleukin-1 (IL-1): A cytokine that is released early in an immune system response by monocytes and macrophages. It stimulates T-cell proliferation and protein synthesis. Another effect of IL-1 is that it causes fever.

Interleukin-2 (IL-2): A cytokine secreted by Th1 CD4 cells to stimulate CD8 cytotoxic T lymphocytes. IL-2 also increases the proliferation and maturation of the CD4 cells themselves. During HIV infection, IL-2 production gradually declines. Commercially, IL-2 is produced by recombinant DNA technology and is approved by the FDA for the treatment of metastatic renal (i.e., kidney) cell cancer. Recent data suggest that therapy with subcutaneous IL-2, in combination with antiretroviral drugs, has the potential to halt the usual progression of HIV disease by maintaining an individual's CD4+ T-cell count in the normal range for prolonged periods of time.

Interleukin-4 (IL-4): A cytokine secreted by Th2 CD4 cells that promotes antibody production by stimulating B cells to proliferate and mature.

Interleukin-12 (IL-12): A cytokine released by macrophages in response to infection that promotes the activation of cell-mediated immunity. Specifically, IL-12 triggers the maturation of Th1 CD4 cells, specific cytotoxic T lymphocyte responses, and an increase in the activity of NK cells. IL-12 is under study as an immunotherapy in HIV infection.

Interstitial: Relating to or situated in the small, narrow spaces between tissues or parts of an organ.

Intramuscular (IM): Injected directly into a muscle.

Intrapartum: Time during labor and delivery.

Intravenous (IV): 1. Of or pertaining to the inside of a vein, as of a thrombus. 2. An injection made directly into a vein.

Intravenous Immunoglobulin (IVIG): A sterile solution of concentrated antibodies extracted from healthy people. IVIG is used to prevent bacterial infections in persons with low or abnormal antibody production. IVIG is injected into a vein.

Intravitreal: Within the eye.

Investigational New Drug (IND): The status of an experimental drug after the FDA agrees that it can be tested in humans.

In Vitro: (In glass.) An artificial environment created outside a living organism (e.g., a test tube or culture plate) used in experimental research to study a disease or process.

In Vivo: (In life.) Studies conducted within living organisms (e.g., animal or human studies).

IRB: See Institutional Review Board.

Isolate: An individual (as a spore or a single organism), viable part of an organism (as a cell), or a strain that has been separated (as from diseased tissue, contaminated water, or the air) from the whole. Also, a pure culture produced from such an isolate. A particular strain of HIV taken from a patient.

ITP: See Immune Thrombocytopenic Purpura.

IVIG: See Intravenous Immune Globulin.

Jaundice: Yellow pigmentation of the skin, mucous membranes, whites of the eyes, and body fluids caused by elevated blood levels of bilirubin. The condition is associated with either liver or gallbladder disease or excessive destruction of red blood cells.

JC Virus: See Progressive Multifocal Leukoencephalopathy; Papilloma.

Kaposi's Sarcoma (KS): An AIDS-defining illness consisting of individual cancerous lesions caused by an overgrowth of blood vessels. KS typically appears as pink or purple painless spots or nodules on the surface of the skin or oral cavity. KS also can occur internally, especially in the intestines, lymph nodes, and lungs, and in this case is life threatening. The cancer may spread and also attack the eyes. There has been considerable speculation that KS is not a spontaneous cancer but is sparked by a virus. A species of herpes virus—also referred to as Kaposi's Sarcoma herpes virus (KSHV) or HHV-8—similar to the Epstein-Barr virus is currently under extensive investigation.

Up to now, KS has been treated with alpha interferon, radiation therapy (outside the oral cavity), and various systemic and intralesional cancer chemotherapies.

Karnofsky Score: A score between 0 and 100 assigned by a clinician based on observations of a patient's ability to perform common tasks. Thus, 100 signifies normal physical abilities with no evidence of disease. Decreasing numbers indicate a reduced ability to perform activities of daily living.

Killer T-cells: Because viruses lurk inside host (e.g., human) cells where antibodies cannot reach them, the only way they can be eliminated is by killing the infected host cell. To do this, the immune system uses a kind of white blood cell, called killer T-cells. These cells act only when they encounter another cell that carries a marker (i.e., a protein) that links it to a foreign protein, that of the invading virus. Killer T-cells can themselves become infected by HIV or other viruses, or transformed by cancer. Also known as cytotoxic T-cells (or cytotoxic T lymphocytes). See NK (natural killer) Cells; Null Cells; T-cells.

KSHV: Kaposi's Sarcoma Herpes Virus. See Kaposi's Sarcoma.

Kupffer Cells: Specialized macrophages in the liver. See Macrophage.

LAI: HIV-1 isolate used in HIV vaccine development. LAI is also referred to as IIIB or LAV. LAI belongs to clade B, the clade to which most HIV-1 found in the U.S. and Europe belongs. See Clade; Isolate.

LAK Cells: Lymphocytes transformed in the laboratory into lymphokine activated killer cells, which attack tumor cells.

Langerhans Cells: Dendritic cells in the skin that pick up an antigen and transport it to the lymph nodes.

LAS: See Lymphadenopathy Syndrome.

Latency: The period when an infecting organism is in the body but is not producing any clinically noticeable ill effects or symptoms. In HIV disease, clinical latency is an asymptomatic period in the early years of HIV infection. The period of latency is characterized in the peripheral blood by near-normal CD4+ T-cell counts. Recent research indicates that HIV remains quite active in the lymph nodes during this period. Cellular latency is the period after HIV has integrated its genome into a cell's DNA but has not yet begun to replicate.

Lentivirus: Slow virus characterized by a long interval between infection and the onset of symptoms. HIV is a lentivirus, as is the simian immunodeficiency virus (SIV) that infects non-human primates.

Lesion: A general term to describe an area of altered tissue (e.g., the infected patch or sore in a skin disease).

Leukocytes: Any of the various white blood cells that together make up the immune system. Neutrophils, lymphocytes, and monocytes are all leukocytes.

Leukocytosis: An abnormally high number of leukocytes in the blood. This condition can occur during many types of infection and inflammation.

Leukopenia: A decrease in the number of white blood cells. The threshold value for leukopenia is usually taken as less than 5,000 white blood cells per cubic millimeter of blood.

Leukoplakia: See Oral Hairy Leukoplakia.

LFT: See Liver Function Test.

LIP: See Lymphoid Interstitial Pneumonitis.

Lipid: Any of a group of fats and fatlike compounds, including sterols, fatty acids, and many other substances.

Lipodystrophy: A disturbance in the way the body produces, uses, and distributes fat. Lipodystrophy is also referred to as buffalo hump, protease paunch, or Crixivan potbelly. In HIV disease, lipodystrophy has come to refer to a group of symptoms that seem to be related to the use of protease inhibitor and NRTI drugs. How protease inhibitors and NRTIs may cause or trigger lipodystrophy is not yet known. Lipodystrophy symptoms involve the loss of the thin layer of fat under the skin, making veins seem to protrude; wasting of the face and limbs; and the accumulation of fat on the abdomen (both under the skin and within the abdominal cavity) or between the shoulder blades. Women may also experience narrowing of the hips and enlargement of the breasts. Hyperlipidemia and insulin resistance are frequently associated with lipodystrophy. Also called lipodystrophy syndrome, pseudo-Cushing's syndrome.

Liposomes: A spherical particle in an aqueous (watery) medium (e.g., inside a cell) formed by a lipid bilayer enclosing an aqueous compartment. Microscopic globules of lipids are manufactured to enclose medications. The fatty layer of the liposome is supposed to protect and confine the enclosed drug until the liposome binds with the outer membrane of target cells. By delivering treatments directly to the cells needing them, drug efficacy may be increased while overall toxicity is reduced.

Live Vector Vaccine: As pertaining to HIV, a vaccine that uses an attenuated (i.e., weakened) virus or bacterium to carry pieces of HIV into the body to directly stimulate a cell-mediated immune response.

Liver Function Test (LFT): A test that measures the blood serum level of any of several enzymes (e.g., SGOT and SGPT) produced by the liver. An elevated liver function test is a sign of possible liver damage.

Log: Changes in viral load are often reported as logarithmic or log changes. This mathematical term denotes a change in value of what is being measured by a factor of 10. For example, if the baseline viral load by PCR were 20,000 copies/mL plasma, then a 1-log increase equals a 10-fold (10 times) increase, or 200,000 copies/mL plasma. A 2-log increase equals 2,000,000 copies/mL plasma, or a 100-fold increase.

Long Terminal Repeat Sequence (LTR): The genetic material at each end of the HIV genome. When the HIV genome is integrated into a cell's own genome, the LTR interacts with cellular and viral factors to trigger the transcription of the HIV-integrated HIV DNA genes into an RNA form that is packaged in new virus particles. Activation of LTR is a major step in triggering HIV replication.

Long-Term Nonprogressors: Individuals who have been living with HIV for at least 7 to 12 years (different authors use different time spans) and have stable CD4+ T-cell counts of 600 or more cells per cubic millimeter of blood, no HIV-related diseases, and no previous antiretroviral therapy. Data suggest that this phenomenon is associated with the maintenance of the integrity of the lymphoid tissues and with less virus trapping in the lymph nodes than is seen in other individuals living with HIV.

LTR: See Long Terminal Repeat Sequence.

Lumbar: Lower back region. Of, relating to, or constituting the vertebrae between the thoracic vertebrae and the sacrum region. The sacrum is the triangular bone made up of five fused vertebrae and forming the posterior section of the pelvis. The thorax is the part of the human body between the neck and the diaphragm, partially encased by the ribs and containing the heart and lungs (i.e., the chest).

Lumbar Puncture: A procedure in which cerebrospinal fluid from the subarachnoid space in the lumbar region is tapped for examination. Also known as spinal tap.

Lymph: A transparent, slightly yellow fluid that carries lymphocytes. Lymph is derived from tissue fluids collected from all parts of the body and is returned to the blood via lymphatic vessels.

Lymph Nodes: Small, bean-sized organs of the immune system, distributed widely throughout the body. Lymph fluid is filtered through the lymph nodes in which all types of lymphocytes take up temporary residence. Antigens that enter the body find their way into lymph or blood and are filtered out by the lymph nodes or spleen, respectively, for attack by the immune system.

Lymphadenopathy Syndrome (LAS): Swollen, firm, and possibly tender lymph nodes. The cause may range from an infection such as HIV, the flu, or mononucleosis to lymphoma (cancer of the lymph nodes).

Lymphatic Vessels: A body-wide network of channels, similar to the blood vessels, that transport lymph to the immune organs and into the bloodstream.

Lymphocyte: A white blood cell. Present in the blood, lymph, and lymphoid tissue. See B Lymphocytes; T-cells.

Lymphoid Interstitial Pneumonitis (LIP): A type of pneumonia that affects 35 to 40% of children with AIDS, and which causes hardening of the lung membranes involved in absorbing oxygen. LIP is an AIDS-defining illness in children. The cause of LIP is not clear. There is no established therapy for LIP, but the use of corticosteroids for progressive LIP has been advocated.

Lymphoid Organs: Include tonsils, adenoids, lymph nodes, spleen, thymus, and other tissues. These organs act as the body's filtering system, trapping invaders (foreign particles, e.g., bacteria and viruses) and presenting them to squadrons of immune cells that congregate there. Within these lymphoid tissues, immune activity is concentrated in regions called germinal centers, where the thread-like tentacles of follicular dendritic cells (FDCs) form networks that trap invaders.

Lymphoid Tissue: See Lymphoid Organs.

Lymphokines: 1. Products of the lymphatic cells that stimulate the production of disease-fighting agents and the activities of other lymphatic cells. Among the lymphokines are gamma interferon and interleukin-2. 2. Non-antibody mediators of immune responses, released by activated lymphocytes.

Lymphoma: Cancer of the lymphoid tissues. Lymphomas are often described as being large cell or small cell types, cleaved or non-cleaved, or diffuse or nodular. The different types often have different prognoses (i.e., prospect of survival or recovery). Lymphomas can also be referred to by the organs where they are active, such as CNS lymphomas, which are in the central nervous system, and GI lymphomas, which are in the gastrointestinal tract. The types of lymphomas most commonly associated with HIV infection are called non-Hodgkin's lymphomas or B cell lymphomas. In these types of cancers, certain cells of the lymphatic system grow abnormally. They divide rapidly, growing into tumors.

Lymphopenia: A relative or absolute reduction in the number of lymphocytes in the circulating blood.

Lymphoproliferative Response: A specific immune response that entails rapid T-cell replication. Standard antigens, such as tetanus toxoid, that elicit this response, are used in lab tests of immunocompetency.

Lysis: Rupture and destruction of a cell.

MAC: See Mycobacterium Avium Complex.

Macrophage: A large immune cell that devours invading pathogens and other intruders. Stimulates other immune cells by presenting them with small pieces of the invader. Macrophages can harbor large quantities of HIV without being killed, acting as reservoirs of the virus.

Macrophage-Tropic Virus: HIV strains that preferentially infect macrophages in cell culture experiments. They readily fuse with cells that have both CD4 and CCR5 molecules on their surfaces, whereas the same viral isolates fail to fuse with cells expressing only CD4. These isolates are the main strains found in patients during the symptom-free stage of HIV disease.

Magnetic Resonance Imaging (MRI): A noninvasive, non-x-ray diagnostic technique that provides computer-generated images of the body's internal tissues and organs.

MAI: See Mycobacterium Avium Complex.

Maintenance Therapy: Also referred to as secondary prophylaxis. A therapy that prevents reoccurrence of an infection that has been brought under control.

Major Histocompatibility Complex (MHC): Two classes of molecules on cell surfaces. MHC class I molecules exist on all cells, and hold and present foreign antigens to CD8 cytotoxic T lymphocytes if the cell is infected by a virus or other microbe. MHC class II molecules are the billboards of the immune system. Peptides derived from foreign proteins are inserted into MHC's binding groove and displayed on the surface of antigen-presenting cells. These peptides are then recognized by T lymphocytes so that the immune system is alerted to the presence of foreign material. See Histocompatibility Testing.

Malabsorption Syndrome: Decreased intestinal absorption resulting in loss of appetite, muscle pain, and weight loss. See AIDS Wasting Syndrome.

Malaise: A generalized, nonspecific feeling of discomfort.

Malignant: Refers to cells or tumors growing in an uncontrolled fashion. Such growths may spread to and disrupt nearby normal tissue, or reach distant sites via the bloodstream. By definition, cancers are always malignant, and the term malignancy implies cancer. See Metastasis.

Mast Cell: A granulocyte found in tissue. The contents of the mast cells, along with those of basophils, are responsible for the symptoms of allergy.

MEDLINEplus: Contains extensive information from the National Institutes of Health and other trusted sources on about 500 diseases and conditions. There are also lists of hospitals and physicians, a medical encyclopedia and dictionaries, health information in Spanish, extensive information on prescription and nonprescription drugs, health information from the media, and links to thousands of clinical trials. Internet address: http://www.nlm.nih.gov/medlineplus/aids.html.

Mega-HAART: Also referred to as multi-drug rescue therapy. Salvage or rescue regimens containing 6 or more antiretroviral drugs for patients who have had previous treatment. The hypothesis is that patients with multiple drugs exposure and failures are unlikely to be infected with virus that is resistant to all drugs in the rescue regimen.

Memory T-cells: A subset of T lymphocytes that have been exposed to specific antigens and can then proliferate (i.e., reproduce) on subsequent immune system encounters with the same antigen.

Meninges: Membranes surrounding the brain or spinal cord. Part of the so-called blood-brain barrier. See Meningitis.

Meningitis: An inflammation of the meninges (membranes surrounding the brain or spinal cord), which may be caused by a bacterium, fungus, or virus. See Cryptococcal Meningitis; Central Nervous System.

Messenger RNA: Also referred to as mRNA. An RNA (ribonucleic acid) that carries the genetic code for a particular protein from the DNA in the cell's nucleus to a ribosome in the cytoplasm and acts as a template, or pattern, for the formation of that protein.

Metabolism: The chemical changes in living cells by which energy is provided for vital processes and activities and new material is assimilated.

Metastasis: The spread of a disease (e.g., cancer) from an original site to other sites in the body.

MHC: See Major Histocompatibility Complex.

Microbes: Microscopic living organisms, including bacteria, protozoa, viruses, and fungi.

Microbicide: An agent (e.g., a chemical or antibiotic) that destroys microbes. Research is being carried out to evaluate the use of rectal and vaginal microbicides to inhibit the transmission of sexually transmitted diseases, including HIV.

Microsporidiosis: An intestinal infection that causes diarrhea and wasting in persons with HIV. It results from two different species of microsporidia, a protozoal parasite. In HIV infection, it generally occurs when CD4+ T-cell counts fall below 100. See Pathogen; Protozoa; AIDS Wasting Syndrome.

Mitochondria: Organelles (particles of a living substance) within the cytoplasm of the cells, that serve as a source of energy for the cell.

Mitochondrial Toxicity: Also referred to as mitochondrial dysfunction. A possible side effect of certain anti-HIV drugs, primarily NRTIs, that results in mitochondrial damage. This damage can cause symptoms in the heart, nerves, muscles, pancreas, kidney, and liver, and it can also cause changes in lab tests. Some of the common conditions related to mitochondrial toxicity include myopathy, peripheral neuropathy, pancreatitis, thrombocytopenia, anemia, and neutropenia. Mitochondrial damage can lead to lactic acidosis and hepatitic steatosis (fatty liver). It also may play a role in lipodystrophy.

Molecule: The smallest particle of a compound that has all the chemical properties of that compound. Molecules are made up of two or more atoms, either of the same element or of two or more different elements.

Molluscum Contagiosum: A disease of the skin and mucous membranes caused by a poxvirus (*molluscum contagiosum* virus, MCV) infection. It is characterized by pearly white or flesh-colored papules (bumps) on the face, neck, and genital region. In persons living with HIV, *molluscum contagiosum* is often a progressive disease, resistant to treatment. When CD4+ cells fall below 200, the lesions tend to proliferate and spread.

Monocyte: A large white blood cell that ingests microbes or other cells and foreign particles. When a monocyte enters tissues, it develops into a macrophage.

Mononeuritis Multiplex (MM): A rare type of neuropathy that has been described with HIV infection. It may fall into two different settings. One type occurs during the early period of the infection and has a more benign outcome. The second form occurs later and is more aggressive, leading to progressive paralysis and death in some patients. It has been suggested that MM is related to multifocal cytomegalovirus (CMV) infection.

Monovalent Vaccine: A vaccine that is specific for only one antigen.

Morbidity: The condition of being diseased or sick; also the incidence of disease or rate of sickness.

MRI: See Magnetic Resonance Imaging.

Mucocutaneous: Anything that concerns or pertains to mucous membranes and the skin (e.g., mouth, eyes, vagina, lips, or anal area).

Mucosa: See Mucous Membrane.

Mucosal Immunity: Resistance to infection across the mucous membranes. Dependent on immune cells and antibodies present in the lining of the urogenital tract, gastrointestinal tract, and other parts of the body exposed to the outside world.

Mucous Membrane: Moist layer of tissue lining the digestive, respiratory, urinary, and reproductive tracts—all the body cavities with openings to the outside world except the ears.

Multi-Drug Rescue Therapy: See Mega-HAART.

Multiple Drug-Resistant Tuberculosis (MDR-TB): A strain of TB that does not respond to two or more standard anti-TB drugs. MDR-TB usually occurs when treatment is interrupted, thus allowing organisms in which mutations for drug resistance have occurred to proliferate. See Tuberculosis.

Mutation: In biology, a sudden change in a gene or unit of hereditary material that results in a new inheritable characteristic. As related to HIV: During the course of HIV disease, mutated HIV strains may emerge in an infected individual. These mutated strains may differ widely in their ability to infect and kill different cell types, as well as in their rate of replication. Of course, HIV does not mutate into another type of virus.

Myalgia: Diffuse muscle pain or tenderness, usually accompanied by malaise (vague feeling of discomfort or weakness).

Mycobacterium: Any bacterium of the genus Mycobacterium or a closely related genus.

Mycobacterium Avium Complex (MAC): 1. A common opportunistic infection caused by two very similar mycobacterial organisms, Mycobacterium avium and Mycobacterium intracellulare (MAI), found in soil and dust particles. 2. A bacterial infection that can be localized (limited to a specific organ or area of the body) or disseminated throughout the body. It is a life-threatening disease, although new therapies offer promise for both prevention and treatment. MAC disease is extremely rare in persons who are not infected with HIV. It generally occurs when the CD4+ T-cell count falls below 50.

Mycosis: Any disease caused by a fungus.

Myelin: A substance that sheathes nerve cells, acting as an electric insulator that facilitates the conduction of nerve impulses. See Chronic Idiopathic Demyelinating Polyneuropathy.

Myelopathy: Any disease of the spinal cord.

Myelosuppression: Suppression of bone marrow activity, causing decreased production of red blood cells (anemia), white blood cells (leukopenia), or platelets (thrombocytopenia). Myelosuppression is a side effect of some drugs, such as AZT.

Myelotoxic: Destructive to bone marrow.

Myocardial: Refers to the heart's muscle mass.

Myopathy: Progressive muscle weakness. Myopathy may arise as a toxic reaction to AZT or as a consequence of the HIV infection itself.

Nadir: The lowest level to which viral load falls after starting antiretroviral treatment. Studies have shown that the nadir of the viral load is the best predictor of long-term viral suppression.

NAT: See Nucleic Acid Test.

National AIDS Hotline: See CDC National AIDS Hotline.

National Cancer Institute (NCI): An institute of the National Institutes of Health (NIH) with the overall mission of conducting and supporting research, training, and disseminating health information with respect to the causes, diagnosis, and treatment of cancer. NCI also performs these functions for HIV-related cancers. Internet address: http://www.nci.nih.gov.

National Institute of Allergy and Infectious Diseases (NIAID): An NIH institute that conducts and supports research to study the causes of allergic, immunologic, and infectious diseases, and to develop better means of preventing, diagnosing, and treating illnesses. NIAID is responsible for the federally funded, national basic research program in AIDS. It supports basic research, epidemiology, and natural history studies; blood screening tests; drug discovery and development; vaccine development and testing; and treatment studies, some directly and some through contracts and cooperative agreements with other institutions. It administers the networks of the Adult AIDS Clinical Trials Group (AACTG) and the Pediatric AIDS Clinical Trials Group testing units at hospitals around the country. NIAID also administers the Community Programs for Clinical Research on AIDS (CPCRA), a community-based network of AIDS treatment research centers. Internet address: http://www.niaid.nih.gov.

National Institute of Child Health and Human Development (NICHD): An NIH institute that conducts and supports research on the reproductive, developmental, and behavioral processes that determine the health of children, adults, families, and populations. Thus, NICHD supports clinical research related to the transmission of HIV from infected mothers to their offspring, the progression of disease in HIV-infected infants and children, and the testing of potential therapies and preventatives for this population. Internet address: http://www.nichd.nih.gov.

National Institutes of Health (NIH): A multi-institute agency of the U.S. Department of Health and Human Services, NIH is the federal focal point for health research. It conducts research in its own laboratories and supports research in universities, medical schools, hospitals, and research institutions throughout this country and abroad. Internet address: http://www.nih.gov.

National Library Of Medicine (NLM): An NIH institute, NLM is the world's largest medical library. The library collects materials in all areas of biomedicine and health care, as well as works on biomedical aspects of technology, the humanities, and the physical, life, and social sciences. In the HIV/AIDS area, NLM provides electronic and print information services, including the online services AIDSLINE, AIDSTRIALS, and AIDSDRUGS. Internet address: http://www.nlm.nih.gov.

National Prevention Information Network (NPIN): See CDC National Prevention Information Network.

Natural History Study: Study of the natural development of something (such as an organism or a disease) over a period of time.

Natural Killer Cells (NK Cells): A type of lymphocyte. Like cytotoxic T-cells, NK cells attack and kill tumor cells and protect against a wide variety of infectious microbes. They are natural killers because they do not need additional stimulation or need to recognize a specific antigen in order to attack and kill. Persons with immunodeficiencies such as those caused by HIV infection have a decrease in natural killer cell activity. See Antigen; B Lymphocytes; T-cells; Null Cell.

NCI: See National Cancer Institute.

NDA: See New Drug Application.

Nebulized: See Aerosolized.

NEF: (nef) One of the regulatory genes of HIV. Three HIV regulatory genes—tat, rev, and nef—and three so-called auxiliary genes—vif, vpr, and vpu—contain information necessary for the production of proteins that control the virus; ability to infect a cell, produce new copies of itself, or cause disease. See rev; tat.

Neonatal: Concerning the first 6 weeks of life after birth.

Neoplasm: An abnormal and uncontrolled growth of tissue; a tumor.

Nephrotoxic: Poisonous to the kidneys.

Neuralgia: A sharp, shooting pain along a nerve pathway.

Neurological Complications of AIDS: See Central Nervous System (CNS) Damage.

Neuropathy: The name given to a group of disorders involving nerves. Symptoms range from a tingling sensation or numbness in the toes and fingers to paralysis. It is estimated that 35% of persons with HIV disease have some form of neuropathy. See Peripheral Neuropathy.

Neutralization: The process by which an antibody binds to specific antigens, thereby neutralizing the microorganism.

Neutralizing Antibody: An antibody that keeps a virus from infecting a cell, usually by blocking receptors on the cell or the virus.

Neutralizing Domain: The section of the HIV envelope protein, gp120, that elicits antibodies with neutralizing activities.

Neutropenia: An abnormal decrease in the number of neutrophils (the most common type of white blood cells) in the blood. The decrease may be relative or absolute. Neutropenia may also be associated with HIV infection or may be drug induced.

Neutrophil: A type of white blood cell (leukocyte) that engulfs and kills foreign micro-organisms such as bacteria.

New Drug Application (NDA): An application submitted by the manufacturer of a drug to the FDA after clinical trials have been completed, for a license to market the drug for a specified indication.

NIAID: See National Institute of Allergy and Infectious Diseases.

NICHD: See National Institute of Child Health and Human Development.

Night Sweats: Extreme sweating during sleep. Although they can occur with other conditions, night sweats are also a symptom of HIV disease.

NIH: See National Institutes of Health.

NK Cell: See Natural Killer Cells.

NLM: See National Library of Medicine.

NNRTI: See Non-Nucleoside Reverse Transcriptase Inhibitors.

Non-Hodgkin's Lymphoma (NHL): A lymphoma made up of B cells and characterized by nodular or diffuse tumors that may appear in the stomach, liver, brain, and bone marrow of persons with HIV. After Kaposi's Sarcoma, NHL is the most common opportunistic cancer in persons with AIDS.

Non-Nucleoside Reverse Transcriptase Inhibitors (NNRTI): A group of structurally diverse compounds that bind to the catalytic site of HIV-1's reverse transcriptase. They are quite specific; unlike the nucleoside reverse transcriptase inhibitors, the NNRTIs have no activity against HIV-2. As noncompetitive inhibitors of reverse transcriptase, their antiviral activity is additive or synergistic with most other anti-retroviral agents. However drug-drug interactions may dictate dosage adjustments with protease inhibitors.

NRTI: See Nucleoside Reverse Transcriptase Inhibitor.

NSAID: A classification of drugs called nonsteroidal anti-inflammatory drugs. NSAIDs reduce inflammation and are used to treat arthritis and mild to moderate pain.

Nucleic Acid: Organic substance found in all living cells, in which the hereditary information is stored and from which it can be transferred. Nucleic acid molecules are long chains that generally occur in combination with proteins. The two chief types are DNA (deoxyribonucleic acid), found mainly in cell nuclei, and RNA (ribonucleic acid), found mostly in cytoplasm. See Gene; Genetic Engineering; Mutation.

Nucleic Acid Test: A technology that allows detection of very small amounts of genetic material (DNA or RNA) in blood, plasma and tissue. A Nucleic Acid Test can detect any number of viruses in blood or blood products, thereby better assuring the safety of the blood supply.

Nucleocapsid: The viral genome is surrounded by a protein coating or shell called the capsid. The genome plus the capsid is called the nucleocapsid.

Nucleoli: Bodies in the nucleus that become enlarged during protein synthesis and contain the DNA template for ribosomal RNA. See Ribonucleic Acid; Ribosome.

Nucleoside: A building block of nucleic acids, DNA, or RNA, the genetic material found in living organisms. Nucleosides are nucleotides without the phosphate groups.

Nucleoside Analog: An artificial copy of a nucleoside. When incorporated into the DNA or RNA of a virus during viral replication, the nucleoside analog acts to prevent production of new virus. Nucleoside analogs may take the place of natural nucleosides, blocking the completion of a viral DNA chain during infection of a new cell by HIV. The HIV enzyme reverse transcriptase is more likely to incorporate the nucleoside analogs into the DNA it is constructing than is the DNA polymerase normally used for DNA creation in cell nuclei.

Nucleoside Reverse Transcriptase Inhibitor (NRTI): A nucleoside analog antiretroviral drug whose chemical structure constitutes a modified version of a natural nucleoside. These compounds suppress replication of retroviruses by interfering with the reverse transcriptase enzyme. The nucleoside analogs cause premature termination of the proviral (viral precursor) DNA chain. All NRTIs require phosphorylation in the host's cells prior to their incorporation into the viral DNA.

Nucleotide: Nucleotides are the building blocks of nucleic acids, DNA, and RNA. Nucleotides are composed of phosphate groups, a five-sided sugar molecule (ribose sugars in RNA, deoxyribose sugars in DNA), and nitrogen-containing bases. These fall into two classes: pyrimidines and purines. A nucleotide without its phosphate group is called a nucleoside.

Nucleotide Analogs: Nucleotide analogs are drugs that are structurally related to nucleotides; they are chemically altered to inhibit production or activity of disease-causing proteins. The chemical structures of these drugs may cause them to replace natural nucleotides in the viral DNA nucleic acid sequence. Nucleotide analogs do not require as much phosphorylation in the host's cells as the nucleoside reverse transcriptase inhibitors to become active drugs.

Nucleus: The central controlling body within a living cell, usually a spherical unit enclosed in a membrane and containing genetic codes for maintaining the life systems of the organism and for issuing commands for growth and reproduction. The nucleus of a cell is essential to such cell functions as reproduction and protein synthesis.

Null Cell: A lymphocyte that develops in the bone marrow and lacks the characteristic surface markers of the B and T lymphocytes. Null cells represent a small proportion of the lymphocyte population. Stimulated by the presence of antibody, null cells can attack certain cellular targets directly and are known as natural killer (NK) cells.

Ocular: Pertaining to the eye or vision.

Office of AIDS Research (OAR): An office within the National Institute of Health (NIH) that is responsible for the scientific, budgetary, legislative, and policy elements of the NIH AIDS research program. Internet address: http://www.nih.gov/od/oar.

Off-Label Use: A drug prescribed for conditions other than those approved by the FDA.

OI: See Opportunistic Infections.

Oncology: The branch of medicine that studies cancers or other tumors.

Open-Label Trial: A clinical trial in which doctors and participants know which drug or vaccine is being administered.

Opportunistic Infections: Illnesses caused by various organisms, some of which usually do not cause disease in persons with normal immune systems. Persons living with advanced HIV infection suffer opportunistic infections of the lungs, brain, eyes, and other organs. Opportunistic infections common in persons diagnosed with AIDS include *Pneumocystis carinii* pneumonia; Kaposi's Sarcoma; cryptosporidiosis; histoplasmosis; other parasitic, viral, and fungal infections; and some types of cancers.

Oral Hairy Leukoplakia (OHL): A whitish lesion that appears on the side of the tongue and inside cheeks. The lesion appears raised, with a ribbed or hairy surface. OHL occurs mainly in persons with declining immunity and may be caused by Epstein-Barr virus infection. OHL was not observed before the HIV epidemic.

Organelle: Any one of various particles of living substance bound within most cells, such as the mitochondria, the Golgi complex, the endoplastic reticulum, the lysosomes, and the centrioles.

Oropharyngeal: Relating to that division of the pharynx between the soft palate and the epiglottis. The pharynx is a tube that connects the mouth and nasal passages with the esophagus, the connection to the stomach. The epiglottis is a thin, valve-like structure that covers the glottis, the opening of the upper part of the larynx (the part of the throat containing the vocal cords), during swallowing.

Orphan Drugs: An FDA category that refers to medications used to treat diseases and conditions that occur rarely. Therefore, there is little financial incentive for the pharmaceutical industry to develop such medications. Orphan drug status gives a manufacturer specific financial incentives to develop and provide such medications.

Osteonecrosis: Also known as avascular necrosis. Generalized death of bone tissue. Recent NIH studies have shown that osteonecrosis of the hip is common among patients with HIV infection. While researchers can't yet pinpoint a specific cause, patients in the NIH studies were more likely to have taken testosterone, lipid-lowering drugs, and corticosteroids, all prescribed therapies for the acute and chronic complications of HIV infection.

Osteopenia: Diminished amount of bone tissue or decreased bone density.

557

P24: (p24) A bullet-shaped core made of another protein that surrounds the viral RNA within the envelope of HIV. The p24 antigen test looks for the presence of this protein in a patient's blood. A positive result for the p24 antigen suggests active HIV replication. p24 found in the peripheral blood is also thought to correlate with the amount of virus in the peripheral blood. Measurement of p24 levels in the blood has been used to monitor viral activity, although this is not considered a very accurate method due to the existence of the p24 antibody that binds with the antigen and makes it undetectable. See Branched DNA Assay.

Package Insert: A document, approved by the FDA and furnished by the manufacturer of a drug, for use when dispensing the drug (i.e., inserted into the package). The document indicates approved uses, contraindications, and potential side effects.

Palliative: A treatment that provides symptomatic relief but not a cure.

Palliative Care: Palliative care is an approach to life-threatening chronic illnesses, especially at the end of life. Palliative care combines active and compassionate therapies to comfort and support patients and their families who are living with life-ending illness. Palliative care strives to meet physical needs through pain relief and maintaining quality of life while emphasizing the patient's and family's rights to participate in informed discussion and to make choices. This patient—and family—centered approach uses the skills of interdisciplinary team members to provide a comprehensive continuum of care including spiritual and emotional needs.

Pancreas: A gland situated near the stomach that secretes a digestive fluid into the intestine through one or more ducts and also secretes the hormone insulin.

Pancreatitis: Inflammation of the pancreas that can produce severe pain and debilitating illness. Its onset can be predicted by rises in blood levels of the pancreatic enzyme, amylase.

Pancytopenia: Deficiency of all cell elements of the blood.

Pandemic: A disease prevalent throughout an entire country, continent, or the whole world. See Epidemic.

Pap Smear: A method for the early detection of cancer and other abnormalities of the female genital tract, especially of the cervix.

Papilloma: 1. A benign tumor (as a wart, condyloma, or polyp) resulting from an overgrowth of epithelial tissue on papillae of vascularized connective tissue (as of the skin). 2. An epithelial tumor caused by a virus. See Condyloma; Epithelium; JC Virus.

Parallel Track: A system of distributing experimental drugs to patients who are unable to participate in ongoing clinical efficacy trials and have no other treatment options. See Clinical Trial.

Parasite: A plant or animal that lives and feeds on or within another living organism (host), causing some degree of harm to the host organism.

Parenteral: A route other than in or through the digestive system. For example, parenteral can pertain to blood being drawn from a vein in the arm or introduced into that vein via a transfusion (intravenous), or to injection of medications or vaccines through the skin (subcutaneous) or into the muscle (intramuscular).

Paresthesia: Abnormal sensations such as burning, tingling, or a pins-and-needles feeling. Paresthesia may constitute the first group of symptoms of peripheral neuropathy, or it may be a limited drug side effect that does not worsen with time. Circumoral paresthesia affects the area around the mouth.

Passive Immunity: Also referred to as acquired immunity. Resistance resulting from previous exposure to an infectious agent or antigen may be active or passive. Passive immunity can be acquired from the transfer of antibodies from another person or from an animal, either naturally—as from mother to fetus or to the newborn via breast milk—or by intentional inoculation (vaccination).

Passive Immunotherapy: Process in which individuals with advanced disease (who have low levels of HIV antibody production) are infused with plasma rich in HIV antibodies or an immunoglobulin concentrate (HIVIG) from such plasma. The plasma is obtained from asymptomatic HIV-positive individuals with high levels of HIV antibodies.

Pathogen: Any disease-producing microorganism or material.

Pathogenesis: The origin and development of a disease.

PCP: See *Pneumocystis carinii* Pneumonia.

PCR: See Polymerase Chain Reaction.

Pediatric AIDS Clinical Trials Group (PACTG): This is the pre-eminent organization in the world for evaluating treatments for HIV-infected children and adolescents, and for developing new approaches for the interruption of mother-to-infant transmission. It has set the standards of care for children infected with HIV and for the interruption of vertical transmission. Internet address: http://pactg.s-3.com.

Pelvic Inflammatory Disease (PID): Gynecological condition caused by an infection (usually sexually transmitted) that spreads from the vagina to the upper parts of a woman's reproductive tract in the pelvic cavity. PID takes different courses in different women, but can cause abscesses and constant pain almost anywhere in the genital tract. If left untreated, it can cause infertility or more frequent periods. Severe cases may even spread to the liver and kidneys, causing dangerous internal bleeding and death.

Peptide: (Also polypeptide.) Biochemical formed by the linkage of up to about 50 amino acids to form a chain. Longer chains are called proteins. The amino acids are coupled by a peptide bond, a special linkage in which the nitrogen atom of one amino acid binds to the carboxyl carbon atom of another. Many peptides, such as the hormones vasopressin and ACTH, have physiological or antibacterial activity.

Perianal: Around the anus.

Perinatal: Events that occur at or around the time of birth.

Perinatal Transmission: Transmission of a pathogen, such as HIV, from mother to baby before, during, or after the birth process. Ninety percent of children reported with AIDS acquired HIV infection from their HIV-infected mothers.

Peripheral Neuritis: Inflammation of terminal nerves or the nerve endings, usually associated with pain, muscle wasting, and loss of reflexes.

Peripheral Neuropathy: Condition characterized by sensory loss, pain, muscle weakness, and wasting of muscle in the hands or legs and feet. It may start with burning or tingling sensations or numbness in the toes and fingers. In severe cases, paralysis may result. Peripheral neuropathy may arise from an HIV-related condition or be the side effect of certain drugs, some of the nucleoside analogs in particular.

Persistent Generalized Lymphadenopathy (PGL): Chronic, diffuse, noncancerous lymph node enlargement. Typically it has been found in persons with persistent bacterial, viral, or fungal infections. PGL in HIV infection is a condition in which lymph nodes are chronically swollen in at least two areas of the body for 3 months or more with no obvious cause other than the HIV infection.

PGL: See Persistent Generalized Lymphadenopathy.

Phagocyte: A cell that is able to ingest and destroy foreign matter, including bacteria.

Phagocytosis: The process of ingesting and destroying a virus or other foreign matter by phagocytes. See Macrophage; Monocyte.

pharmacokinetics: The processes (in a living organism) of absorption, distribution, metabolism, and excretion of a drug or vaccine.

Phase I Trials: Involve the initial introduction of an investigational new drug into humans. Phase I trials are closely monitored and may be conducted in patients or in healthy volunteers. The studies are designed to determine the metabolism and pharmacologic actions of the drug in humans, safety, side effects associated with increasing doses, and if possible, early evidence of effectiveness. The trials also can include studies of structure-activity relationships, mechanisms of action in humans, use of the investigational drug as research tools to explore biological phenomena, or disease processes. The total number of patients included in Phase I studies varies but is generally in the range of 20 to 80. Sufficient information should be obtained in the trial to permit design of well-controlled, scientifically valid Phase II studies.

Phase II Trials: Include controlled clinical studies of effectiveness of the drug for a particular indication or indications in patients with the disease or condition under study, and determination of common, short-term side effects and risks associated with the drug. Phase II studies are typically well controlled, closely monitored, and usually involve no more than several hundred patients.

Phase III Trials: Expanded controlled and uncontrolled studies. They are performed after preliminary evidence of drug effectiveness has been obtained. They are intended to gather additional information about effectiveness and safety that is needed to evaluate the overall benefit-risk relationship of the drug and to provide an adequate basis for physician labeling. These studies usually include anywhere from several hundred to several thousand subjects.

Phase IV Trials: Post-marketing studies, carried out after licensure of the drug. Generally, a Phase IV trial is a randomized, controlled trial that is designed to evaluate the long-term safety and efficacy of a drug for a given indication. Phase IV trials are important in evaluating AIDS drugs because many drugs for HIV infection have been given accelerated approval with small amounts of clinical data about the drugs' effectiveness.

Phenotypic Assay: A procedure whereby sample DNA of a patient's HIV is tested against various antiretroviral drugs to see if the virus is susceptible or resistant to these drugs. See Resistance.

Photosensitivity: Heightened skin response to sunlight or ultraviolet light (rapid burning when exposed to the sun).

Pituitary Gland: Small, oval endocrine gland that lies at the base of the brain. It is called the master gland because the other endocrine glands depend on its secretions for stimulation.

Placebo: An inactive substance (may look like the real medication) against which investigational treatments are compared for efficacy and safety. See Placebo Controlled Study.

Placebo Controlled Study: A method of investigation of drugs in which an inactive substance (placebo) is given to one group of patients, while the drug being tested is given to another group. The results obtained in the two groups are then compared to see if the investigational treatment is more effective in treating the condition.

Placebo Effect: A physical or emotional change, occurring after a substance is taken or administered, that is not the result of any special property of the substance. The change may be beneficial, reflecting the expectations of the patient and, often, the expectations of the person giving the substance.

Plasma: The liquid part of the blood and lymph that contains nutrients, electrolytes (dissolved salts), gases, albumin, clotting factors, wastes, and hormones.

Plasma Cells: Large antibody-producing cells that develop from B cells. See Antibodies; B Lymphocytes.

Platelets: Active agents of inflammation that are released when damage occurs to a blood vessel. The platelets stick to the vascular walls, forming clots to prevent the loss of blood. Thus, it is important to have adequate numbers of normally functioning platelets to maintain effective coagulation (clotting) of the blood. Some persons living with HIV develop thrombocytopenia, a condition characterized by a platelet count of less than 100,000 platelets per cubic millimeter of blood.

PML: See Progressive Multifocal Leukoencephalopathy.

***Pneumocystis Carinii* Pneumonia (PCP):** An infection of the lungs caused by *Pneumocystis carinii*, which is thought to be a protozoa but may be more closely related to a fungus. *P. carinii* grows rapidly in the lungs of persons with AIDS and is a frequent AIDS-related cause of death. *P. carinii* infection sometimes may occur elsewhere in the body (skin, eye, spleen, liver, or heart).

POL: (pol) A gene of HIV that codes for the enzymes protease, reverse transcriptase, and integrase.

Polymerase: Any of several enzymes that catalyzes the formation of DNA or RNA from precursor substances in the presence of preexisting DNA or RNA acting as templates (i.e., patterns).

Polymerase Chain Reaction (PCR): A laboratory process that selects a DNA segment from a mixture of DNA chains and rapidly replicates it to create a large, readily analyzed sample of a piece of DNA. As related to HIV: a sensitive laboratory technique that can detect and quantify HIV in a person's blood or lymph nodes (also called RT-PCR). It is an FDA-approved test to measure viral load.

Polyneuritis: Inflammation of many nerves at once.

Polypeptide: See Peptide.

Polyvalent Vaccine: A vaccine that is active against multiple viral strains.

Post-Exposure Prophylaxis (PEP): As it relates to HIV disease, a potentially preventative treatment using antiretroviral drugs to treat individuals within 72 hours of a high-risk exposure (e.g., needlestick injury, unprotected sex, needle sharing).

PPD Test: See Purified Protein Derivative.

Preclinical: Refers to the testing of experimental drugs in the test tube or in animals—the testing that occurs before trials in humans may be carried out.

Preconception Counseling: Recommended by the American College of Obstetrics and Gynecology for all women of childbearing age as a component of their primary medical care. The purpose of preconception care is to identify risk factors for adverse maternal or fetal outcome, provide education and counseling targeted to the patient's individual needs, and treat or stabilize medical conditions prior to conception in order to optimize maternal and fetal outcomes.

Precursor Cells: Cells that, via natural processes, form other cells.

Prevalence: A measure of the proportion of people in a population affected with a particular disease at a given time.

Primary HIV Infection: See Acute HIV Infection.

Primary Isolate: HIV taken from an infected individual (as opposed to grown in laboratory cultures).

Proctitis: Inflammation of the rectum.

Prodrome: A symptom that indicates the onset of a disease.

Prodrug: An inactive or partially active drug that is metabolically changed in the body to an active drug.

Progressive Multifocal Leukoencephalopathy (PML): A rapidly debilitating opportunistic infection caused by the JC virus that infects brain tissue and causes damage to the brain and the spinal cord. Symptoms vary from patient to patient but include loss of muscle control, paralysis, blindness, problems with speech, and an altered mental state. PML can lead to coma and death.

Prophylactic Drug: A drug that helps to prevent a disease or initial infection. See Prophylaxis.

Prophylaxis: Treatment to prevent the onset of a particular disease (primary prophylaxis), or the recurrence of symptoms in an existing infection that has been brought under control (secondary prophylaxis, maintenance therapy).

Protease: An enzyme that breaks down proteins into their component peptides. HIV's protease enzyme breaks apart long strands of viral protein into the separate proteins making up the viral core. The enzyme acts as new virus particles are budding off a cell membrane. Protease is the first HIV protein whose three-dimensional structure has been characterized. See Proteins.

Protease Inhibitors: Antiviral drugs that act by inhibiting the virus' protease enzyme, thereby preventing viral replication. Specifically, these drugs block the protease enzyme from breaking apart long strands of viral proteins to make the smaller, active HIV proteins that comprise the virion. If the larger HIV proteins are not broken apart, they cannot assemble themselves into new functional HIV particles.

Protease-Sparing Regimen: An antiretroviral drug regimen that does not include a protease inhibitor.

Proteins: Highly complex organic compounds found naturally in all living cells. Proteins are a source of heat and energy to the body. They are essential for growth, the building of new tissue, and the repair of injured tissue.

Protocol: The detailed plan for conducting a clinical trial. It states the trial's rationale, purpose, drug or vaccine dosages, length of study, routes of administration, who may participate (see Inclusion/Exclusion Criteria), and other aspects of trial design.

Protozoa: Large group of one-celled (unicellular) animals, including amoebas. Some protozoa cause parasitic diseases in persons with AIDS, notably toxoplasmosis and cryptosporidiosis. See *Pneumocystis carinii* Pneumonia.

provirus: Viral genetic material, in the form of DNA that has been integrated into the host genome. HIV, when it is dormant in human cells, is in a proviral form.

Pruritus: Itching.

Pseudo-Cushing's Syndrome: Also referred to as lipodystrophy; syndrome characterized by changes in bodily fat distribution that could be a side effect of HAART therapy, especially when HAART includes protease inhibitors.

Pseudovirion: A virus-like particle.

PubMed: A service of the National Library of Medicine, it provides access to over 11 million MEDLINE citations back to the mid-1960's and additional life science journals. PubMed includes links to many sites providing full text articles and other related resources. Internet site: http://www.ncbi.nlm.nih.gov/entrez/query.fcgi.

Pulmonary: Pertaining to the lungs.

Purified Protein Derivative (PPD): Material used in the tuberculin skin test (TST); the most common test for exposure to Mycobacterium tuberculosis, the bacterium that causes tuberculosis (TB). PPD is sometimes used synonymously with TST. In the PPD test, a small amount of protein from TB is injected under the skin. If patients have been previously infected, they will mount a delayed-type hypersensitivity reaction, characterized by a hard red bump called an induration.

PWA: Person with AIDS. Also known as PLWA, person living with AIDS.

Radiology: The science of diagnosis and/or treatment of disease using radioactive substances, including x-rays, radioactive isotopes, ionizing radiation, and CT scans.

Randomized Trial: A study in which participants are randomly (i.e., by chance) assigned to one of two or more treatment arms or regimens of a clinical trial. Occasionally placebos are utilized. Randomization minimizes the differences among groups by equally distributing people with particular characteristics among all the trial arms.

Rebound: An increase in viral load following a previous decrease due to anti-HIV therapy.

Receptor: A molecule on the surface of a cell that serves as a recognition or binding site for antigens, antibodies, or other cellular or immunological components.

Recombinant: An organism whose genome contains integrated genetic material from a different organism. Also used in relation to compounds produced by laboratory or industrial cultures of genetically engineered living cells. The cells' genes have been altered to give the capability of producing large quantities of the desired compound for use as a medical treatment. Recombinant compounds often are altered versions of naturally occurring substances.

Recombinant DNA: See Biotechnology: Genetic Engineering.

Recombinant DNA Technology: See Genetic Engineering.

Refractory: Referring to a disease that does not readily respond to treatment.

Regulatory Genes: As related to HIV: Three regulatory HIV genes—tat, rev, and nef—and three so-called auxiliary genes—vif, vpr, and vpu—contain information for the production of proteins that regulate the ability of the virus to infect a cell, produce new copies of the virus, or cause disease. See nef; rev; tat.

Regulatory T-cells: T-cells that direct other immune cells to perform special functions. The chief regulatory cell, the CD4+ T-cell or T-helper cell, is the chief target of HIV.

Remissions: The lessening in the severity of symptoms or duration of an outbreak of a disease.

Renal: Pertaining to the kidneys.

Rescue Therapy: See Salvage Therapy.

Resistance: Reduction in a pathogen's sensitivity to a particular drug. Resistance is thought to result usually from a genetic mutation. In HIV, such mutations can change the structure of viral enzymes and proteins so that an antiviral drug can no longer bind with them as well as it used to. Resistance detected by searching a pathogen's genetic makeup for mutations thought to confer lower susceptibility is called genotypic resistance. Resistance that is found by successfully growing laboratory cultures of the pathogen in the presence of a drug is called phenotypic resistance.

Resistance Testing: See genotypic assay; phenotypic assay.

Retina: Light-sensitive tissue at the back of the eye that transmits visual impulses via the optic nerve to the brain. See Retinitis.

Retinal Detachment: Condition in which a portion of the retina becomes separated from the inner wall of the eye. In AIDS patients, it can result from retinal disease such as cytomegalovirus (CMV) retinitis. The condition can rapidly lead to vision loss but is treatable by adding silicone to the vitreous humor of the eye to increase the pressure on the retina.

Retinitis: Inflammation of the retina, linked in AIDS to cytomegalovirus (CMV) infection. Untreated, it can lead to blindness.

Retrovirus: A type of virus that, when not infecting a cell, stores its genetic information on a single-stranded RNA molecule instead of the more usual double-stranded DNA. HIV is an example of a retrovirus. After a retrovirus penetrates a cell, it constructs a DNA version of its genes using a special enzyme called reverse transcriptase. This DNA then becomes part of the cell's genetic material.

REV: (rev) One of the regulatory genes of HIV. Three HIV regulatory genes—tat, rev, and nef—and three so-called auxiliary genes—vif, vpr, and vpu—contain information necessary for the production of proteins that control the virus's ability to infect a cell, produce new copies of the virus, or cause disease. See nef; tat.

Reverse Transcriptase: This enzyme of HIV and other retroviruses converts the single-stranded viral RNA into DNA, the form in which the cell carries its genes. Some antiviral drugs approved by the FDA for the treatment of HIV infection work by interfering with this stage of the viral life cycle. They are referred to as nucleoside reverse transcriptase inhibitors (NRTIs).

Ribonucleic Acid (RNA): A nucleic acid, found mostly in the cytoplasm of cells (rather than the nucleus) that is important in the synthesis of proteins. The amount of RNA varies from cell to cell. RNA, like the structurally similar DNA, is a chain made up of subunits called nucleotides. Some viruses, such as HIV, carry RNA instead of the more usual genetic material DNA. See Cytoplasm; Retrovirus.

Ribosome: A cytoplasmic organelle, composed of ribonucleic acid and protein, that functions in the synthesis of protein. Ribosomes interact with messenger RNA (mRNA) and transfer RNA to join together amino acid units into a polypeptide chain according to the sequence determined by the genetic code.

RNA: See Ribonucleic Acid.

Route of Administration: See Administration.

RTI: (Reverse Transcriptase Inhibitors) See Reverse Transcriptase.

RT-PCR: (Reverse Transcriptase Polymerase Chain Reaction) An FDA-approved test to measure viral load. The test is also known as PCR (Polymerase Chain Reaction). See Polymerase Chain Reaction.

Ryan White C.A.R.E. Act: Through the Ryan White Comprehensive AIDS Resources Emergency (C.A.R.E.) Act, health care and support services are provided for persons living with HIV/AIDS. The Health Resources and Services Administration (HRSA) administers this Act. The metropolitan areas most affected by the HIV epidemic are awarded Title I grants to improve and expand health care. Title II grants to states and territories support essential health care and support services for persons living with HIV/AIDS, including health insurance and AIDS Drug Assistance Programs. Title III(b) supports early intervention in clinical settings such as community and migrant health centers, health care for the homeless programs, and Native Hawaiian health programs. Title IV supports services for women, children, adolescents, and families affected by the HIV epidemic. Part F of the Act supports Special Projects of National Significance (SPNS) and AIDS Education and Training Centers (AETCs). Internet address: http://hab.hrsa.gov/history.htm.

Salmonella: A family of gram-negative bacteria, found in under-cooked poultry or eggs, that are a common cause of food poisoning, and that can cause serious disseminated disease in HIV-infected persons.

Salvage Therapy: Also referred to as rescue therapy. A treatment effort for people whose antiretroviral regimens have failed at least two times and who have had extensive prior exposure to antiretroviral agents. Some use these terms when any patient's HAART regimen has failed. In this case, failed refers to the inability of a drug to achieve and sustain low viral loads.

SAMHSA: See Substance Abuse and Mental Health Services Administration.

Sarcoma: A malignant (cancerous) tumor of the skin and soft tissue.

Seborrheic Dermatitis: A chronic inflammatory disease of the skin of unknown cause or origin, characterized by moderate erythema; dry, moist, or greasy scaling; and yellow crusted patches on various areas, including the mid-parts of the face, ears, supraorbital regions (above the orbit of the eye), umbilicus (the navel), genitalia, and especially the scalp.

Secondary Prophylaxis: See Maintenance Therapy.

Sepsis: The presence of harmful micro-organisms or associated toxins in the blood.

Seroconversion: The development of antibodies to a particular antigen. When people develop antibodies to HIV, they seroconvert from antibody-negative to antibody-positive. It may take from as little as 1 week to several months or more after infection with HIV for antibodies to the virus to develop. After antibodies to HIV appear in the blood, a person should test positive on antibody tests. See Incubation Period; Window Period.

Serologic Test: Any number of tests that are performed on the clear fluid portion of blood. Often refers to a test that determines the presence of antibodies to antigens such as viruses.

Seroprevalence: As related to HIV infection, the proportion of persons who have serologic (i.e., pertaining to serum) evidence of HIV infection at any given time. See Serum.

Serostatus: Results of a blood test for specific antibodies.

Serum: The clear, thin, and sticky fluid portion of the blood that remains after coagulation (clotting). Serum contains no blood cells, platelets, or fibrinogen.

Set Point: The measurable holding point or balance between the virus and the body's immune system reported as the viral load measurement. The viral set point is established within a few weeks to months after infection and is thought to remain steady for an indefinite period of time. Set points are thought to determine how long it will take for disease progression to occur.

Sexually Transmitted Disease (STD): Also called venereal disease (VD) (an older public health term) or sexually transmitted infections (STIs). Sexually transmitted diseases are infections spread by the transfer of organisms from person to person during sexual contact. In addition to the traditional STDs (syphilis and gonorrhea), the spectrum of STDs now includes HIV infection, which causes AIDS; *Chlamydia trachomatis* infections; human papilloma virus (HPV) infection; genital herpes; chancroid; genital mycoplasmas; hepatitis B; *trichomoniasis*; enteric infections; and ectoparasitic diseases (i.e., diseases caused by organisms that live on the outside of the host's body). The complexity and scope of STDs have increased dramatically since the 1980s; more than 20 micro-organisms and syndromes are now recognized as belonging in this category.

SGOT: (Serum Glutamic Oxaloacetic Transaminase) Also known as AST (aspartate aminotransaminase), a liver enzyme that plays a role in protein metabolism, such as SGPT. Elevated serum levels of SGOT are a sign of liver damage from disease or drugs.

SGPT: (Serum Glutamic Pyruvate Transaminase) Also known as ALT (alanine aminotransaminase), a liver enzyme that plays a role in protein metabolism like SGOT. Elevated serum levels of SGPT are a sign of liver damage from disease or drugs.

Shingles: See *Herpes Varicella Zoster* Virus.

SHIV: Genetically engineered hybrid virus having an HIV envelope and an SIV core. See Genetic Engineering; Hybrid; Simian Immunodeficiency Virus (SIV).

Side Effects: The actions or effects of a drug (or vaccine) other than those desired. The term usually refers to undesired or negative effects, such as headache, skin irritation, or liver damage. Experimental drugs must be evaluated for both immediate and long-term side effects.

Simian Immunodeficiency Virus (SIV): An HIV-like virus that infects monkeys, chimpanzees, and other non-human primates.

Sinusitis: Inflammation of the nasal cavity and sinuses.

SIT: See Structured Intermittent Therapy.

SIV: See Simian Immunodeficiency Virus.

Special Projects of National Significance (SPNS): The SPNS Program is the research and demonstration program of the Ryan White C.A.R.E. Act. The program's mission is to advance knowledge and skills in health and support services for persons with HIV/AIDS. The authorizing legislation specifies three objectives for this program: (1) to assess the effectiveness of particular models of care, (2) to support innovative program design, and (3) to promote replication of effective models.

Spinal Tap: See Lumbar Puncture.

Spleen: Large lymphatic organ in the upper left of the abdominal cavity with several functions: trapping of foreign matter in the blood, destruction of degraded red blood cells and foreign matter by macrophages, formation of new lymphocytes and antibody production, and storage of excess red blood cells.

Splenomegaly: An enlarged spleen.

Sputum Analysis: Method of detecting certain infections (especially tuberculosis) by culturing of sputum—the mucus matter that collects in the respiratory and upper digestive passages and is expelled by coughing.

Standards of Care: Treatment regimen or medical management based on state-of-the-art patient care.

Staphylococcus: Type of bacteria that may cause various types of infections.

STD: See Sexually Transmitted Disease.

Stem Cells: Cells from which all blood cells derive. Bone marrow is rich in stem cells. Clones of stem cells may become any one of the repertoires of immune cells depending upon exposure to specific cytokines and hormones.

Steroid: Member of a large family of structurally similar lipid substances. Steroid molecules have a basic skeleton consisting of four interconnected carbon rings. Different classes of steroids have different functions. All the natural sex hormones are steroids. Anabolic steroids increase muscle mass. Anti-inflammatory steroids (or corticosteroids) can reduce swelling, pain, and other manifestations of inflammation.

Stevens-Johnson Syndrome: A severe and sometimes fatal form of erythema multiforme that is characterized by severe skin manifestations; conjunctivitis (eye inflammation), which often results in blindness; Vincent's angina (trench mouth); and ulceration of the genitals and anus.

STI: See Structured Treatment Interruption.

Stomatitis: Any of numerous inflammatory diseases of the mouth (e.g., canker sores, thrush, fever blisters) having various causes, such as mechanical trauma, irritants, allergy, vitamin deficiency, or infection.

Strain: Subgroup of a species (also called taxon).

Stratification: A layered configuration.

Structured Intermittent Therapy (SIT): Carefully planned periods or regimens of intermittent therapy that might sustain viral control while reducing costs of treatment. See Structured Treatment Interruption.

Structured Treatment Interruption (STI): STI is the planned interruption of treatment by discontinuation of all antiretroviral drugs. There are four reasons to consider STI: (1) to provide a drug holiday to patients to relieve them of the inconvenience and toxicity of unsuccessful antiretroviral therapy and to improve the response to salvage therapy by allowing the emergence of wild-type virus; (2) to re-immunize the patient to HIV in the hopes of regaining immunologic control through a regenerated HIV-specific immune response; (3) to decrease the cumulative exposure to antiretroviral agents, reducing toxicity and cost and improving quality of life; and (4) to discontinue antiretroviral drugs during the first trimester of pregnancy.

Study Endpoint: A primary or secondary outcome used to judge the effectiveness of a treatment.

Subarachnoid Space: The space through which the spinal fluid circulates.

Subclinical Infection: An infection, or phase of infection, without readily apparent symptoms or signs of disease.

Subcutaneous (SQ): Beneath the skin or introduced beneath the skin (e.g., subcutaneous injections).

Substance Abuse and Mental Health Services Administration (SAMHSA): An agency of the U.S. Department of Health and Human

Services. SAMHSA's mission within the Nation's health system is to improve the quality and availability of prevention, treatment, and rehabilitation services in order to reduce illness, death, disability, and cost to society resulting from substance abuse and mental illnesses. Internet address: http://www.samhsa.gov.

Subunit HIV Vaccine: A genetically engineered vaccine that is based on only part of the HIV molecule. See Genetic Engineering.

Sulfa Drug: A sulfonamide drug used to treat bacterial infections. These drugs inhibit the action of p-aminobenzoic acid, a substance bacteria need in order to reproduce.

Sulfonamides: Synthetic derivatives of p-aminobenzene sulfonamide. See Sulfa Drug.

Superantigen: Investigators have proposed that a molecule known as a superantigen, made by either HIV or an unrelated agent, may stimulate massive quantities of CD4+ T-cells at once, rendering them highly susceptible to HIV infection and subsequent cell death. See Antigen.

Suppressor T-cells: (T8, CD8) Subset of T-cells that halts antibody production and other immune responses.

Surrogate Markers: Variables (measures) that are followed in clinical trials when the variable of the primary interest cannot conveniently be observed in a direct manner. Two commonly used surrogate markers in HIV studies are CD4+ T-cell counts and quantitative plasma HIV RNA (viral load).

Surveillance: See Epidemiologic Surveillance.

Susceptible: Vulnerable or predisposed to a disease or infection.

Symptoms: Any perceptible, subjective change in the body or its functions that indicates disease or phases of disease, as reported by the patient.

Syncytia: (Giant Cells) Dysfunctional multicellular clumps formed by cell-to-cell fusion. Cells infected with HIV may also fuse with nearby uninfected cells, forming balloon-like giant cells called syncytia. In test tube experiments, these giant cells have been associated with the death of uninfected cells. The presence of so-called syncytia-inducing variants of HIV has been correlated with rapid disease progression in HIV-infected individuals.

573

Syndrome: A group of symptoms as reported by the patient and signs as detected in an examination that together are characteristic of a specific condition.

Synergism, Synergistic: An interaction between two or more treatments (e.g., drugs) that produces or enhances an effect that is greater than the sum of the effects produced by the individual treatments.

Synthesis: 1. In chemistry, the formation of a compound from simpler compounds or elements. 2. The production of a substance (e.g., as in protein synthesis) by the union of chemical elements, groups, or simpler compounds, or by the degradation (i.e., breaking down) of a complex compound.

Syphilis: A primarily sexually transmitted disease resulting from infection with the spirochete (a bacterium), *Treponema pallidum*. Syphilis can also be acquired in the uterus during pregnancy.

Systemic: Concerning or affecting the body as a whole. A systemic therapy is one that the entire body is exposed to, rather than just the target tissues affected by a disease.

TAT: (tat) One of the regulatory genes of HIV. Three HIV regulatory genes—tat, rev, and nef—and three so-called auxiliary genes—vif, vpr, and vpu—contain information necessary for the production of proteins that control the virus' ability to infect a cell, produce new copies of the virus, or cause disease. The tat gene is thought to enhance virus replication. See nef; rev.

Tanner Staging: A way to determine where an adolescent is in the spectrum of sexual development, regardless of chronological age. In HIV treatment, Tanner staging is used to determine which treatment regimen to follow, either adult, adolescent, or pediatric.

TB: See Tuberculosis.

T-cells: (T Lymphocytes) T-cells are white blood cells derived from the thymus gland that participate in a variety of cell-mediated immune reactions. Three fundamentally different types of T-cells are recognized: helper, killer, and suppressor. They are the immune system's border police, responsible for finding infected or cancerous cells. The killer T-cell receptors (TCR) bind to an infected cell's distress signal—a combination of one of the cell's own proteins and a tiny fragment of the invader's protein. The bits of foreign protein are made with the help of enzymes inside the infected cell that break down the pathogens into protein fragments (peptides), which are then picked up by the major histocompatibility complex (MHC) and carried through the cell membrane.

T4 Cell: (Also called T-helper cell.) Antibody-triggered immune cells that seek and attack invading micro-organisms. Macrophages summon T4 cells to the infection site. There the T4 cell reproduces and secretes its potent lymphokines that stimulate B cells to produce antibodies, signal natural killer or cytotoxic (cell-killing) T-cells, and summon other macrophages to the infection site. In healthy immune systems, T4 cells are twice as common as T8 cells. If a person has AIDS, the proportion is often reversed. The virus enters a T4 cell through its receptor protein and encodes its genetic information into the host cell's DNA, making T-cells virtual viral factories. HIV-infected T4 cells may not die, but rather may cease to function. They also begin to secrete a substance known as soluble suppressor factor that inhibits the functioning of unaffected T-cells.

T8 Cell: (killer cells) Immune cells that shut down the immune response after it has effectively wiped out invading organisms. Sensitive to high concentrations of circulating lymphokines, T8 cells release their own lymphokines when an immune response has achieved its goal, signaling all other components of the immune system to cease their coordinated attack. A number of B lymphocytes remain in circulation in order to fend off a possible repeat attack by the invading micro-organism. With HIV, however, the immune system's response does not work. T4 cells are dysfunctional, lymphokines proliferate in the bloodstream, and T8 cells compound the problem by interpreting the oversupply of lymphokines to mean that the immune system has effectively eliminated the invader. So while HIV is multiplying in infected CD4 cells, T8 cells are simultaneously attempting to further shut down the immune system. The stage is set for normally repressed infectious agents, such as PCP or CMV, to proliferate unhindered and to cause disease. See Cytotoxic T Lymphocyte.

Template: A gauge, pattern, or mold used as a guide to the form of the piece being made. In biology, a molecule—such as DNA—that serves as a pattern for the generation of another macromolecule (e.g., messenger RNA). See Ribonucleic Acid.

Teratogenicity: The production of physical defects in offspring in utero (i.e., causing birth defects). Teratogenicity is a potential side effect of some drugs, such as thalidomide.

Terry Beirn Community Programs for Clinical Research on AIDS: See Community Programs for Clinical Research on AIDS.

Testosterone: Naturally occurring male hormone. When administered as a drug it can cause gain in lean body mass, increased sex drive, and possibly aggressive behavior. Many men with HIV infection have low testosterone levels.

Therapeutic HIV Vaccine: Also called treatment vaccine. A vaccine designed to boost the immune response to HIV infection. A therapeutic vaccine is different from a preventive vaccine, which is designed to prevent an infection or disease from becoming established in a person.

Thrombocytopenia: A decreased number of blood platelets (cells important for blood clotting). See Platelets; Immune Thrombocytopenia Purpura.

Thrush: Sore patches in the mouth caused by the fungus *Candida albicans*. Thrush is one of the most frequent early symptoms or signs of an immune disorder. The fungus commonly lives in the mouth, but only causes problems when the body's resistance is reduced either by antibiotics that have reduced the number of competitive organisms in the mouth, or by an immune deficiency such as HIV disease. See Candidiasis.

Thymosin: A polypeptide hormone of the thymus gland that influences the maturation of T-cells destined for an active role in cell-mediated immunity.

Thymus: A mass of glandular tissue (lymphoid organ) found in the upper chest under the breastbone in humans. The thymus is essential to the development of the body's system of immunity beginning in fetal life (i.e., before birth). The thymus processes white blood cells (lymphocytes), which kill foreign cells and stimulate other immune cells to produce antibodies. An important function of the thymus is to remove lymphocytes that react to proteins produced by the body (self-antigens), thus preventing autoimmune disease. The gland grows throughout childhood until puberty and then gradually decreases in size. See Thymosin.

Tissue: A collection of similar cells acting together to perform a particular function. There are four basic tissues in the body: epithelial, connective, muscle, and nerve.

Titer: (Also titre.) A laboratory measurement of the amount—or concentration—of a given compound in solution.

T Lymphocyte Proliferation Assay: Measures the strength of response of T memory cells, a subgroup of T lymphocytes, to HIV and other micro-organisms.

T Lymphocytes: See T-cells.

Toxicity: The extent, quality, or degree of being poisonous or harmful to the body.

Toxoplasmic Encephalitis: See Toxoplasmosis.

Toxoplasmosis: Toxoplasmosis is an infection that is caused by the protozoan parasite, *Toxoplasma gondii*. The parasite is carried by cats, birds, and other animals, and is found in soil contaminated by cat feces and in meat, particularly pork. The parasite can infect the lungs, retina of the eye, heart, pancreas, liver, colon, and testes. Once *T. gondii* invades the body, it remains there, but the immune system in a healthy person usually prevents the parasite from causing disease. If the immune system becomes severely damaged, as in HIV-infected persons, or is suppressed by drugs, *T. gondii* can begin to multiply and cause severe disease. In HIV-infected persons, the most common site of toxoplasmosis is the brain. When *T. gondii* invades the brain, causing inflammation, the condition is called toxoplasmic encephalitis. While the disease in HIV-infected persons can generally be treated with some success, lifelong therapy is required to prevent its reoccurrence.

Transaminase: A liver enzyme. A laboratory test that measures transaminase levels is used to assess the functioning of the liver.

Transplacental: Across or through the placenta. Usually refers to the exchange of nutrients, waste products, and other materials (e.g. drugs) between the developing fetus and the mother.

Transcription: The process of constructing a messenger RNA molecule, using a DNA molecule as a template, with the resulting transfer of genetic information to the messenger RNA. As related to HIV: The process by which the provirus produces new viruses. RNA copies, called messenger RNA, must be made that can be read by the host cell's protein-making machinery. Cellular enzymes, including RNA polymerase II, facilitate transcription. The viral genes may partly control this process. For example, tat encodes a protein that accelerates the transcription process by binding to a section of the newly made viral RNA. See Integration; Ribonucleic Acid.

Transfusion: 1. The process of transfusing fluid (such as blood) into a vein. 2. The transfer of compatible whole blood or blood products from one individual to another.

Translation: As related to HIV: The process by which HIV messenger RNA is processed in a cell's nucleus and transported to the cytoplasm, the component of the cell outside of the nucleus. In the cytoplasm, the cell's protein-making machinery translates the messenger RNA into viral proteins and enzymes.

Transmission: In the context of HIV disease: HIV is spread most commonly by sexual contact with an infected partner. The virus can enter the body through the mucosal lining of the vagina, vulva, penis, rectum, or, rarely, the mouth during sex. The likelihood of transmission is increased by factors that may damage these linings, especially other sexually transmitted diseases that cause ulcers or inflammation. HIV also is spread through contact with infected blood, most often by the sharing of drug needles or syringes contaminated with minute quantities of blood containing the virus. Children can contract HIV from their infected mothers during either pregnancy or birth, or postnatally, through breast-feeding. In developed countries, HIV is now rarely transmitted by transfusion of blood or blood products because of screening measures.

Treatment IND: IND stands for Investigational New Drug application, which is part of the process to get approval from the FDA for marketing a new prescription drug in the U.S. It makes promising new drugs available to desperately ill patients as early in the drug development process as possible. Treatment INDs are made available to patients before general marketing begins, typically during Phase III studies. To be considered for a treatment IND a patient cannot be eligible to be in the definitive clinical trial.

Triglyceride: A compound made up of a fatty acid (such as oleic, palmitic, or stearic acid) and glycerol. Triglycerides make up most animal and vegetable fats and are the basic water-insoluble substances (lipids) that appear in the blood where they circulate. In the blood they are bound to proteins, forming high- and low-density lipoproteins. Elevations of triglyceride levels (particularly in association with elevated cholesterol) have been correlated with the development of atherosclerosis, the underlying cause of some heart diseases and stroke. In relation to HIV disease, there are some patients receiving combination therapies who develop significant elevation in their triglyceride levels.

T Suppressor Cells: T lymphocytes responsible for turning the immune response off after an infection is cleared. They are a subset of the CD8+ lymphocytes.

Tuberculin Skin Test (TST): A purified protein derivative (PPD) of the tubercle *bacilli*, called tuberculin, is introduced into the skin by scratch, puncture, or intradermal injection. If a raised, red, or hard zone forms surrounding the test site, the person is said to be sensitive to tuberculin, and the test is read as positive.

Tuberculosis (TB): A bacterial infection caused by *Mycobacterium tuberculosis*. TB bacteria are spread by airborne droplets expelled from the lungs when a person with active TB coughs, sneezes, or speaks. Exposure to these droplets can lead to infection in the air sacs of the lungs. The immune defenses of healthy people usually prevent TB infection from spreading beyond a very small area of the lungs. If the body's immune system is impaired because of HIV infection, aging, malnutrition, or other factors, the TB bacterium may begin to spread more widely in the lungs or to other tissues. TB is seen with increasing frequency among HIV-infected persons. Most cases of TB occur in the lungs (pulmonary TB). However, the disease may also occur in the larynx, lymph nodes, brain, kidneys, or bones (extrapulmonary TB). Extrapulmonary TB infections are more common among persons living with HIV. See Multiple Drug Resistant TB.

Tumor Necrosis Factor (TNF): A cytokine, produced by macrophages, which helps activate T-cells. It also may stimulate HIV activity. TNF levels are high in persons with HIV infection, and the molecule is suspected to play a part in HIV-related wasting, neuropathy, and dementia. TNF triggers a biochemical pathway that leads to the programmed form of cell suicide known as apoptosis. It also activates a key molecule that can block this very pathway, and it sets up a delicate life-death balance within the cell.

V3 Loop: Section of the gp120 protein on the surface of HIV. Appears to be important in stimulating neutralizing antibodies.

Vaccination: Inoculation of a substance (i.e., the vaccine) into the body for the purpose of producing active immunity against a disease. See Vaccine.

Vaccine: A substance that contains antigenic components from an infectious micro-organism. By stimulating an immune response—but not the disease—it protects against subsequent infection by that organism. There can be preventive vaccines (e.g., measles or mumps) as well as therapeutic (treatment) vaccines. See Therapeutic HIV Vaccine; Antigen.

Vaccinia: A cowpox virus, formerly used in human smallpox vaccines. Employed as a vector in HIV vaccine research to transport HIV genes into the body. See Vaccination; Vector.

Vaginal Candidiasis: Infection of the vagina caused by the yeast-like fungus *Candida* (especially *Candida albicans*). Symptoms include, pain, itching, redness, and white patches in the vaginal wall. It can occur in all women, but it is especially common in women with HIV infection. The usual treatment is a cream applied locally to the vagina. Women with HIV infection may experience frequent re-occurrence of symptoms and may require systemic medications in order to treat these symptoms successfully. See Candidiasis.

Valley Fever: See Coccidioidomycosis.

Variable Region: The part of an antibody's structure that differs from one antibody to another.

Varicella Zoster Virus (VZV): A virus in the herpes family that causes chicken pox during childhood and may reactivate later in life to cause shingles in immunosuppressed individuals.

Vector: A nonpathogenic bacterium or virus used to transport an antigen into the body to stimulate protective immunity (e.g., in vaccine).

Vertical Transmission: Transmission of a pathogen such as HIV from mother to fetus or baby during pregnancy or birth. See Perinatal Transmission.

Viral Burden: The amount of HIV in the circulating blood. Monitoring a person's viral burden is important because of the apparent correlation between the amount of virus in the blood and the severity of the disease: sicker patients generally have more virus than those with less advanced disease. A new, sensitive, rapid test—called the viral load assay for HIV-1 infection—can be used to monitor the HIV viral burden. This procedure may help clinicians to decide when to give anti-HIV therapy or to switch drugs. It may also help investigators determine more quickly if experimental HIV therapies are effective. See Viral Load Test; Polymerase Chain Reaction; Branched DNA Assay.

Viral Core: Typically a virus contains an RNA (ribonucleic acid) or DNA (deoxyribonucleic acid) core of genetic material surrounded by a protein coat. As related to HIV: Within HIV's envelope is a bullet-shaped core made of another protein, p24, that surrounds the viral RNA. Each strand of HIV RNA contains the virus' nine genes. Three of these (gag, pol, and env) are structural genes that contain information needed to make structural proteins. The env gene, for example, codes for gp160, a protein that is later broken down to gp120 and gp41. See Surrogate Marker.

Viral Culture: A laboratory method for growing viruses.

Viral Envelope: As related to HIV: HIV is spherical in shape with a diameter of 1/10,000 of a millimeter. The outer coat, or envelope, is composed of two layers of fat-like molecules called lipids, taken from the membranes of human cells. Embedded in the envelope are numerous cellular proteins, as well as mushroom-shaped HIV proteins that protrude from the surface. Each mushroom is thought to consist of four gp41 molecules embedded in the envelope. The virus uses these proteins to attach to and infect cells.

Viral Load Test: In relation to HIV: Test that measures the quantity of HIV RNA in the blood. Results are expressed as the number of copies per milliliter of blood plasma. Research indicates that viral load is a better predictor of the risk of HIV disease progression than the CD4 count. The lower the viral load, the longer the time to AIDS diagnosis and the longer the survival time. Viral load testing for HIV infection is being used to determine when to initiate and/or change therapy. See Viral Burden.

Viremia: The presence of virus in the bloodstream. See Sepsis.

Viricide: Any agent that destroys or inactivates a virus.

Virion: A virus particle existing freely outside a host cell. A mature virus.

Virology: The study of viruses and viral disease.

Virus: Organism composed mainly of nucleic acid within a protein coat. When viruses enter a living plant, animal, or bacterial cell, they make use of the host cell's chemical energy, protein, and nucleic acid-synthesizing ability to replicate themselves. After the infected host cell makes viral components and virus particles are released, the host cell is often dissolved. Some viruses do not kill cells but transform them into a cancerous state. Some cause illness and then seem to disappear, while remaining latent and later causing another, sometimes much more severe, form of disease. In humans, viruses cause measles, mumps, yellow fever, poliomyelitis, influenza, and the common cold, among others. Some viral infections can be treated with drugs.

Visceral: Pertaining to the major internal organs.

Wasting Syndrome: See AIDS Wasting Syndrome.

Western Blot: A laboratory test for specific antibodies to confirm repeatedly reactive results on the HIV ELISA or EIA tests. In the U.S.,

Western Blot is the validation test used most often for confirmation of these other tests.

White Blood Cells: See Leukocytes.

Wild-Type Virus: The original type of HIV, unchanged by having developed any resistance to antiretroviral drugs. Also, 1. the prevalent type of a virus in the host population before genetic manipulation or mutation; 2. virus that is isolated from a host as opposed to one grown in a laboratory culture. See Primary Isolates.

Window Period: Time from infection with HIV until antibodies are detected.

Women's Interagency HIV Study (WIHS): A multicenter, prospective study that was established in August 1993 to carry out comprehensive investigations of the impact of HIV infection in women. The rationale for establishing the WIHS was to investigate the clinical, laboratory, and psychosocial aspects of HIV infection in women.

Yeast Infection: See Candidiasis.

Zinc Fingers: Chains of amino acids found in cellular protein which bind to DNA or messenger RNA, and play important roles in a cell's life cycle. They are called zinc fingers because they capture a zinc ion, which contributes to the array's binding to RNA or DNA. There are two zinc fingers in HIV's nucleocapsid. Zinc fingers are involved in binding and packaging viral RNA into new virions budding from an infected host cell. The nucleocapsid protein and the zinc fingers also play a role during the process of reverse transcription. See Reverse Transcriptase.

Zinc Finger Inhibitors: A class of experimental anti-HIV drugs which prevents the nucleocapsid part of the gag protein of HIV—which contains the zinc finger amino acid structures—from capturing and packaging new HIV genetic material into newly budding virions.

Chapter 72

Finding Reliable HIV/AIDS Information on the Internet

With a new HIV/AIDS treatment issue in the news each day, it is difficult for people living with HIV/AIDS and the health professionals who care for them to keep up with the latest breakthroughs. The purpose of this chapter is to inform those who need to stay current about where to go for the most accurate and up-to-date information about treatment and research. Searching for quality HIV/AIDS Web sites is an efficient, inexpensive, and powerful way to find current information. Newspapers and television may break current developments, but often more in-depth information on the same topics—on the same day—can be found on a reputable HIV/AIDS Web site. It may take 6-12 months for new information to appear in a printed medical journal or newsletter, but some researchers, drug companies, HIV/AIDS organizations, and government agencies release important information on the Internet within days. Additionally, many treatment newsletters are published on the Internet.

HIV/AIDS Treatment Web Sites

Following is a list of HIV/AIDS treatment Web sites, selected for quality and uniqueness. The main Web sites.

Excerpted from "How to Find Reliable HIV/AIDS Treatment Information on the Internet," from the National Library of Medicine, prepared by the Medical Education and Outreach Group, Oak Ridge Institute for Science and Education, February 2002; available online at http://www.orau.gov/meo/manuals/treatment/02-sites.pdf.

Adult AIDS Clinical Trials Group (AACTG)

http://aactg.s-3.com

The AACTG, the largest AIDS clinical trials organization in the world, assists in setting standards of care for HIV infection and related opportunistic diseases. The AACTG also provides data for the approval of therapeutic agents, and treatment and prevention strategies for opportunistic infections and malignancies. The management and core members of the AACTG consist of clinical scientists in the field of HIV/AIDS therapeutic research. The AACTG is funded by the Division of AIDS of the National Institute of Allergy and Infectious Diseases, part of the National Institutes of Health. This site would be of interest to clinicians conducting HIV/AIDS treatment research trials.

AIDS 2002: XIV International AIDS Conference

http://www.aids2000.org/IE_Home.asp

The XIV International AIDS Conference was held in Barcelona, Spain, July 7-12, 2002.

AIDS Action Committee of Massachusetts, Inc.

http://www.aac.org

The AIDS Action Committee of Massachusetts, Inc. is a New England service organization. It provides services, educates, and is an advocate for people living with HIV/AIDS. Most of the committee's income is derived from non-government sources, including foundations, corporations, private donations, and special events. Individual donors are the largest source of financial support.

AIDS Clinical Trials Information Service (ACTIS)

http://www.aidsinfo.nih.gov

ACTIS provides resource information on federally and privately funded clinical trials for adults and children. Certain sections of the site can be viewed in either a general or technical format. The Food and Drug Administration, the Centers for Disease Control and Prevention (CDC), the National Institute for Allergy and Infectious Diseases (NIAID), and the National Library of Medicine sponsor this site. This is probably the best site for government information on HIV/AIDS clinical trials. Some of the information on this site is in Spanish.

You can hear information or leave a message in Spanish by calling the toll-free number listed on the web site.

AIDS Education Global Information System (AEGIS)

http://www.aegis.org

AEGIS is a nonprofit charitable and educational corporation. The AEGIS Web site is managed by the Sisters of St. Elizabeth of Hungary in San Juan Capistrano, California. Its purpose is to encourage understanding and knowledge that will lead to better care, prevention, and a cure for HIV/AIDS. This, probably the largest, HIV/AIDS Web site is updated on a regular basis. A wealth and wide variety of information ranging from legal issues to reference materials on HIV/AIDS is available. The emphasis is on inclusion of all HIV/AIDS resources rather than selectively reviewing a smaller number of items.

Funding comes from Boehringer Ingelheim/Roxane Laboratories, the National Library of Medicine, and other private sources. Some information is also in Spanish. Although much of the information on this site is older, the news sources can be searched for the latest information.

AIDS Nutrition Services Alliances (ANSA)

http://www.aidsnutrition.org

The AIDS Nutrition Service Alliance is a collaboration of nonprofit organizations that provide nutrition services for people living with HIV/AIDS. The mission of ANSA is to enhance the quality of life of people living with HIV/AIDS (PLWAs) by information sharing, technical assistance, education and advocacy, pooling resources, and collaboration. The home page contains links to over 30 fact sheets on topics related to nutrition and HIV treatment.

AIDS Treatment Data Network

http://www.aidsinfonyc.org/network

The AIDS Treatment Data Network (commonly called the Network) is a national, not-for-profit, community-based organization. Treatment education and counseling services for men, women, and children with AIDS and HIV are supported by extensive, comprehensive, and up-to-date informational databases about AIDS treatments, research studies, services, and accessing care. Each link from the home page shows the date it was updated. Includes information in Spanish.

AIDScience

http://www.aidscience.com

AIDScience is an online information service from the American Association for the Advancement of Science, the world's largest general science organization. AIDScience provides scientists and researchers with current and accurate data on HIV prevention strategies and vaccine research. This Web site is funded by a grant from the National Institute of Mental Health.

Aidsinfonyc.org

http://aidsinfonyc.org

Aidsinfonyc.org is a series of information pages for people living with HIV/AIDS. The information is provided by community-based organizations. The Web site is supported by grants from nonprofit organizations and by donations from private organizations. Most of the information on this site seems current, but check the dates on each item.

AIDSMAP

http://www.aidsmap.com

The National AIDS Manual (NAM Publications), in collaboration with the British HIV Association, produces this site. NAM is a community-based organization located in the United Kingdom. Its mission is to develop and disseminate independent, accurate, accessible, and up-to-date HIV treatment information. NAM publishes a monthly newsletter entitled *AIDS Treatment Update*. Information is produced in both book form and as searchable databases. The Web sites can be searched in six languages. A medical advisory panel reviews the materials on the site. This site is supported by the International HIV/AIDS Alliance, Crusaid, the London HIV Commissioners Consortium, the United Kingdom Department of Health, the British HIV Association, the European Commission, the Elton John AIDS Foundation, UNAIDS, and numerous pharmaceutical companies.

AIDSmeds.com

http://www.aidsmeds.com

The mission of AIDSmeds is to provide people living with HIV the necessary information they need to make informed treatment decisions. A physician experienced in the treatment of HIV/AIDS reviews the content of this site. The organization is HIV-positive owned and operated. Sponsored by pharmaceutical and retail companies.

AIDS.ORG

http://aids.org

AIDS.Org (formerly known as Immunet) is a nonprofit organization dedicated to distributing HIV/AIDS information over the Internet. AIDS.ORG includes the *AIDS Treatment News* archive, accredited Continuing Medical Education (CME) programs, Direct AIDS Alternative Information Resources (DAAIR), the AIDS BookStore with over 3,000 titles, independent AIDS book reviews, medical conference listings and abstracts, a resource directory, hotline phone numbers, and links to information on other Web sites. You can register to receive updates about the site via e-mail. Supported by various computer companies and HIV/AIDS organizations. Some resources are available in Spanish.

AIDSTRIALS and AIDSDRUGS

http://www.aidsinfo.nih.gov

The AIDSTRIALS (AIDS Clinical Trials) database was created by the Specialized Information Services Division of the National Library of Medicine (NLM). It provides information about AIDS-related studies of experimental treatments conducted under the Food and Drug Administration's (FDA's) investigational new drug (IND) regulations. AIDSTRIALS contains information about clinical trials of agents undergoing evaluation for use against AIDS, HIV infection, and AIDS-related opportunistic diseases such as *Pneumocystis carinii* pneumonia (PCP). Detailed information is supplied by the National Institute for Allergy and Infectious Diseases (NIAID) for trials sponsored by the National Institutes of Health (NIH). Information about non-NIH-funded trials undergoing tests for efficacy is furnished by FDA. The companion database, AIDSDRUGS, contains descriptive information about the agents being tested in clinical trials. AIDSTRIALS and AIDSDRUGS are produced as part of the AIDS Clinical Trials Information Service

(ACTIS). The information contained in AIDSTRIALS includes the title of the trial, the trial purpose, the agent being tested, the trial phase, diseases studied, patient inclusion and exclusion criteria, trial locations, and whether the trial is open or closed. Details of the treatment regimen may also be included. The file may be used to identify trials testing a particular agent or to find open trials in a specific location. If additional information is required about the trial, all records contain a telephone number for contacting the specific trial site or sponsor. If additional information about the agent being tested is required, the AIDSDRUGS database may be searched using either the drug name, accession number contained in the trial record, or the number of the protocol. AIDSDRUGS may be searched to find out about a new drug, and then AIDSTRIALS may be accessed to search for trials using that drug.

After a search of AIDSTRIALS, a user may switch to the AIDSDRUGS database and view descriptive information about the agent used in the clinical trial, such as synonyms for the name including trade names, the standard chemical name, pharmacology, contraindications, adverse reactions, manufacturer, and physical/chemical properties such as molecular composition, formula, and weight. It is easy to coordinate searches between databases since the Substance Identification number from AIDSDRUGS is present in the AIDSTRIALS record and the protocol numbers from AIDSTRIALS are carried in AIDSDRUGS. As new trials are added to AIDSTRIALS, information is compiled about the agents and records are added to AIDSDRUGS. AIDSTRIALS and AIDSDRUGS are available free of charge, 24 hours a day, seven days a week.

The Alternative Medicine HomePage

http://www.pitt.edu/~cbw/altm.html

The Alternative Medicine HomePage is a jump station for sources of information on unconventional, unorthodox, unproven, alternative, complementary, innovative, and integrative therapies.

amfAR (American Foundation for AIDS Research)

http://www.amfar.org

The American Foundation for AIDS Research (amfAR) is a nonprofit organization dedicated to the support of HIV/AIDS research, AIDS prevention, treatment education, and the advocacy of sound AIDS-related public policy. The organization's mission is to prevent HIV infection and the disease and death associated with it, along with protecting the human rights of people with HIV/AIDS. Funding sources include voluntary contributions from individuals, foundations, and corporations.

Bastyr University AIDS Research Center (BUARC)

http://www.bastyr.edu/research/buarc

This research center was formed in 1994 with a grant from the National Institutes of Health's National Institute of Allergy and Infectious Diseases and the National Center on Complementary and Alternative Medicine (NCCAM). The center was established to document the use of alternative medicine in HIV/AIDS treatment, to screen and evaluate alternative medicine therapies, and to offer support to the medical field in evaluation of alternative therapies. The BUARC Web site provides information on the scientific activities in progress.

The Body

http://www.thebody.com

The Body's mission is to use the Web to lower barriers between patients and clinicians, demystify HIV/AIDS and its treatment, improve patients' quality of life, and foster community through human connection. The Body is a service of Body Health Resources Corporation and is sponsored in part by several drug companies. The Board of Advisers reviews links. Most of the information on this site is updated frequently. Links are organized in a logical, coherent manner. This is one of the larger HIV/AIDS Web sites, containing information on many topics. Users may want to click on Comprehensive Site Map to see the 250 topic areas.

Canadian HIV Trials Network

http://www.hivnet.ubc.ca/ctn.html

The Canadian HIV Trials Network (CTN) is a nonprofit clinical trials research organization committed to developing treatments, vaccines, and a cure for HIV/AIDS. The CTN is federally funded by Health Canada and jointly sponsored by the University of British Columbia and St. Paul's Hospital in Vancouver. The Network is comprised of a national headquarters in Vancouver, six regional offices in five regions, and over two dozen satellite sites. Information is available in English and French.

Center for Mental Health Research on AIDS (CMHRA)

http://www.nimh.nih.gov/oa

Since 1983, the National Institute of Mental Health (NIMH) CMHRA has supported research activities related to the primary and secondary prevention of AIDS and the neurobehavioral sequelae that develop as a result of HIV infection.

Centers for Disease Control and Prevention (CDC)

Division of HIV/AIDS Prevention (DHAP)

http://www.cdc.gov/hiv/dhap.htm

This is the Web site for CDC's National Center for HIV, STD and TB Prevention, Divisions of HIV/AIDS Prevention. It contains links to statistical, prevention, and treatment information on HIV/AIDS. You can subscribe to receive e-mail notification when the site is updated. Many items are also available in Spanish.

CenterWatch Clinical Trials Listing Service

http://www.centerwatch.com

CenterWatch is a publishing company focusing on the clinical trials industry. The CenterWatch site provides information to patients and their advocates about ongoing clinical trials seeking study volunteers. Over 41,000 clinical trials are listed on the site. Clinical trial resources are available for patients as well as research professionals. The site offers a notification service for new clinical trials and drugs approved by the FDA. Detailed profiles of more than 150 clinical research centers are listed. CenterWatch is a division of the Medical Economics Company.

ClinicalTrials.gov

http://clinicaltrials.gov

ClinicalTrials.gov is designed to provide patients, family members, health care professionals, and members of the public easy access to information on clinical trials for a wide range of diseases and conditions. The National Library of Medicine (NLM), an office of the U.S. National Institutes of Health (NIH), has developed this site in close and ongoing collaboration with all NIH Institutes and the Food and Drug

Administration (FDA). This site currently contains approximately 5,500 clinical studies sponsored primarily by the NIH. Additional studies from other federal agencies and the pharmaceutical industry are anticipated, and will be included on this site. As new features and designs are developed, they will be incorporated into ClinicalTrials.gov.

DIRLINE®

http://dirline.nlm.nih.gov

DIRLINE (Directory of Information Resources Online) is a free online database created by the Specialized Information Services Division of the National Library of Medicine (NLM). It contains location and descriptive information about a wide variety of organizations, including publications, holdings, and services provided that may not be readily available in other bibliographic databases. DIRLINE contains approximately 10,000 records and focuses primarily on health and biomedicine, although it also provides limited coverage of some other special interests. These information resources fall into many categories, including federal, state, and local government agencies; information and referral centers; professional societies; self-help groups and voluntary associations; academic and research institutions and their programs; information systems; and research facilities. Topics include HIV/AIDS (about 1,000 records), maternal and child health, most diseases and conditions including genetic and other rare diseases, health services research, and technology assessment.

Elizabeth Glaser Pediatric AIDS Foundation

http://www.pedaids.org

The Elizabeth Glaser Pediatric AIDS Foundation is a nonprofit organization. Its goals are to find therapies to prevent transmission from an infected mother to her newborn, to prolong and improve the lives of children with HIV, and to eliminate HIV in infected children.

Food and Drug Administration (FDA) HIV and AIDS Activities

http://www.fda.gov/oashi/aids/hiv.html

The FDA's HIV/AIDS Program in the Office of Special Health Issues works with outside individuals and advocacy groups on issues related to HIV/AIDS, informs the HIV-affected community of activities and policies at FDA related to HIV/AIDS, represents patient and community views and concerns to the agency, serves as a resource for HIV/AIDS-related information, explains the regulatory processes affecting development and approval of new therapies, represents FDA at a range of public and government meetings related to serious and life-threatening illnesses, and assists in development of federal government policies and regulations related to HIV/AIDS.

Gay Men's Health Crisis (GMHC)

http://www.gmhc.org

GMHC is the oldest and largest not-for-profit AIDS organization in the U.S. GMHC offers hands-on support services to more than 9,500 men, women, and children with AIDS and their families in New York City annually, as well as education and advocacy for hundreds of thousands nationwide. Some information is available in Spanish.

Health Resources and Services Administration (HRSA)

HIV/AIDS Services

http://hab.hrsa.gov

This is the Web site of HRSA's HIV/AIDS Bureau. One of four bureaus of HRSA, it is the largest single source (except for the Medicaid program) of federal funding for HIV/AIDS care for low-income, uninsured, and underinsured individuals.

HIV InSite

http://hivinsite.ucsf.edu

HIV InSite is a project of the University of California, San Francisco (UCSF). Within UCSF, the project is a collaboration among the San Francisco Veterans Affairs Medical Center, the Positive Health Program at San Francisco General Hospital, and the Center for AIDS Prevention Studies of UCSF's AIDS Research Institute. The home page of this site contains recent news items. The editorial process at this site is independent of financial sponsors, which include MERCK, Agouron, Roche, Stempel Foundation, Ortho Biotech, Boehringer-Ingelheim, and GlaxoSmithKline. This is an information-dense site created primarily for clinicians.

HIV/AIDS Dietetic Practice Group

http://hivaidsdpg.org

The HIV/AIDS Dietetic Practice Group (DPG) is part of the American Dietetic Association. The group was founded in response to the overwhelming evidence that nutrition was an important factor in the treatment of HIV disease. The mission of HIV/AIDS DPG is to share information regarding the nutritional management of HIV, provide an avenue for national research projects, and advocate for nutrition intervention for all persons living with HIV. *Positive Communication* is the group's peer reviewed quarterly publication, but it is not posted to the Web site.

HIV/AIDS Treatment Information Service (ATIS)

http://www.aidsinfo.nih.gov

ATIS is a project of the Department of Health and Human Services, and is managed by the National Library of Medicine. It is co-sponsored by the National Institutes of Health; the Health Care Financing Administration, Medicare, Medicaid, and SCHIP Agency; the Health Resources and Services Administration; and Centers for Disease Control and Prevention (CDC). ATIS provides the most recent information about federally approved treatment guidelines for HIV and AIDS. Most of the information on this site is from the U.S. Public Health Service (PHS) or CDC. One can request e-mail notification of new features and publications on the Web site, including treatment guidelines.

HIVandHepatitis.com™

http://www.hivandhepatitis.com

The objective of HIVandHepatitis.com is to develop an online publication that provides accurate and timely treatment information to people living with HIV/AIDS, hepatitis B, hepatitis C, and co-infection. The staff consists of individuals who have years of combined experience in publishing, community education, and HIV treatment advocacy. The Medical Editor has a medical degree and is experienced in HIV/AIDS treatment, research, and education. This site is financially supported by grants from pharmaceutical companies and the majority of information is current. This site is dense with information, much of it written, and all of it reviewed, by medical doctors.

Hivcme.com

http://www.hivcme.com/index.html

Hivcme.com is an online HIV continuing medical education (CME) library. This site provides health care professionals access to accredited HIV CME materials on up-to-date treatment issues. The Healthcare Consortium, a nonprofit organization committed to improving the quality of medical care for HIV-infected individuals, provides support for this site.

HIVDENT

http://www.hivdent.org

HIVDENT is a not-for-profit coalition of health care professionals committed to assuring access to high quality oral health care services for adults, adolescents, and children living with HIV. HIVDENT disseminates treatment information and shares expertise in advocacy, development, training, integration, and evaluation of oral health services for the HIV-infected population. The Web site contains several sections on the oral manifestations of HIV (including a large picture gallery) and information on infection control, postexposure protocols, pediatric/adolescent care, medications, funding, and other resources. Support is provided through non-restricted educational grants and support from Bristol-Myers Squibb Immunology, Colgate Oral Pharmaceuticals, and the Grady Health System.

Hivfitness.org

http://www.hivfitness.org

The mission of hivfitness is to provide exercise and nutrition information to HIV-infected individuals and health care providers. The editor of this site is an Advanced Certified Personal Fitness Trainer and dietetic professional. Some information is available in Spanish. A menu on the left side of the page shows links organized into categories.

International Association of Physicians in AIDS Care (IAPAC)

http://www.iapac.org

The IAPAC Web site serves as a member resource and a public service for physicians and other healthcare professionals, nongovernmental and governmental agencies, communities of faith, and others throughout the world who care for and about the people infected and affected by the intersecting pandemics of life-threatening infectious diseases, poverty, and dehumanization. Much of the information on this site is not current; therefore, it is not recommended as a resource unless it is updated.

International Bibliographic Information on Dietary Supplements (IBIDS)

http://ods.od.nih.gov/databases/ibids.html

The IBIDS database is a cooperative project of the Office of Dietary Supplements (ODS) at the National Institutes of Health (NIH), and the Food and Nutrition Information Center at the National Agricultural Library of the U.S. Department of Agriculture. IBIDS was launched specifically to assist health care providers, researchers, and the general public with locating scientific information on dietary supplements.

Johns Hopkins AIDS Service

http://www.hopkins-aids.edu

This is the Web site of the faculty of Johns Hopkins University, Division of Infectious Diseases. The home page contains current news articles and a question/answer of the week.

Journal of the American Medical Association (JAMA)

HIV/AIDS Resource Center

http://www.ama-assn.org/special/hiv

The *JAMA* HIV/AIDS Resource Center is designed for physicians and other health professionals. The site is produced and maintained by *JAMA* editors and staff under the direction of an editorial review board of leading HIV/AIDS authorities. The primary selection criterion is the quality of the science.

Medem Medical Library

http://www.medem.com/MedLB/medlib_entry.cfm

Medem is an organization of professional medical societies. The Medical Library includes peer-reviewed (by physicians, probably, but not spelled out as such) patient education information from its partner societies, including the American Medical Association, the American Academy of Pediatrics, the American College of Allergy, Asthma & Immunology, and other sources. Under "Diseases and Conditions" on the home page, there is an HIV/AIDS link.

MEDLINEplus®

http://medlineplus.gov

MEDLINEplus is the National Library of Medicine's (NLM's) Web site for consumer health information. NLM's experienced staff of information experts review hundreds of government and non-government publications, brochures, databases, and Web sites in order to link the public with the most reliable and authoritative information. MEDLINEplus is available on the World Wide Web from the NLM home page (http://www.nlm.nih.gov) or directly at MEDLINEplus (http://medlineplus.gov). MEDLINEplus is not meant to be an exhaustive list of every health Web resource. It is a selective list of appropriate, authoritative health information sources. MEDLINEplus includes mostly U.S. resources. International sites may be included at a later date.

The National AIDS Treatment Advocacy Project (NATAP)

http://www.natap.org

NATAP is a nonprofit organization dedicated to educating the diverse communities affected by HIV on the latest HIV treatments and advocating on treatment and policy issues for people with HIV. NATAP posts summary reports of conferences and conducts free community forums, usually at the New York University (NYU) Medical Center, to bridge the gap between the very latest research and the community by bringing in speakers who are conducting cutting-edge research. Proceedings from these forums are also posted to the NATAP Web site.

National Center for Complementary and Alternative Medicine

http://nccam.nih.gov

The National Center for Complementary and Alternative Medicine (NCCAM) at the National Institutes of Health (NIH) conducts and supports basic and applied research and training and disseminates information on complementary and alternative medicine to practitioners and the public. The NCCAM does not serve as a referral agency for various alternative medical treatments or individual practitioners. The NCCAM facilitates and conducts biomedical research.

National HIV/AIDS Clinicians' Consultation Center (NCCC)

[Formerly the Community Provider AIDS Training (CPAT) Web site]

http://www.ucsf.edu/hivcntr

The NCCC is funded by the University of California, San Francisco (USCF) and the Health Resources and Services Administration (HRSA). It is an AIDS Education and Training Centers clinical resource for health care providers from the USCF at San Francisco General Hospital. NCCC includes the National HIV Telephone Consultation Service (Warmline) and the National Clinician's Post-Exposure Prophylaxis Hotline (PEPline). These national services continue as programs of the AIDS Education and Training Centers (ETC) of the HIV/AIDS Bureau of HRSA, with additional funding from CDC.

National Institute of Allergy and Infectious Diseases (NIAID)

Division of Acquired Immunodeficiency Syndrome (DAIDS)

http://www.niaid.nih.gov/daids

The mission of DAIDS is to increase basic knowledge of the pathogenesis, natural history, and transmission of HIV disease and to support research that promotes progress in its detection, treatment, and prevention. DAIDS accomplishes this through planning, implementing, managing, and evaluating programs in (1) fundamental basic research, (2) discovery and development of therapies for HIV infection and its complications, and (3) discovery and development of vaccines and other prevention strategies.

National Institutes of Health (NIH) Office of AIDS Research (OAR)

http://www.nih.gov/od/oar

OAR is located within the Office of the Director of NIH and is responsible for the scientific, budgetary, legislative, and policy elements of the NIH AIDS research program. Congress has provided broad authority to the OAR to plan, coordinate, evaluate, and fund all NIH AIDS research. The OAR is responsible for the development of an annual comprehensive plan and budget for all NIH AIDS research. OAR supports trans-NIH Coordinating Committees to assist in these efforts in the following areas of program emphasis that have to do with treatment.

National Library of Medicine (NLM), National Institutes of Health (NIH)

U.S. Department of Human Services (DHHS)

http://www.nlm.nih.gov

The NLM is the world's largest medical library. NLM's online AIDS resources and other NLM databases are searchable at libraries, other institutions, and via personal computers.

National Minority AIDS Council (NMAC)

http://www.nmac.org

NMAC, established in 1987, is dedicated to developing leadership within communities of color to address the challenge of HIV/AIDS. NMAC sponsors the U.S. Conference on AIDS and the North American AIDS Treatment Action Forum each year, along with regional training for community-based organizations. This site lacks a site map or a search utility, which would assist the user in finding information. Some of the information is not current. NMAC has many useful publications, but most of them are not posted on the Web site.

National Pediatric AIDS Network (NPAN)

http://www.npan.org

NPAN is a nonprofit organization that works collaboratively with a number of other HIV/AIDS information providers to provide an extensive resource page of Web links for information on children and adolescents with HIV/AIDS. If you are interested in HIV/AIDS treatment for children and adolescents, this page is highly recommended as a guide to resources on the Internet.

National Prevention Information Network (NPIN)

http://www.cdcnpin.org

The Centers for Disease Control and Prevention's (CDC's) National Prevention Information Network is a reference, referral, and distribution service for information on HIV/AIDS, sexually transmitted diseases, and tuberculosis. This Web site is supported by the CDC and replaced the CDC National AIDS Clearinghouse.

New Mexico AIDS InfoNet

http://www.aidsinfonet.org

The New Mexico AIDS InfoNet is a project of the New Mexico AIDS Education and Training Center in the Infectious Diseases Division of the University of New Mexico School of Medicine. The InfoNet was originally designed to make information on HIV/AIDS services and treatments easily accessible in both English and Spanish for residents of New Mexico. Some InfoNet Fact Sheets have information that is specific to New Mexico; national references are provided when relevant. Major project funding has been provided by the National Library of Medicine; the New Mexico Department of Health, Public Health Division; and the Levi Strauss Foundation. Additional support has been provided by several pharmaceutical companies.

Pediatric AIDS Clinical Trials Group

http://pactg.s-3.com

The Pediatric AIDS Clinical Trials Group (PACTG) is a collaborative effort of the National Institute of Allergy and Infectious Diseases (NIAD) and the National Institute for Child Health and Human Development (NICHD). The PACTG specializes in evaluating treatments for HIV-infected children, developing new approaches for the interruption of mother-to-infant transmission, and establishing standards of care for children infected with HIV. This site would be of interest to clinicians conducting HIV/AIDS treatment research trials.

Physicians Research Network (PRN)

http://www.prn.org

The mission of this not-for-profit organization is to provide peer support to health care providers who treat people with HIV disease. The organization works to improve the diagnosis, management, and prevention of all aspects of HIV disease and to enhance the skills of providers. Clinical reports and scientific meeting summaries are published in a monthly journal entitled *The PRN Report*. Physicians review the content of the site. Several pharmaceutical companies provide unrestricted educational grants to support the site. The home page contains links to *PRN Reports* (reports on HIV/AIDS treatment), *PRN Notebook Online*™ (their newsletter on HIV/AIDS treatment), *PRN News Capsules* (current news Reports), and Provider Resources.

Project Inform (PI)

http://www.ProjectInform.org

Project Inform is a national, nonprofit, community-based organization based in San Francisco working to end the AIDS epidemic. Its mission is to provide vital information on the diagnosis and treatment of HIV to HIV-infected individuals, their caregivers, and their health care and service providers; to advocate enlightened regulatory, research, and funding policies affecting the development of, access to, and delivery of effective treatments, as well as to fund innovative research opportunities; to inspire people to make informed choices amid uncertainty, and to choose hope over despair. Funded by individuals, corporate and private foundations, individual bequests, and government sources. Some items are in Spanish.

PubMed®

http://pubmed.gov

PubMed is the National Library of Medicine's Web search interface that provides access to over 10 million journal article abstracts/citations in MEDLINE, PreMEDLINE, and other related databases with links to participating online journals. The online journal providers usually charge a fee to read the entire journal article, but viewing the abstracts is free through PubMed. PubMed is also the free Web interface to search AIDS journal article abstracts/citations. To limit your search to only items in the AIDS subset of MEDLINE, click on the word "Limits" under the search box. On the lower right of the screen, click on the arrow to the right of "Subsets" and select "AIDS." Click in the search box and type in your search terms.

San Francisco AIDS Foundation (SFAF)

http://www.sfaf.org

The goal of the San Francisco AIDS Foundation is to provide treatment information, support services, and advocacy for people living with HIV disease. The organization was founded in 1982. *The Bulletin of Experimental Treatment for AIDS (BETA)* and *Treatment Flash* are treatment journals published by the Foundation. Resources on the site are available in Spanish. The San Francisco AIDS Foundation receives most of its funding from government grants and private donations.

Sci.med.aids FAQ

http://www.aids.wustl.edu

Sci.med.aids is an international newsgroup on AIDS, a USENET newsgroup that discusses AIDS and HIV. A gateway forwards articles posted to sci.med.aids to a listserv mailing list called AIDS. The thousands of sci.med.aids readers include people with HIV infections, published authors, researchers, public health officials, and interested individuals. It is carried in several countries, particularly in the Americas and Europe. Sci.med.aids is moderated by a team. When readers submit an article, it must be approved by two members of the moderation team before it will be posted to the newsgroup. The sci.med.aids "FAQ" answers frequently asked questions about AIDS and the sci.med.aids newsgroup. The moderators try to keep things as up to date and accurate as possible. However, readers of the site may post updates to the moderators. Some sections may contain information that is not current.

Social Security Administration (SSA)

http://www.ssa.gov

"Social Security Online" is the official home page of the SSA. Information on disability benefits is helpful to HIV/AIDS patients.

The University of North Carolina AIDS Clinical Trials Unit

http://www.med.unc.edu/medicine/hivaidsc

The University of North Carolina AIDS Clinical Trials Unit is dedicated to conducting research on HIV infection and providing access to promising treatment to persons living with HIV. The program provides access to clinical studies researching antiretroviral therapies, immunomodulators, HIV-related malignancies, wasting syndrome, neurological complications, gastrointestinal illnesses, and many others. In addition to conducting research, the staff provides treatment consultation for health care providers. The program was established in 1987. The National Institutes of Health is a sponsor of the program. Funding is also accepted from pharmaceutical companies. This page is geared toward clinicians.

Veterans Administration AIDS Information Center

http://vhaaidsinfo.cio.med.va.gov

The AIDS Service Division of the Department of Veterans Affairs (VA) sponsors the VA AIDS Information Center, which provides up-to-date HIV/AIDS treatment information to physicians, researchers, social workers, counselors, and other health care professionals. Information is provided by electronic communication, including a biweekly AIDS Information Newsletter.

Veterans Administration (VA) AIDS Service

http://vhaaidsinfo.cio.med.va.gov

The VA AIDS Service is a division of the Department of Veterans Affairs. The program is responsible for planning, coordinating, implementing, and evaluating HIV/AIDS clinical programs for all of the VA health care system. Their mission is to provide the highest quality of care to VA patients with HIV infection. The program staff has broad expertise in the VA medical system and in HIV care and research. The program disseminates information through their biweekly newsletter, *AIDS News Service*.

Chapter 73

National Organizations Providing HIV/AIDS Services

AIDS Action Council
1906 Sunderland Place NW
Washington, DC 20036
Tel: 202-530-8030
Fax: 202-530-8031
Internet: http://
www.aidsaction.org

AIDS Policy Center for Children, Youth and Families
1600 K Street NW, Suite 300
Washington, DC 20006
Tel: 202-785-3564
Toll Free: 888-917-AIDS
Fax: 202-785-3579
E-Mail: info@aids-alliance.org
Internet: http://
www.aidspolicycenter.org

American Foundation for AIDS Research (AmFar)
120Wall Street, 13th Floor
New York, NY 10005-3902
Tel: 212-806-1600
Fax: 212-806-1601
Internet: http://www.amfar.org

Midwest Hispanic AIDS Coalition
1753 North Damen Avenue
Chicago, IL 60647
Tel: 312-772-8195
Fax: 312-772-8484

"National HIV/AIDS Organizations and Hotlines," Substance Abuse and Mental Health Services Administration (SAMHSA), 1995, available online at http://www.health.org/govpubs/bkd163/15p.htm, cited November 2002; resources verified December 2002.

National Association of People with AIDS

1413 K Street, N.W.
Washington, DC 20005
Tel: 202-898-0414
Fax: 202-898-0435
Internet: http://www.napwa.org
E-Mail: napwa@napwa.org

National Episcopal AIDS Coalition

520 Clinton Avenue
Brooklyn, NY 11238-2211
Tel: 718-857-9445

National Leadership Coalition on AIDS

1730 M Street, N.W.
Suite 905
Washington, DC 20036
Tel: 202-429-0930
Fax: 202-872-1977
Internet: http://www.dccare.org/
spnlca.htm

National Minority AIDS Council (NMAC)

1931 13th Street, NW
Washington, DC 20009
Tel: 202-483-6622
Fax: 202-483-1135
Internet: http://www.nmac.org

National Native American AIDS Prevention Center (NNAAPC)

436 14th Street
Suite 1020
Oakland, CA 94612
Tel: 510-444-2051
Fax: 510-444-1593
Internet: http://www.nnaapc.org
E-Mail: information@nnaapc.org

National Pediatric HIV Resource Center

30 Bergen Street, ADMC #4
Newark, NJ 07103
Toll Free: 800-362-0071
Tel: 973-972-0410
Fax: 973-972-0399
Internet: http://
www.pedhivaids.org

Chapter 74

National Religious AIDS Organizations and Hotlines

This chapter provides a sample of national organizations which offer extensive or specialized AIDS-related services for the religious community. This information is designed to support, not replace, the relationship that exists between you and your doctor.

AIDS Advocacy in African American Churches Project
611 Pennsylvania Ave. S.E.
Suite 359
Washington, DC 20003
Tel: 202-546-8587
Fax: 202-546-8867

AIDS Ministry Network of the United Methodist Church
General Board of Global Ministries
475 Riverside Drive
Room 330
New York, NY 10115
Tel: 212-870-3870
TDD: 212-870-3709
Fax: 212-870-3624
Internet: http://gbgm-umc.org/health/aids
E-Mail: aidsmin@gbgm-umc.org

The organizations listed in this chapter were originally compiled by HIV InfoWeb, formerly a service of the AIDS Education Global Information Service (AEGIS). With their permission, the list has been updated and all contact information was verified and updated in December 2002.

Christian AIDS Services Alliance
P.O. Box 3612
San Rafael, CA 94912-3612
Tel: 415-454-1017

The Congress of National Black Churches
2000 L Street NW
Suite 225
Washington, DC 20036-4962
Tel: 202-296-5657
Fax: 202-296-4939
Internet: http://www.cnbc.org

Lutheran AIDS Network
625 4th Avenue South
Minneapolis, MN 55415
Internet: http://
www.lutheranaids.net
E-Mail: info@lutheranaids.net

National Catholic AIDS Network
P.O. Box 422984
San Francisco, CA 94142-2984
Tel: 707-874-3031
Fax: 707-874-1433
Internet: http://www.ncan.org
E-Mail: info@ncan.org

National Episcopal AIDS Coalition
520 Clinton Avenue
Brooklyn, NY 11238-2211
Tel: 718-857-9445
Internet: http://www.neac.org

Presbyterian AIDS Network
3060A Presbyterian Center
100 Witherspoon St.
Louisville, KY 40202-1396
Tel: 502-569-5794
Internet: http://www.virtual-arts.com/stage/pan

Seventh-Day Adventist Kinship International
P.O. Box 7320
Laguna Niguel, CA 92607
Tel: 714-248-1299
Internet: http://
www.sdakinship.org
E-Mail: office@sdakinship.org

Southern Baptist Convention
Christian Life Commission
901 Commerce
Suite 550
Nashville, TN 37203
Tel: 615-244-2495
Internet: http://www.sbc.net

Union of American Hebrew Congregations
633 Third Avenue
New York, NY 10017-6778
Tel: 212-650-4221
Internet: http://www.uahc.org

United Church AIDS/HIV Network
700 Prospect Ave.
Cleveland, OH 44115
Tel: 216-736-3270
Fax: 216-736-3263

Unitarian Universalist Association AIDS Resources Network
717 Westwood Avenue
Lodi, CA 95242
Tel: 209-369-7286
Fax: 209-333-8657

Universal Fellowship of Metropolitan Community Churches AIDS Ministry
5300 Santa Monica Blvd.
Suite 304
Los Angeles, CA 90029
Tel: 213-464-5100
Fax: 213-464-2123
E-Mail: UFMCCHQ@aol.com

Chapter 75

CDC's National AIDS Hotline

The Centers for Disease Control and Prevention's (CDC) National AIDS Hotline is an activity of the Technical Information and Communications Branch, Divisions of HIV/AIDS Prevention, National Center for HIV, STD, and TB Prevention.

The CDC National AIDS Hotline operates toll free, 24 hours a day, 7 days a week. The Hotline offers anonymous, confidential HIV/AIDS information to the American public. Trained information specialists answer questions about HIV infection and AIDS.

The Hotline also provides referrals to appropriate services, including clinics, hospitals, local hotlines, counseling and testing sites, legal services, health departments, support groups, educational organizations, and service agencies throughout the United States. Callers can also order various publications, posters, and other informational materials from the CDC National Prevention Information Network through the Hotline.

Established in February 1983, the CDC National AIDS Hotline was one of the first government services established to respond to the public's questions about the AIDS epidemic. The Hotline is presently the world's largest health information service, receiving an average of about 3,000 calls each day. To date, over 13 million calls have been handled by the Hotline.

"CDC National AIDS Hotline (NAH)," National Center for HIV, STD, and TB Prevention, Centers for Disease Control and Prevention (CDC), December 2000.

The Centers for Disease Control and Prevention's (CDC) National AIDS Hotline

In English
Toll Free: 800-342-AIDS

In Spanish
Toll Free: 800-344-7432

For the Deaf
TTY: 800-243-7889

Index

Index

Page numbers followed by 'n' indicate a footnote. Page numbers in *italics* indicate a table or illustration.

A

AACTG *see* Adult AIDS Clinical Trials Group
abacavir (ABC) 64, 119, 127, 142, 373
ABC *see* abacavir
Abelcet (amphotericin) 120
ABLC (amphotericin) 120
ABT-538 *see* ritonavir
acidophilus 313
acquired immune deficiency syndrome (AIDS)
  caretakers 269–89
  defined 495
  overview 3–11, 61–69, 237–44, 495
  research 427–38, 465–67
  statistics 471–73
  see also human immunodeficiency virus
acquired immunity *see* passive immunity
ACTIS *see* AIDS Clinical Trials Information Service

active immunity, defined 495–96
acupuncture
  AIDS treatment 157–59
  defined 496
acute HIV infection, defined 496
Acute HIV Infection and Early Diseases Research Program (AIEDRP), defined 496
acyclovir 315
ADAP *see* AIDS Drug Assistance Programs
ADC *see* AIDS dementia complex
ADCC *see* antibody-dependent cell-mediated cytotoxicity
adenopathy, defined 496
adherence, defined 496
adjuvant, defined 496
administration, defined 496–97
adolescents
  HIV/AIDS statistics 472, 489–92
  oral sex 39–40
Adult AIDS Clinical Trials Group (AACTG), defined 497
Adult AIDS Clinical Trials Group (AACTG), Web site address 584
adverse event, defined 497
adverse reactions
  defined 497
  described 457

613

AEGIS *see* AIDS Education Global Information System

aerosolized, defined 497

AETC *see* AIDS Education and Training Centers

affected community, defined 497

Africa
HIV-2 infections 28
HIV/AIDS statistics 471
HIV prevention measures 423–24, 441
sexually transmitted diseases 396–97

agammaglobulinemia, defined 497

Agency for Healthcare Research and Quality (AHRQ), defined 497–98

Agenerase (amprenavir) 9, 64, 119, 130, 143, 378–79

AHRQ *see* Agency for Healthcare Research and Quality

AIDS *see* acquired immune deficiency syndrome

AIDS 2002: XIV International AIDS Conference, Web site address 584

AIDS Action Committee of Massachusetts, Inc., Web site address 584

AIDS Action Council, contact information 603

"AIDS: Activism and Advocacy" (FDA) 61n

AIDS Advocacy in African American Churches Project, contact information 605

AIDScience, Web site address 586

AIDS Clinical Trials Information Service (ACTIS), defined 498

AIDS Clinical Trials Information Service (ACTIS), Web site address 584

AIDS dementia complex (ADC)
caretakers 284–85
defined 498
overview 211–13

AIDS Drug Assistance Programs (ADAP), defined 498

AIDSDrugs, defined 498

AIDSDRUGS, Web site address 587

AIDS Education and Training Centers (AETC), defined 498–99

AIDS Education Global Information System (AEGIS), Web site address 585

AIDSinfo, HAART publication 133n

Aidsinfonyc.org, Web site address 586

AIDSLINE, defined 499

AIDSMAP, Web site address 586

AIDSmeds.com, Web site address 587

AIDS Ministry Network of the United Methodist Church, contact information 605

AIDS Nutrition Services Alliances (ANSA)
nutrition publications 251n
Web site address 585

AIDS.ORG, Web site address 587

AIDS Policy Center for Children, Youth and Families, contact information 603

AIDS-related cancers, defined 499

AIDS-related complex (ARC), defined 499

AIDS Research Advisory Committee (ARAC), defined 499

AIDS Service Organization (ASO), defined 499

AIDS Treatment Data Network, Web site address 585

AIDSTrials, defined 499

AIDSTRIALS, Web site address 587

AIDSVAX 66, 443–48

AIDS wasting syndrome *see* wasting syndrome

AIEDRP *see* Acute HIV Infection and Early Diseases Research Program

alanine aminotransferase activity test, hepatitis exposure 60

alcohol use
drug interactions 229
hepatitis C virus 181, 183

alitretinoin 119

alkaline phosphatase, defined 500

alopecia, defined 500

alpha interferon
defined 500
hepatitis 182
Kaposi's sarcoma 10

alprazolam 227

"Alternative and Complementary Therapies" (New Mexico AIDS InfoNet) 157n

alternative medicine
  AIDS treatment 157–60
  defined 500
The Alternative Medicine HomePage,
  Web site address 588
alveolar, defined 500
AmBisome (amphotericin) 120
amebiasis, defined 500
American Association of Blood Banks,
  Web site address 52
American Foundation for AIDS Research (AmFAR)
  contact information 603
  Web site address 588
American Red Cross, Web site address 52
AmFAR *see* American Foundation for
  AIDS Research
amino acids, defined 500
amphotericin 120, 218
amprenavir 9, 64, 119, 130, 143, 378–79
amyl nitrate, drug interactions 229, 233
anaphylactic shock, defined 501
anemia, defined 501
anergy
  defined 501
  described 24
angiogenesis, defined 501
angiomatosis, defined 501
anilingus
  defined 39
  HIV infection 41
animals
  AIDS health precautions 265–68,
    276–77
  cryptosporidiosis 173–74
  mycobacterium avium complex dis-
    ease 194
anorexia
  defined 501
  treatment 161
ANSA *see* AIDS Nutrition Services
  Alliances
Ansamycin (rifabutin) 125
antenatal, defined 501
antibiotic, defined 501
antibodies
  defined 501
  HIV infection 74

antibody-dependent cell-mediated
  cytotoxicity (ADCC), defined 501
antibody-mediated immunity, defined
  501
antifungal, defined 501
antigen, defined 502
antigen presentation, defined 502
antigen-presenting cell (APC), defined 502
antineoplastic, defined 502
antiprotozoal, defined 502
antiretroviral drugs
  children 353–54, 372–81
  clinical trial 458–60
  cryptosporidiosis 173
  defined 502
  described 9, 21, 114–15
  drug interactions 230
  HAART 133, 136
  HIV prevention 399–402
antisense drugs, defined 502
antitioxins, defined 502
antiviral, defined 502
antiviral drugs
  described 17
  pregnancy 344
APC *see* antigen-presenting cell
aphasia, defined 502
aphthous ulcer, defined 502
Apmrenavir (agenerase) 119
apoptosis
  defined 502–3
  described 23
approved drugs, defined 503
ARC *see* AIDS-related complex
ARM, defined 503
arthralgia, defined 503
ASO *see* AIDS Service Organization
aspergillosis, defined 503
assembly and budding
  defined 503
  described 18
asymptomatic, defined 503
ataxia, defined 503
atazanavir 130
ATIS *see* HIV/AIDS Treatment Information Service
atorvastatin 188
atovaquone 120, 144

"Attacking AIDS with a 'Cocktail' Therapy: Drug Combo Sends Deaths Plummeting" (Henkel) 141n
attenuated, defined 503
atypia, defined 324
autoantibody, defined 504
autoimmunization, defined 504
autoinoculation, defined 504
autologous, defined 504
auxiliary genes, described 553, 566
avascular necrosis (AVN), defined 504
AVN *see* avascular necrosis
ayurveda 157
Azidothymidine (zidovudine) 127
azithromycin 120, 144, 194–95
AZT *see* zidovudine

B

"Backgrounder: HIV Infection in Infants and Children" (NIAID) 351n
bactericidal, defined 504
bacteriostatic, defined 504
bacterium, defined 504
Bactrim (sulfamethoxazole/ trimethoprim) 126, 144, 240, 384
baculovirus, defined 504
Barret, Bob 93
baseline, defined 504
baseline metabolism, described 221–22
basophil, defined 504
Bastyr University AIDS Research Center (BUARC), Web site address 589
Bay Area Young Positives, contact information 326
B cell lymphoma *see* lymphoma
B-cells *see* B-lymphocytes
bDNA test *see* branched DNA assay
Terry Beirn Community Programs for Clinical Research on AIDS, described 514–15
see also Community Programs for Clinical Research on AIDS
benzodiazepines 227, 233
beta 2 microglobulin, defined 505

BFR *see* body fat redistribution syndrome
Biaxin (clarithromycin) 120, 144
Bicillin 315
bilirubin, defined 505
binding antibody, defined 505
bioavailability, defined 505
biological response modifier (BMR), defined 505
biopsy, defined 505
biotechnology, defined 505
BI-RG-587 (nevirapine) 125
biting, HIV infection 37
blinded study, defined 505
BLIPS, defined 506
blood-brain barrier, defined 506
see also meninges
"Blood Safety: The Importance of Donor Screening and Testing" (CDC) 47n
blood supply safety 47–52, 242
blood transfusions
HIV-2 infection 29
HIV infection 4, 33
B-lymphocytes (B-cells)
defined 506
described 21
The Body, Web site address 589
body fat redistribution syndrome (BFR), defined 525
body fluids, defined 506
bone marrow, defined 506
bone marrow suppression, defined 506
booster, defined 506
branched DNA assay (bDNA test), defined 506507
breakthrough infection, defined 507
breastfeeding, HIV infection 4, 60
BRM *see* biological response modifier
bronchoscopy, defined 507
brown bag medicine checkup, described 226
BUARC *see* Bastyr University AIDS Research Center
budding *see* assembly and budding
buffalo hump *see* lipodystrophy
Bullers, Anne Christiansen 61n
Burkitt's lymphoma, defined 507

C

cachexia, defined 507
Canadian HIV Trials Network, Web site address 589
cancers, AIDS 14
candida
  defined 507
  marijuana use 163
candidiasis
  defined 507
  treatment 10
capsid, described 15
carcinoma-in-situ (CIS), defined 324
cardinogen, defined 507
caretakers, AIDS patients 269–89
CAT scan *see* computed tomography
CBC *see* complete blood count
CBCT *see* community-based clinical trial
CBO *see* community-based organization
CCR5
  defined 508
  described 16
CD4 cells
  defined 508
  described 16
CD4+ cells
  gender difference 340–42
  HIV infection 19
CD4+ count, described 77
CD4+ T-cells
  AIDS 6–7, 14
  described 5, 13, 16–17
  HIV infection 21–22
  opportunistic infections 10
CD8 cells
  defined 508
CD8+ T-cells
  described 19, 22
CDC *see* Centers for Disease Control and Prevention
CDC-NAH *see* CDC National AIDS Hotline
"CDC National AIDS Hotline (NAH)" (CDC) 609n
CDC National AIDS Hotline (CDC-NAH), defined 508

CDC National Prevention Information Network (CDC-NPIN), defined 508–9
CDC-NPIN *see* CDC National Prevention Information Network
"CDC's HIV/AIDS Prevention Activities" (NCHSTP) 417n
"CDC's International Activities Support Global HIV Prevention Efforts" (NCHSTP) 417n
ceftriaxone 218, 315
cell lines, defined 509
cell-mediated immunity (CMI) defined 509
cellular immunity *see* cell-mediated immunity
Center for Mental Health Research on AIDS (CMHRA), Web site address 590
Centers for Disease Control and Prevention (CDC)
  described 509
  HIV prevention strategy 417–26
  HIV testing recommendations 100
  hotlines 102
  National AIDS Hotline 610
  publications
    AIDS hotline 609n
    blood supply safety 47n
    clinical trials 451n
    drug-associated HIV transmission 43n
  Web site address 590
Centers for Medicare and Medicaid Services (CMS), described 509–10
central nervous system (CNS)
  defined 509
  HIV infection 24—25
central nervous system damage, defined 509
central nervous system lymphoma, described 218–19
cerebral, defined 510
cerebrospinal fluid (CSF) defined 510
cervical cancer, defined 510
cervical dysplasia
  defined 510
  HIV infection 308–9, 317–18

cervical intraepithelial neoplasia (CIN), defined 324–25, 510
cervicitis, HIV infection 317
cervix, defined 510
challenge, defined 510
chancroid, defined 510
chemokines, defined 511
chemoprophylaxis, defined 511
chemotherapy, defined 511
chickenpox, AIDS caretakers 275
children
  hepatitis 184
  HIV-2 infection 29, 30–31
  HIV/AIDS statistics 471–72
  HIV infection 348
  HIV infection determination 296
  HIV infection symptoms 5–6
  opportunistic infections 7
  Pneumocystis carinii pneumonia 10
  see also pediatric AIDS
chiropractic 157
chlamydia
  defined 511
  HIV infection 398
Christian AIDS Services Alliance, contact information 606
chronic idiopathic demyelinating polyneuropathy (CIPD), defined 511
cidofovir 120, 144, 315
CIN see cervical intraepithelial neoplasia
CIPD see chronic idiopathic demyelinating polyneuropathy
CIPRA see Comprehensive International Program of Research on AIDS
ciproflaxacin 262
circumoral paresthesia, defined 511
clade, defined 511–12
clarithromycin 120, 144, 194–95
clindamycin 217
clinical, defined 512
clinical alert, defined 512
clinical endpoint see endpoint
clinical latency, defined 512
clinical practice guidelines, defined 512

clinical trials
  defined 512–13
  described 430–31, 451–58
  HIV/AIDS research 458–64
ClinicalTrials.gov
  described 513
  Web site address 590
clonazepam 227
clone, defined 513
clotting factor, HIV infection 33
CMHRA see Center for Mental Health Research on AIDS
CMI see cell-mediated immunity
CMS see Centers for Medicare and Medicaid Services
CMV see cytomegalovirus
CMV retinitis see cytomegalovirus retinitis
CNS see central nervous system
cocaine, drug interactions 230
Coccidioides immitis 513
coccidioidomycosis, defined 513
"Cocktails and Party Favors" (Potochnic) 225n
cocktail therapy see drug cocktails
codon, defined 513
cofactors, defined 513
cognitive impairment, defined 514
cohort, defined 514
colitis, defined 514
colposcopy 320–21
"Combination Therapy with IL-2 Plus Antiretroviral Drugs to Treat HIV Infection" (CDC) 451n
Combivir (lamivudine/zidovudine) 124, 143
community-based clinical trial (CBCT), defined 514
community-based organization (CBO), defined 514
Community Programs for Clinical Research on AIDS (CPCRA), described 514–15
compassionate use, defined 515
complement, defined 515
complementary and alternative therapy
  AIDS treatment 157–60
  defined 515

complement cascade, defined 515
complete blood count (CBC), defined 515
Comprehensive International Program of Research on AIDS (CIPRA) 439–42
computed tomography (CAT scan; CT scan), defined 517
condoms
   HIV infection prevention 11, 38, 411–16
   see also female condom
"Condoms: Barriers to Bad News" (Nordenberg) 411n
Condyloma acuminatum, defined 515
The Congress of National Black Churches, contact information 606
contagious, defined 515–16
contraindication, defined 516
controlled trials, defined 516
Cooke, David A. 27n
core, defined 516
co-receptors, defined 516
correlates of immunity, defined 516
correlates of protection, defined 516
Cotrim (trimethoprim-sulfamethoxazole) 240, 374
counseling
   hepatitis 183
   HIV tests 73, 84–85, 97–111
   see also preconception counseling
CPCRA *see* Community Programs for Clinical Research on AIDS
creatinine, defined 516
Crixivan (indinavir) 9, 64, 123, 130, 143, 231, 246, 321, 379
Crixivan potbelly 144
   see also lipodystrophy
cross-resistance, defined 516
cryotherapy, defined 516
cryptococcal meningitis
   defined 516–17
   described 218
cryptococcosis, defined 517
cryptococcus neoformans, defined 517
cryptosporidiosis
   defined 517
   household pets 265
   overview 171–76

Cryptosporidium parvum, defined 517
crystal methamphetamine, drug interactions 230
CSF *see* cerebrospinal fluid
CTL *see* cytotoxic T lymphocyte
CT scan *see* computed tomography
cunnilingus
   defined 39
   HIV infection 41
cutaneous, defined 517
CXCR4 cell molecule, defined 517–18
cytokines, defined 518
cytomegalovirus (CMV)
   defined 518
   HIV infection 20
   overview 177–78
   treatment 10
cytomegalovirus retinitis
   defined 518
cytopenia, defined 518
cytotoxic, defined 518
cytotoxic T lymphocyte (CTL), defined 518
Cytovene (ganciclovir) 123, 144

D

d4T *see* stavudine
DAIDS *see* Division of Acquired Immunodeficiency Syndrome
Data Safety and Monitoring Board (DSMB), described 518–19
daunorubicin 145
daunorubicin-liposomal 120
DaunoXone (daunorubicin-liposomal) 120
ddC *see* Dideoxycytidine; Hivid; zalcitabine
ddI *see* didanosine
DDS *see* Disability Determination Service
death process, AIDS 287–88
Delaney, Martin 63, 68
delavirdine (DLV) 9, 65, 121, 143, 230, 376
deletion, defined 519
dementia, defined 519
   see also AIDS dementia complex

demyelination, defined 519
dendrite, defined 519
dentists, HIV infection 34
dentritic cells, defined 519
deoxyribonucleic acid (DNA)
   defined 519
   described 14–15
depression, HIV infection 245–49
"Depression and HIV/AIDS" (NIMH)
   245n
desensitization, defined 520
desert fever, defined 513
DHHS *see* US Department of Health
   and Human Service; US Department of Health and Human Services
DHPG (ganciclovir) 123
diabetes mellitus
   defined 520
   lipodystrophy 185
   protease inhibitors 130
diagnosis, defined 520
diarrhea, defined 520
diazepam 227, 229
didanosine (ddI) 9, 64, 121, 142, 366,
   373–74
dideooxyinosine 9
Dideoxycytidine (zalcitabine) 127,
   375
Dideoxyinosine (didanosine) 9, 121
diet and nutrition
   clinical trial 461–62
   HIV/AIDS 251–55, 278
Diflucan (fluconazole) 122
diplopia, defined 520
DIRLINE, Web site address 591
Disability Determination Service
   (DDS), described 294–96
disseminated, defined 520
Division of Acquired Immunodeficiency Sydrome (DAIDS/
   NIAID), described 520–21
DLV *see* delavirdine
DMP-266 *see* efavirenz
DNA *see* deoxyribonucleic acid
domain, defined 521
dose-ranging study, defined 521
dose-response relationship, defined
   521

double-blind study, defined 521
Doxil (doxorubicin hydrochloride-
   liposomal) 121
doxorubicin 145
doxorubicin hydrochloride-liposomal
   121
dronabinol 121, 145, 161, 165–67, 222
"Drug-Associated HIV Transmission
   Continues in the United States"
   (CDC) 43n
drug cocktails, described 65–66
drug-drug interactions
   defined 521
   overview 225–34
drug-food interactions 254–55
drug holiday *see* pulsed therapy;
   structured intermittent therapy
"Drug Interactions" (Project Inform)
   225n
drug resistance
   defined 521
   described 129–30
drug use
   HIV infection 4, 43–45, 107
   protease inhibitors 132
DSMB *see* Data Safety and Monitoring Board
dysplasia, defined 325, 521
dyspnea, defined 521

E

EBV *see* Epstein-Barr Virus
ecstasy, drug interactions 230–31
education
   HIV infection 44–45
   HIV prevention 392
efavirenz 9, 65, 121, 143, 322, 343,
   377
efficacy, defined 521
EIA *see* enzyme immunoassay
ELISA *see* enzyme-linked
   immunosorbent assay
emotional concerns, AIDS caretakers
   273–74
empirical, defined 522
encephalitis, defined 522
   see also toxoplasma encephalitis

endemic, defined 522
endogenous, defined 522
endoscopy, defined 522
endotoxin, defined 522
endpoint, defined 522
end-stage disease, defined 522
Entamoeba histolytica 500
enteric, defined 522
enteritis, defined 522
entry inhibitors, defined 522
env
  defined 522
  described 15–16
envelope, defined 522–23
enzyme, defined 523
enzyme immunoassay (EIA), described
  79–81
enzyme-linked immunosorbent assay
  (ELISA)
  defined 522
  described 74, 105
eosinophil, defined 523
eosinophilic folliculitis, defined 523
epidemic
  defined 523
  HIV 14
epidemiologic surveillance, defined
  523
epidemiology, defined 523
epithelium, defined 524
epitope, defined 524
Epivir (lamivudine) 64, 127, 190–91,
  374
EPO (erythropoietin) 122
Epogen (erythropoietin) 122
Epstein-Barr Virus (EBV) 218, 524
ERT *see* estrogen replacement
  therapy
erythema, defined 524
erythema multiforme, defined 524
erythrocytes, defined 524
erythropoietin 122
estrogen replacement therapy (ERT),
  HIV infection 332
ethnic factors
  AIDS 3
  HIV infection 348, 404
  HIV transmission 43
etiology, defined 524

exclusion criteria, defined 524
exogenous, defined 524
exotoxin, defined 524
expanded access, defined 524
expanded access protocol, described
  454
experimental drug, defined 525
expression syndrome, defined 525
expression system, defined 525

F

famciclovir 122, 315
family issues
  HIV infection 35
  pediatric AIDS 354
Famvir (famciclovir) 122, 315
fat redistribution, defined 525
fat redistribution syndrome, defined
  525
fatty liver *see* hepatic steatosis
Fauci, Anthony 142, 146
FDA *see* US Food and Drug Administration
FDC *see* follicular dendritic cells
feline immunodeficiency virus (FIV),
  described 15
fellatio
  defined 39
  HIV infection 40–41
female condom 414–15
financial considerations
  HIV counseling 109–10
  HIV infection prevention 392
5-fluorouracil 309
floaters, defined 525
fluconazole 10, 122, 218, 313
fluoxetine 231
Fogarty International Foundation,
  Web site address 52
folinic acid 144
follicular dendritic cells (FDC)
  defined 525
  described 21–22
fomivirsen sodium injection 122
"Food and Medication Interactions
  Can Be Very Harmful" (AIDS Nutrition Services Alliances) 251n

food safety, HIV infection 257–60, 278
Fortovase (saquinavir) 64, 130, 381
foscarnet 10, 122, 144, 315
Foscavir (foscarnet) 122, 144, 315
"Frequently Asked Questions and Answers about Co-infection with HIV and Hepatitis C Virus" (NCHSTP) 179m
functional antibody, defined 525
fungal infections, treatment 10
fungus
   defined 525
   marijuana 163
fusin *see* CXCR4
fusion inhibitor, defined 525–26
fusion mechanism, defined 526

G

gag
   defined 526
   described 15
Gamimune N (immune globulin) 123
gamma globulin 123, 526
gamma interferon, defined 526
ganciclovir 10, 123, 144, 178, 226
ganglion, defined 526
GART *see* genotypic antiretroviral resistance test
gastrointestinal (GI), defined 526
Gay Men's Health Crisis (GMHC), Web site address 592
G-CSF *see* granulocyte-colony stimulating factor; Neupogen
gemfibrozil 188
"Gender Difference in Viral Load" (Project Inform) 339n
gender factor
   HIV/AIDS statistics 472
   viral load 339–42
"General Nutrition Recommendations" (AIDS Nutrition Services Alliances) 251n
genes
   defined 526
   HIV infection 553
gene therapy, defined 526
genetic engineering, defined 526–27

genital herpes 314–15
genital warts, defined 515
genitourinary tract, defined 527
genome, defined 527
genotypic antiretroviral resistance test (GART)
   defined 526
genotypic assay, defined 527
gential ulcer disease, defined 527
Geraci, Anthony 216
Geraty, Edward 93
germinal centers, defined 527
GHB, drug interactions 229, 230–31
GI *see* gastrointestinal
giant cells *see* syncytia
giardiasis, defined 527
Elizabeth Glaser Pediatric AIDS Foundation, Web site address 591
"Global AIDS Program Technical Strategies Overview: 2.3 Blood Safety" (CDC) 47n
globulins, defined 527
"Glossary of HIV/AIDS-Related Terms" (DHHS) 495n
Glucophage (metformin) 188
glycoprotein, defined 527
glycoprotein 41 (gp41)
   defined 528
   described 15, 16
glycoprotein 120 (gp120)
   defined 528
   described 16
glycoprotein 160 (gp160)
   defined 528
   described 16, 444–45
glycoprotein molecules, described 523
GM-CSF *see* granulocyte macrophage-colony stimulating factor
GMHC *see* Gay Men's Health Crisis
gonorrhea, defined 527
gp41 *see* glycoprotein 41
gp120 *see* glycoprotein 120
gp160 *see* glycoprotein 160
granulocyte, defined 528
granulocyte-colony stimulating factor (G-CSF), defined 528
granulocyte macrophage-colony stimulating factor (GM-CSF), defined 528

granulocytopenia, defined 528
"Guidelines for the Use of Antiretroviral Agents in Pediatric HIV Infection" (NIH) 357n
"A Guide to Social Security and SSI Disability Benefits for People with HIV Infection" (SSA) 291n
Gutman, Steven 92, 94, 96
"GYN Conditions in Women with HIV" (Project Inform) 311n

H

HAART *see* highly active antiretroviral therapy
Haemophilus ducreyi bacterium 510
hairy leukoplakia *see* oral hairy leukoplakia
Halcion (triazolam) 229
half-life, defined 528
HAM/TSP *see* HTLV-I-associated myelopathy/tropical spastic paraparesis
HCFA (Health Care Financing Administration) *see* Centers for Medicare and Medicaid Services
HCSUS *see* HIV Cost and Services Utilization Study
HCV *see* hepatitis C virus
Health Care Financing Administration (HCFA) *see* Centers for Medicare and Medicaid Services
health care workers
  blood exposure 53–60
  HIV/AIDS statistics 475–76
  HIV infection 34
Healthcommunities.com, Inc., HIV tests publication 73n
Health Resources and Services Administration (HRSA)
  described 528–29
  Web site address 592
HELLP syndrome, defined 529
helper ratio, defined 529
helper T-cells
  defined 529
  described 98
  see also CD4+ T-cells; T4 lymphocyte cells

hematocrit, defined 529
hematotoxic, defined 529
hemoglobin, defined 529
hemolysis, defined 529
hemophilia, defined 529–30
Henkel, John 141n
Henry, Keith 62, 67
hepatic, defined 530
hepatic steatosis (fatty liver)
  defined 530
  mitochondrial toxicity 549
hepatitis, defined 530
hepatitis B virus (HBV), blood exposure 53–60
hepatitis C/co-infection with HIV
  defined 530
  overview 179–84
hepatitis C virus (HCV), blood exposure 53–60
hepatomegaly, defined 530
herb therapy 157
heroin, drug interactions 232
herpes simplex virus, HIV infection 314–15
herpes simplex virus 1 (HSV-1), defined 531
herpes simplex virus 2 (HSV-2), defined 531
herpes varicella zoster virus, defined 531
herpes viruses, defined 530–31
HGH *see* human growth hormone
highly active antiretroviral therapy (HAART)
  alcohol use 229
  defined 531
  described 10, 21, 114–16, 389–90
  overview 133–40
  protease boosting 130
histocompatibility testing, defined 531
histoplasmosis, defined 531
HIV *see* human immunodeficiency virus
HIV-1 *see* human immunodeficiency virus type 1
HIV-2 *see* human immunodeficiency virus type 2
"HIV/AIDS among Hispanics in the United States" (NCHSTP) 481n

"HIV/AIDS among U.S. Women: Minority and Young Women at Continuing Risk" (NCHSTP) 485n
"HIV/AIDS and U.S. Women Who Have Sex with Women (WSW)" (NCHSTP) 407n
HIV/AIDS Dietetic Practice Group, Web site address 593
"HIV/AIDS Statistics" (NIAID) 471n
HIV/AIDS Treatment Information Service (ATIS), Web site address 593
HIVandHepatitis.com, Web site address 593
"HIV and Its Treatment: What You Should Know" (AIDSinfo) 133n
"HIV and Older Age" (Project Inform) 327n
HIV antibody tests, described 98
  see also immunofluorescence assay; Western blot test
HIV-associated dementia *see* AIDS dementia complex
Hivcme.com, Web site address 594
HIV Cost and Services Utilization Study (HCSUS)
  defined 532
  described 532
HIVDENT, Web site address 594
Hivfitness.org, Web site address 594
Hivid (zalcitabine) 64, 127, 375
HIV infection
  described 19–22
  diagnosis 7–8
  hotline information 102–3, 111
  overview 3–11
  prevention 10–11, 389–426
  primary, defined 564
  symptoms 5–6
  treatment 8–10, 113–17
  see also human immunodeficiency virus
HIV InSite, Web site address 592
HIV Prevention Trials Network (HPTN), defined 532
HIV-related tuberculosis *see* tuberculosis
HIV set point, defined 532
HIV treatment plan, described 136–40

HIV Vaccine Trials Network (HVTN), defined 532
HIV viral load *see* viral load test
HIV wasting syndrome *see* wasting syndrome
HLA *see* human leukocyte antigens
Hodgkin's disease, defined 533
holistic medicine, defined 533
  see also alternative medicine
"Home Diagnostic Tests: The Ultimate House Call?" (Lewis) 91n
homeopathy 157
home test kits, HIV infection 91–96, 102–3
homologous, defined 533
homosexuality
  HIV/AIDS statistics 478–79, 482–83
  HIV prevention 403–9
hormone replacement therapy, HIV infection 320, 327–38
hormones, defined 533
hospice care, AIDS 286–87
host, defined 533
host factors, defined 533
household pets *see* animals
"How Safe Is the Blood Supply in the United States?" (CDC) 47n
"How to Find Reliable HIV/AIDS Treatment Information on the Internet" (National Library of Medicine) 583n
HPMPC *see* cidofovir
HPTN *see* HIV Prevention Trials Network
HPV *see* human papilloma virus
HRSA *see* Health Resources and Services Administration
HSS *see* US Department of Health and Human Services
HSV-1 *see* herpes simplex virus 1
HSV-2 *see* herpes simplex virus 2
HTLVI *see* human T-cell lymphotropic virus type I
HTLV-I-associated myelopathy/tropical spastic paraparesis (HAM/TSP), defined 533
human growth hormone (HGH)
  defined 533–34
  wasting syndrome 223

human immunodeficiency virus (HIV)
  cause of AIDS 13–26
  defined 532
  health care workers 53–60
  overview 237–44
  replication cycle 16–18
  research 427–38
  statistics 14, 471–73
  structure 15–16
  transmission 3–5, 18–19
  transmission overview 33–38
  see also acquired immune deficiency
    syndrome; HIV infection
human immunodeficiency virus type
  1 (HIV-1), defined 534
human immunodeficiency virus type
  2 (HIV-2)
  defined 534
  overview 27–31
human leukocyte antigens (HLA), defined 534
human papilloma virus (HPV)
  defined 534
  HIV infection 307–8, 317–18
human T-cell lymphotropic virus type
  I (HTLVI), defined 534
human T-cell lymphotropic virus type
  II (HTLVII), defined 535
humoral immunity, defined 501, 535
HVTN *see* HIV Vaccine Trials Network
hypergammaglobulinemia, defined 535
hyperlipidemia, defined 535
hyperplasia, defined 535
hyperthermia, defined 535–36
hypogammaglobulinemia, defined 536
hypogonadism, defined 536
hypothesis, defined 536
hypoxia, defined 536
hyroxyruea, defined 535

I

IAPAC *see* International Association
  of Physicians in AIDS Care
IBIDS *see* International Biblio-
  graphic Information on Dietary
  Supplements
idiopathic thrombocytopenia purpura
  (ITP), defined 536, 537
IDU *see* injection drug users
IDV *see* indinavir
IFA *see* immunofluorescence assay
Ig *see* immunoglobulin
IgA *see* immunoglobulin A
IgD *see* immunoglobulin D
IgE *see* immunoglobulin E
IgG *see* immunoglobulin G
IGIV (immune globulin) 123
IgM *see* immunoglobulin M
IHS *see* Indian Health Service
IIIB, defined 543
IL-1 *see* interleukin-1
IL-2 *see* interleukin-2
IL-4 *see* interleukin-4
IL-12 *see* interleukin-12
IM *see* intramuscular
immune complex, defined 536
immune deficiency
  defined 536
  HIV infection 25
immune globulin, 56, 123
immune response, defined 536
immune system
  defined 536–37
  described 322–24
immune system cell loss theories 23–
  24
immunity, defined 537
immunization, defined 537
  see also vaccination
immunocompetent, defined 537
immunocompromised, defined 537
immunodeficiency, defined 537
immunofluorescence assay (IFA), described 79
immunogen, defined 537
immunogenicity, defined 537
immunoglobulin (Ig), defined 537
immunoglobulin A (IgA), defined 537
immunoglobulin D (IgD), defined 537
immunoglobulin E (IgE), defined 538
immunoglobulin G (IgD), defined 538
immunoglobulin M (IgM) defined
  538
immunomodulator, defined 538
immunostimulant, defined 538

immunosuppression
  AIDS 14
  defined 538
immunotherapy, defined 538
immunotoxin, defined 538
incidence, defined 538
inclusion criteria, defined 524
inclusion/exclusion criteria, defined 538
incubation period, defined 538
IND *see* investigational new drug
Indian Health Service (IHS), defined 538–39
indinavir (IDV) 9, 64, 123, 130, 133, 143, 189, 231, 246, 321, 379
infection
  AIDS caretakers 274–75
  defined 539
infectious, defined 539
informed consent
  defined 539
  described 455–56
infusion, defined 539
injection drug users (IDU)
  hepatitis C 179, 183
  HIV infection 43–45, 392
  HIV prevention 403
inoculation, defined 539
insect bites, HIV infection 5, 34, 37–38
institutional review board (IRB), defined 540
integrase
  defined 540
  described 17
integrase inhibitors, defined 540
integration
  defined 540
  described 17
intensification, defined 540
intent to treat, defined 540
interferon, defined 540–41
interferon alfa2a 123
interferon alfa2b 123
interferon alpha, defined 500
interleukin-1 (IL-1), defined 541
interleukin-2 (IL-2)
  clinical trial 458–60
  defined 541

interleukin-4 (IL-4), defined 541
interleukin-6 (IL-6), described 17
interleukin-12 (IL-12), defined 541
interleukins, defined 541
International Association of Physicians in AIDS Care (IAPAC), Web site address 594
International Bibliographic Information on Dietary Supplements (IBIDS), Web site address 595
interstitial, defined 541
intramuscular (IM), defined 541
intrapartum, defined 541
intravenous (IV), defined 541
intravenous immunoglobulin (IVIG), defined 542
intravitreal, defined 542
"An Introduction to Clinical Trials" (CDC) 451n
Intron-A (interferon alpha) 123, 145
investigational new drug (IND), defined 542
Invirase (saquinavir) 9, 125, 143, 381
in vitro, defined 542
in vivo, defined 542
IRB *see* institutional review board
isolate, defined 542
ITP *see* idiopathic thrombocytopenia purpura
itraconazole 124
IV *see* intravenous
IVIG *see* intravenous immunoglobulin

J

JAMA *see* Journal of the American Medical Association
jaundice, defined 542
JC virus *see* papilloma; progressive multifocal leukoencephalopathy
Johns Hopkins AIDS Service, Web site address 595
Journal of the American Medical Association (JAMA), Web site address 595

K

Kaletra (lopinavir; ritonavir) 9, 124, 130, 379–80
Kaposi's sarcoma (KS)
  defined 542–43
  described 7
  overview 207–10
  treatment 10
Kaposi's sarcoma herpes virus (KSHV) *see* Kaposi's sarcoma
"Kaposi's Sarcoma (PDQ): Treatment" (NCI) 207n
Karnofsky score, defined 543
ketamine, drug interactions 232
killer cells *see* T8 lymphocyte cells
killer T-cells, defined 543
  see also CD8+ T-cells
kissing, HIV infection 4, 36
Klacid (clarithromycin) 120
Klein, Richard 142, 143
Klonopin (clonazepam) 227
KS *see* Kaposi's sarcoma
KSHV (Kaposi's sarcoma herpes virus) *see* Kaposi's sarcoma
Kupffer cells, defined 543

L

LAI, defined 543
LAK cells, defined 543
lamivudine (3TC) 9, 57, 64, 124, 127, 142, 190–91, 345, 366, 374
  see also Combivir; Epivir; trizivir
Langerhans cells, defined 543
LAS *see* lymphadenopathy syndrome
latency, defined 543
latex condoms *see* condoms
LAV, defined 543
Lazarus effect, described 142
lentiviruses
  defined 544
  described 15
lesion, defined 544
leucovorin 126, 144
leukocytes (white blood cells), defined 544

leukocytosis, defined 544
leukopenia, defined 499, 544
Lewis, Carol 91n
LFT *see* liver function test
LIP *see* lymphoid interstitial pneumonitis
lipid rafts, described 15
lipids
  defined 544
  described 15
Lipitor (atorvastatin) 188
lipodystrophy
  defined 544
  overview 185–91
"Lipodystrophy" (Project Inform) 185n
lipodystrophy syndrome
  defined 525
  HAART 134
liposomes, defined 544–45
liver enzyme test *see* alanine aminotransferase activity test
liver function test (LFT), defined 546
liver toxicity, protease inhibitors 131
live vector vaccine, defined 546
living wills 287
"Living with AIDS - 20 Years Later" (Bullers) 61n
log, defined 546
long terminal repeat sequence (LTR)
  defined 546
  described 16
long-term nonprogressors, defined 545
Lopid (gemfibrozil) 188
lopinavir 9, 124, 130, 133, 379–80
LTR *see* long terminal repeat sequence
lumbar, defined 545
lumbar puncture (spinal tap), defined 546
Lutheran AIDS Network, contact information 606
Lyle, Dave 95
lymph, defined 546
lymphadenopathy syndrome (LAS), defined 499, 546
lymphatic vessels, defined 546

lymph nodes
    defined 546
    HIV infection 21–22
lymphoid interstitial pneumonitis
    (LIP), defined 546
lymphoid organs, defined 546
lymphokines, defined 546–47
lymphomas
    AIDS 14
    defined 547
lymphopenia, defined 547
lymphoproliferative response, defined
    547
lypodystrophy, protease inhibitors 131
lysis, defined 547
lysosomes, described 25

M

MAC *see* mycobacterium avium com-
    plex
macrophages
    defined 547
    HIV infection 25
macrophage-tropic virus, defined 547
magnetic resonance imaging (MRI),
    defined 547
MAI *see* mycobacterium
    intracellulare
maintenance therapy, defined 547
major histocompatibility complex
    (MHC), defined 548
malabsoption syndrome, defined 548
malaise, defined 548
malignant, defined 548
marijuana use
    AIDS treatment 161–68
    drug interactions 232–33
Marinol (dronabinol) 121, 145, 161,
    165–67, 232–33
massage 157
mast cell, defined 548
MDR-TB *see* multiple drug-resistant
    tuberculosis
Medem Medical Library, Web site ad-
    dress 595
Medicaid 299–300
medical marijuana *see* marijuana use

"Medical Marijuana" (Project Inform)
    161n
Medicare 299–301
meditation 157
MEDLINEplus, Web site address 596
Megace (megestrol acetate) 124
Megace (megestrol) 145
mega-HAART, defined 548
megestrol acetate 124, 145, 222
memory T-cells, defined 548
meninges, defined 548
meningitis, defined 549
menopause, HIV infection 319–20,
    327–38
menstrual irregularity
    AIDS 305–7
    HIV infection 318–19
men who have sex with men *see*
    homosexuality
Mepron (atovaquone) 120, 144
messenger RNA
    defined 549
    described 17
metabolism, defined 549
metastasis, defined 549
metformin 188
MHC *see* major histocompatibility
    complex
microbes, defined 549
microbicide, defined 549
microsporidiosis, defined 549
    see also pathogen; protozoa; wasting
        syndrome
Midwest Hispanic AIDS Coalition,
    contact information 603
mitochondria, defined 549
mitochondrial toxicity, defined 549
MK-639 *see* indinavir
MM *see* mononeuritis multiplex
molecule, defined 549
molluscum contagiosum, defined 550
monocyte, defined 550
mononeuritis multiplex (MM), de-
    fined 550
monovalent vaccine, defined 550
morbidity, defined 550
MRI *see* magnetic resonance imaging
mucocutaneous, defined 550
mucosa *see* mucous membrane

mucosal immunity, defined 550
mucous membrane, defined 550
multi-drug rescue therapy *see* mega-
    HAART
multiple drug-resistant tuberculosis
    (MDR-TB), defined 550
Murray, Jeffrey S. 64–66
mutation, defined 551
myalgia, defined 551
mycobacterium, defined 551
mycobacterium avium complex
    (MAC)
    defined 551
    household pets 265
    treatment 144
mycobacterium intracellulare (MAI),
    defined 551
Mycobacterium tuberculosis
    described 17, 201, 579
Mycobutin (rifabutin) 125, 144
mycosis, defined 551
myelin, defined 551
myelopathy, defined 551
myelosuppression, defined 551
myelotoxic, defined 551
myocardial, defined 551
myopathy, defined 551

N

nadir, defined 551
nandrolone 223
NAT *see* nucleic acid test
NATAP *see* The National AIDS Treat-
    ment Advocacy Project
The National AIDS Treatment Advo-
    cacy Project (NATAP), Web site ad-
    dress 596
National Association of People with
    AIDS, contact information 604
National Cancer Institute (NCI)
    described 435, 552
    Kaposi's sarcoma publication 207n
National Catholic AIDS Network,
    contact information 606
National Center for Chronic Disease
    Prevention and Health Promotion
    (NCCDPHP), described 421

National Center for Complementary
    and Alternative Medicine
    (NCCAM), Web site address 596
National Center for Environmental
    Health's Clinical Biochemistry
    Branch, described 422
National Center for Health Statistics,
    described 422
National Center for HIV, STD, and
    TB Prevention (NCHSTP)
    branches, described 418–21
    publications
        cryptosporidiosis 171n
        cytomegalovirus 177n
        food safety 257n
        hepatitis C 179n
        HIV/AIDS among Hispanics
            481n
        HIV/AIDS among women 485n
        HIV/AIDS among youth 489n
        HIV/AIDS prevention 417n
        HIV prevention 403n, 407n
        household pets 265n
        mycobacterium avium complex
            disease 193n
        pediatric opportunistic infection
            383n
        perinatal HIV prevention 347n
        Pneumocystis Carinii pneumonia
            197n
        Thailand vaccine study 443n
        travel considerations 261n
        tuberculosis 201n
    Web site address 52
National Center for Infectious Dis-
    eases (NCID), described 421
National Center for Research Re-
    sources (NCRR), described 436
National Episcopal AIDS Coalition,
    contact information 604, 606
National Heart Lung and Blood Insti-
    tute (NHLBI)
    described 436
    Web site address 52
National HIV/AIDS Clinician's Con-
    sultation Center (NCCC), Web site
    address 597
"National HIV/AIDS Organization
    and Hotlines" (SAMHSA) 603n

National Insitute on Drug Abuse
(NIDA), described 436
National Insitutes of Health (NIH)
described 552
pediatric AIDS publication 357n
National Institute for Occupational
Safety and Health, described 422
National Institute of Allergy and In-
fectious Diseases (NIAID)
contact information 248
described 435, 552
publications
HIV/AIDS statistics 471n
pediatric AIDS 351n
Web site address 597
National Institute of Child Health
and Human Development (NICHD),
described 436, 552
National Institute of Mental Health
(NIMH)
contact information 247–48
depression publication 245n
described 436
National Leadership Coalition on
AIDS, contact information 604
National Library of Medicine (NLM)
described 552–53
Web site address 598
National Minority AIDS Council
(NMAC)
contact information 604
Web site address 598
National Native American AIDS Pre-
vention Center (NNAAPC), contact
information 604
National Pediatric AIDS Network
(NPAN), Web site address 598
National Pediatric HIV Resource
Center, contact information 604
(NPIN) National Prevention Informa-
tion Network *see* CDC National
Prevention Information Network
National Prevention Information
Network (NPIN), Web site address
598
see also CDC National Prevention
Information Network
Native American healing 157
natural history study, defined 553

natural killer cells (NK cells) 553
NCCC *see* National HIV/AIDS
Clinician's Consultation Center
NCCDPHP *see* National Center for
Chronic Disease Prevention and
Health Promotion
NCHSTP *see* National Center for
HIV, STD, and TB Prevention
NCI *see* National Cancer Institute
NCID *see* National Center for Infec-
tious Diseases
NCRR *see* National Center for Re-
search Resources
NDA *see* new drug application
nebulized *see* aerosolized
NebuPent (pentamidine) 125, 144
"Need for Sustained HIV Prevention
among Men Who Have Sex with
Men" (NCHSTP) 403n
needle sharing
HIV-2 infection 29
HIV infection 4, 33, 55
see also injection drug users
nef
defined 553
described 16, 566
Neisseria gonorrhoeae 527
nelfinavir (NFV) 9, 64, 124, 130, 133,
143, 189, 321, 380
neonatal, defined 553
neoplasm, defined 553
nephrotoxic, defined 553
Neupogen 226
neuralgia, defined 553
neurological complications of AIDS
see central nervous system damage
neuropathy, defined 553
see also peripheral neuropathy
neutralization, defined 554
neutralizing antibody, defined 554
neutralizing domain, defined 554
Neutrexin (trimtrexate glucuronate/
leucovorin) 126, 144
neutropenia
defined 554
treatment 528
neutrophil, defined 554
nevirapine (NVP) 4, 9, 65, 125, 143,
321, 345, 377–78

new drug application (NDA), defined 554

New Mexico AIDS InfoNet
  alternative treatment publication 157n
  Web site address 599

NFV *see* nelfinavir

NHL *see* non-Hodgkin's lymphoma

NHLBI *see* National Heart Lung and Blood Institute

NIAID *see* National Institute of Allergy and Infectious Diseases

NICHD *see* National Institute of Child Health and Human Development

NIDA *see* National Insitute on Drug Abuse

night sweats, defined 554

NIH *see* National Insitutes of Health

NIH Revitalization Act 431

NIMH *see* National Institute of Mental Health

NK cells *see* natural killer cells

NLM *see* National Library of Medicine

NMAC *see* National Minority AIDS Council

NNAAPC *see* National Native American AIDS Prevention Center

NNRTI *see* non-nucleoside reverse transcriptase inhibitors

non-Hodgkin's lymphoma (NHL), defined 554

non-nucleoside reverse transcriptase inhibitors (NNRTI)
  children 364, 376–78
  defined 554–55
  described 9, 65, 143
  lipodystrophy 187

nonoxynil-9, described 413

nonsteroidal anti-inflammatory drugs (NSAID), defined 555

Nordenberg, Tamar 411n

Norvir (ritonavir) 9, 64, 125, 130, 143, 322, 380–81

NPAN *see* National Pediatric AIDS Network

NPIN *see* National Prevention Information Network

NRTI *see* nucleoside reverse transcriptase inhibitors

NSAID *see* nonsteroidal anti-inflammatory drugs

nucleic acid, defined 555

nucleic acid test (NAT), defined 555

nucleocapsid, defined 555

nucleoli, defined 555

nucleoside
  defined 555
  overview 197–99

nucleoside analogs
  defined 555
  described 9, 142

nucleoside reverse transcriptase inhibitors (NRTI)
  defined 555–56
  described 9, 64
  see also reverse transcriptase

nucleotide, defined 556

nucleotide analogs, defined 556

nucleus, defined 556

null cell, defined 556

nutrition *see* diet and nutrition

"Nutrition Intervention in AIDS Wasting" (CDC) 451n

NVP *see* nevirapine

O

OAR *see* Office of AIDS Research

ocular, defined 556

Office of AIDS Research (OAR)
  described 429, 556
  Web site address 597

off-label use, defined 556

OHL *see* oral hairy leukoplakia

OI *see* opportunistic infections

oncology, defined 556

open-label trial, defined 557

opportunistic infections (OI)
  defined 557
  described 6
  pediatric AIDS 352–53
  treatment 10, 225–26

oral hairy leukoplakia (OHL), **defined** 557

oral sex
  described 39–40
  HIV infection 4

organelles
  defined 557
  described 25, 549
oropharyngeal, defined 557
orphan drugs, defined 557
osteonecrosis, defined 557
osteopenia, defined 557
oxandrolone 223

P

p7 protein, described 16
p24 protein
  defined 558
  described 15
package insert, defined 558
paclitaxel 125
PACTG *see* Pediatric AIDS Clinical
  Trials Group
palliative, defined 558
palliative care, defined 558
pancreas, defined 558
pancreatitis, defined 558
pancytopenia, defined 558
pandemic, defined 558
Panretin (alitretinoin) 119
pantretin 145
papilloma, defined 559
Pap plus speculoscopy (PPS) 321
Pap smear
  defined 558
  HIV infection 320–21
parallel track, defined 559
parasite, defined 559
parenteral, defined 559
paresthesia, defined 559
paromomycin 173
paroxetine 231
passive immunity, defined 559
passive immunotherapy, defined 559
pathogen, defined 559
pathogenesis, defined 559
Paxil (paroxetine) 231
PCP *see Pneumocystis carinii* pneumonia
PCR *see* polymerase chain reaction
pediatric AIDS, overview 351–55
  see also children

Pediatric AIDS Clinical Trials Group
  (PACTG), described 560
Pediatric AIDS Clinical Trials Group,
  Web site address 599
Pediatric AIDS Foundation, contact
  information 326
"Pediatric Antiretroviral Drug Information" (NIH) 357n
pelvic inflammatory disease (PID)
  defined 560
  HIV infection 316
penicillin 218, 315
pentamidine 10, 125, 144
PEP *see* post-exposure prophylaxis
peptides, defined 560
  see also amino acids
perianal, defined 560
perinatal, defined 560
perinatal HIV prevention 347–49
perinatal HIV transmission
  defined 560
  HIV infection 361, 392
  see also pregnancy
peripheral neuritis, defined 560
peripheral neuropathy
  defined 560
  overview 215–16
permethrin 262
persistent generalized lymphadenopathy (PGL), defined 560–61
person living with AIDS (PLWA), described 566
person with AIDS (PWA), described 566
perspiration *see* night sweats; sweat
Peterson, Herbert 413–14
pets *see* animals
PGL *see* persistent generalized lymphadenopathy; progressive generalized lymphadenopathy
phagocytes, defined 561
phagocytosis, defined 561
pharmacokinetics, defined 561
phase III trials, defined 561
phase II trials, defined 561
phase I trials, defined 561
phase IV trials, defined 561–62
phenotypic assay, defined 562
PHHPO *see* Public Health Practice
  Program Office

photosensitivity, defined 562
Physicians Research Network (PRN),
    Web site address 599
PI *see* Project Inform
PID *see* pelvic inflammatory disease
pituitary gland, defined 562
placebo
    defined 562
    described 452
placebo controlled study, defined 562
placebo effect, defined 562
plasma, defined 562
plasma cells, defined 562
platelets, defined 562–63
PLWA *see* person living with AIDS
PML *see* progressive multifocal leu-
    koencephalopathy
Pneumocystis carinii pneumonia
    (PCP)
    children 353, 362, 383–85
    defined 563
    HIV infection 20
    treatment 10, 144
pol
    defined 563
    described 15
polarity therapy 157
polymerase, defined 563
polymerase chain reaction (PCR)
    defined 563
    described 75
    pediatric AIDS 351
polyneuritis, defined 563
polypeptide *see* peptide
polyvalent vaccine, defined 563
poppers *see* amyl nitrate
post-exposure prophylaxis (PEP), de-
    fined 563
Potochnic, Meredith A. 225n
PPD *see* purified protein derivative
PPS *see* Pap plus speculoscopy
preclinical, defined 563
preconception counseling, defined 563
precursor cells
    damage 24
    defined 564
pregnancy
    blood exposure 59
    HAART 133, 135–36

pregnancy, continued
    HIV infection 4, 97, 145, 242–43,
        343–45
    HIV tests 85
Presbyterian AIDS Network, contact
    information 606
prevalence, defined 564
"Preventing Infections during Travel:
    A Guide for People with HIV Infec-
    tion" (NCHSTP) 261n
"Preventing Infections from Pets"
    (NCHSTP) 265n
prevention trials, described 453
primary HIV infection, defined 564
primary isolate, defined 564
privacy issues, HIV tests 73, 91–92
PRN *see* Physicians Research Net-
    work
Procrit (erythropoietin) 122
proctitis, defined 564
prodrome, defined 564
prodrug, defined 564
progressive generalized lymphaden-
    opathy (PGL), defined 499
progressive multifocal leukoencephal-
    opathy (PML), defined 564
Project Inform (PI)
    publications
        drug interactions 225n
        gynecological conditions 311n
        HIV and older age 327n
        lipodystrophy 185n
        marijuana use 161n
        pulsed therapy 149n
        viral load gender difference 339n
        women and AIDS 305n
    Web site address 600
Project WISE, contact information 325
prophylactic drug, defined 564
prophylaxis, defined 564
protease, defined 564
protease inhibitors
    children 353, 378–81
    defined 564–65
    described 9, 10, 64, 114
    drug interactions 228, 230–31
    HAART 141
    overview 129–32
protease paunch *see* lipodystrophy

protease-sparing regimen, defined
565
proteins, defined 500, 565
see also amino acids
protocol, defined 565
protocol, described 452
protozoa, defined 565
provirus
defined 565
described 17
Prozac (fluoxetine) 231
pruritis, defined 565
pseudo-Cushing's syndrome, defined
565
see also lipodystrophy
pseudovirion, defined 565
Public Health Practice Program Office (PHHPO)
described 422
Web site address 52
PubMed
described 565
Web site address 600
pulmonary, defined 565
pulsed therapy
HAART 390
overview 149–52
"Pulsed Therapy and Structured Interruptions of Treatment" (Project
Inform) 149n
purified protein derivative (PPD), defined 565–66
PWA *see* person with AIDS
pyrimethamine 217

Q

quality of life trials, described 453
"Questions and Answers on the Thailand Phase III Vaccine Study and
CDC's Collaboration" (NCHTSP)
443

R

racial factor
AIDS 3

racial factor, continued
HIV/AIDS research 431–32
HIV/AIDS statistics 472, 477–79,
481–83
HIV infection 348, 404
HIV transmission 43
radiology, defined 566
randomized trial, defined 566
rapid HIV tests, described 79–86
Reality female condom 414
rebound, defined 566
receptor, defined 566
recombinant, defined 566
recombinant DNA *see* biotechnology;
genetic engineering
recombinant DNA technology *see* genetic engineering
Red Cross *see* American Red Cross
refractory, defined 566
regulatory genes
defined 566
described 16
regulatory T-cells
defined 566
described 566
Reiki 157
relaxation therapy 157
remissions, described 567
renal, described 467
Rescriptor (delavirdine) 9, 65, 121,
143, 376
rescue therapy *see* salvage therapy
resistance, described 567
resistance testing *see* genotypic assay;
phenotypic assay
Restoril (temazepam) 229
retina, defined 567
retinal detachment, defined 567
retinita, defined 567
retinitis, described 177
see also cytomegalovirus
Retrovir (zidovudine) 64, 127, 243,
375–76
retroviruses
defined 567
described 14–15, 291
rev
defined 567
described 16, 553, 566

reverse transcriptase (RT)
defined 567–68
described 9, 64–65
see also non-nucleoside reverse
transcriptase inhibitors; nucleoside reverse transcriptase inhibitors
reverse transcriptase inhibitors (RTI)
described 9, 10, 113–14
protease inhibitors 141, 142
reverse transcriptase polymerase
chain reaction (RT-PCR)
defined 568
reverse transcriptase polymerase chain
reaction (RT-PCR), defined 568
reverse transcription, described 17
Rezulin (troglitazone) 188
ribonucleic acid (RNA), defined 568
see also retroviruses
ribosome, defined 568
rifabutin 125, 144, 194–95
rimming *see* anilingus
ritonavir 9, 64, 124, 125, 130, 133,
143, 230, 231, 322, 379–80, 380–81
RNA *see* ribonucleic acid
Rocephin (ceftriaxone) 315
Roferon-A (interferon alfa-2a) 123
Rosser, Simon 68
route of administration, defined 496–
97, 568
"Routine Testing
(Healthcommunities.com, Inc.) 73n
RTI *see* reverse transcriptase inhibi-
tors
RT-PCR *see* reverse transcriptase
polymerase chain reaction
Ryan White C.A.R.E. Act *see* White
Comprehensive AIDS Resources
Emergency Act

S

"Safe Food and Water: A Guide for
People Living with HIV Infection"
(NCHSTP) 257n
safe sex practices
false complacency 67–68
oral sex 39

St. John's wort 246
saliva, HIV infection 4, 37
salmonella, defined 568–69
salvage therapy, defined 569
SAMHSA *see* Substance Abuse and
Mental Health Services Administration
San Francisco AIDS Foundation
(SFAF), Web site address 600
San Joaquin Valley fever, defined 513
saquinavir (SQV) 9, 64, 125, 130, 133,
143, 189, 231, 381
sarcoma, defined 569
Schacker, Tim 63, 68
Sci.med.aids FAQ, Web site address
601
"Screening Protocol for HIV Vaccine
Studies" (CDC) 451n
screening trials, described 453
seborrheic dermatitis, defined 569
secondary prophylaxis *see* maintenance therapy
sepsis, defined 569
Septra (sulfamethoxazole/
trimethoprim) 126, 144, 240, 384
seroconversion, defined 569
serologic test, defined 569
seronegative, described 105
seroprevalence, defined 569
serostatus, defined 569
Serostim (somatropin) 126, 145
sertraline 231
serum, defined 569
serum glutamic oxaloacetic transaminase (SGOT), defined 570
serum glutamic pyruvate transaminase (SGPT), defined 570
set point, defined 570
Seventh-Day Adventist Kinship International, contact information
606
sexual contact
condom use 411–16
female homosexuality 407–9
HIV infection 33, 39–42, 241–42
male homosexuality 403–5
sexually transmitted diseases (STD)
condom use 412
defined 570

sexually transmitted diseases (STD), continued
   false complacency 67–68
   hepatitis C virus 181
   HIV infection 5, 314–18, 404
   HIV prevention 395–98
   hotline information 102–3, 111
   oral sex 42
SFAF *see* San Francisco AIDS Foundation
SGOT *see* serum glutamic oxaloacetic transaminase
SGPT *see* serum glutamic pyruvate transaminase
shingles
   AIDS caretakers 275
   defined 531
   described 6
   see also herpes varicella zoster virus
SHIV *see* simian HIV infection
side effects
   defined 570
   described 457
side effects, defined 570
SIL *see* squamous intraepithelial lesions
sildenafil 227
simian HIV infection (SHIV), described 570
simian immunodeficiency virus (SIV)
   defined 570
   described 15, 570
Simpson, David 216
sinusitis, defined 570
SIT *see* structured intermittent therapy
SIV *see* simian immunodeficiency virus
slow viruses *see* lentiviruses
SMX (sulfamethoxazole/trimethoprim) 126
Social Security, AIDS 291–302
Social Security Administration (SSA)
   guide to benefits publication 291n
   Web site address 601
Social Security disability insurance (SSDI) 292–93
somatropin 126, 145

Southern Baptist Convention, contact information 606
special projects of national significance (SPNS), defined 571
spermicide 413
spikes, described 15
spinal tap *see* lumbar puncture
spleen, defined 571
splenomegaly, defined 571
SPNS *see* special projects of national significance
Sporanox (itraconazole) 124
sputum analysis, defined 571
squamous intraepithelial lesions (SIL), defined 325
SQV *see* saquinavir
SSDI *see* Social Security disability insurance
SSI *see* Supplemental Security Income
standards of care, defined 571
staphylococcus, defined 571
"Status of Perinatal HIV Prevention: U.S. Declines Continue" (NCHSTP) 347n
stavudine (D4T) 9, 64, 126, 142, 366, 375
STD *see* sexually transmitted diseases
stem cells, defined 571
steroids
   defined 571
   described 223
Stevens-Johnson syndrome, defined 572
STI *see* structured treatment interruption
strain, defined 571
stratification, defined 571
structured intermittent therapy (SIT), defined 572
structured treatment interruption (STI)
   defined 572
   described 152–54
   see also pulsed therapy
study endpoint, defined 571
subarachnoid space, defined 571
subclinical infection, defined 571
subcutaneous (SQ; sub-Q), defined 571

Substance Abuse and Mental Health Services Administration (SAMHSA)
  described 572–73
  hotlines and organizations publication 603n
subtype, defined 511–12
subunit HIV vaccine, defined 573
sulfadiazine 217
sulfa drug, defined 573
sulfamethoxazole 126, 144
sulfonamides, defined 573
superantigen, defined 573
Supplemental Security Income (SSI) 291–94
support groups, HIV infection 107
supportive care trials, described 453
suppressor ratio, defined 529
suppressor T-cells, defined 573
surrogate markers, defined 573
surveillance *see* epidemiologic surveillance
susceptible, defined 573
Sustiva (efavirenz) 9, 65, 121, 143, 322, 343, 377
sweat, HIV infection 37
symptoms, defined 573
syncytia (giant cells), defined 573
syndrome, defined 574
synergism, defined 574
synergistic, defined 574
synthesis, defined 574
syphilis
  defined 574
  described 218
  HIV infection 397
  women 315
syringes, HIV infection 4, 5
systemic, defined 574

T

T4 lymphocyte cells
  defined 508, 575
  described 5, 98
T8 lymphocyte cells, defined 508, 575
Tanner staging
  defined 574
  pediatric HIV infection 363

tat
  defined 574
  described 16, 553, 566
Taxol (paclitaxel) 125
taxon, defined 571
TB *see* tuberculosis
T-cells (T-leukocyte cells), defined 573–74
T-cell test, described 77
tears, HIV infection 37
temazepam 229
template, defined 575
tenovir disoproxil fumarate 127
teratogenicity, defined 575
"Testing for HIV" (Healthcommunities.com, Inc.) 73n
testosterone
  defined 576
  steroids 223
tests
  blood donors 29–30, 48
  hepatitis 182
  hepatitis exposure 60
  HIV infection 7–8, 73–111
  Kaposi's sarcoma 207
  lipodystrophy 186–87
  pediatric AIDS 351–52
Thailand Phase III Vaccine Study 443–50
thalidomide 223
THC 165–68
T-helper cells *see* CD4+ T-cells; T4 lymphocyte cells
therapeutic HIV vaccine, defined 576
3TC *see* lamivudine
thrombocytopenia, defined 576
thrush, defined 576
thymosin, defined 576
thymus, defined 576
tissue, defined 576
titer, defined 576
T lymphocyte proliferation assay, defined 576
T lymphocytes *see* T-cells
TMP/SMX *see* trimethoprim/sulfamethoxazole
TMTX (trimtrexate glucuronate/leucovorin) 126, 144
TNF *see* tumor necrosis factor

tobacco use, HIV infection 107
toxicity, defined 577
toxoplasma encephalitis, described 217
toxoplasmosis
  defined 577
  household pets 265
toxoplasmosis encephalitis *see* toxoplasmosis
transaminase, defined 577
transcription
  defined 577
  described 17
transfusion, defined 577
  see also blood transfusion
translation
  defined 577–78
  described 17–18
transmission, defined 578
transplacental, defined 577
travel considerations, AIDS 261–63
treatment investigational new drug, defined 578
treatment trials, described 453
triazolam 229
triglyceride, defined 578
trimethoprim 126
trimethoprim/sulfamethoxazole (TMP/SMX) 10, 144, 198, 240, 262, 384–85
trimetrexate glucuronate 126
trizivir (abacavir/lamivudine/zidovudine) 127
troglitazone 188
TST *see* tuberculin skin test
T suppressor cells, defined 578
tuberculin skin test (TST), defined 578–79
tuberculosis (TB)
  defined 579
  HIV infection 107, 108
  see also multiple drug-resistant tuberculosis
"Tuberculosis: A Guide for Adults and Adolescents with HIV" (NCHSTP) 201n
tumor necrosis factor (TNF)
  defined 579
  described 17

U

Union of American Hebrew Congregations, contact information 606
Unitarian Universalist Association AIDS Resources Network, contact information 607
United Church AIDS/HIV Network, contact information 606
Universal Fellowship of Metropolitan Community Churches AIDS Ministry, contact information 607
The University of North Carolina AIDS Clinical Trials Unit, Web site address 601
US Department of Health and Human Services (DHHS)
  described 519–20
  glossary 495n
US Food and Drug Administration (FDA)
  AIDS activism publication 61n
  described 525
  HIV and AIDS Activities, Web site address 591

V

V3 loop, defined 579
vaccination
  AIDS 66
  clinical trial 462–64
  defined 579
  hepatitis 57–59, 181–82
  HIV infection 393–94, 434, 443–50
vaccinia, defined 579
vaginal candidiasis
  defined 580
  HIV infection 312–13
valcyte 127
Valcyte (valganciclovir) 127
valganciclovir 127
Valium (diazepam) 227, 229
Valley fever, defined 513
vally fever *see* coccidioidomycosis
variable region, defined 580
varicella zoster virus (VZV)
  defined 531, 580

vector, defined 580
venereal warts, defined 515
verruca acuminata, defined 515
Veterans Administration AIDS Information Center, Web site address 602
Veterans Administration (VA) AIDS Service, Web site address 602
Viagra (sildenafil) 143–44, 227, 233
Videx (didanosine) 64, 121, 373–74
vif
    described 16, 553, 566
Viracept (nelfinavir) 9, 64, 124, 130, 143, 321, 380
viral burden, defined 580
    see also branched DNA assay; polymerase chain reaction; viral load test
viral core
    defined 580
    described 15–16
    see also surrogate markers
viral culture, defined 581
viral envelope
    defined 581
    described 15
viral load test
    defined 581
    described 76–77
    gender difference 339–42
    HAART 134
    overview 87–89
    pulsed therapy 150
    structured treatment interruption 152
Viramune (nevirapine) 9, 65, 125, 143, 321, 377–78
Viread (tenovir disoproxil fumarate) 127
viremia, defined 581
viricide, defined 581
virion
    defined 581
    described 15
virology, defined 581
virus, defined 581
visceral, defined 581
Vistide (cidofovir) 120, 144, 315
visualization 157

vitamin supplements 252–53
Vitrasert (ganciclovir) 123, 144
Vitravene intravitreal injectable (fomivirsen sodium injection) 122
vpr, described 16, 553, 566
vpu, described 16, 553, 566
VZV *see* varicella zoster virus

W

wasting syndrome
    clinical trial 461–62
    defined 500
    overview 221–23
Western blot test
    defined 581–82
    described 74–75, 105
white blood cells *see* leukocytes
Ryan White Comprehensive AIDS Resources Emergency Act
    defined 568
    drug assistance program 498
WHO *see* World Health Organization
WIHS *see* Women's Interagency HIV Study
wild-type virus, defined 582
window period, defined 582
women
    HIV/AIDS research 431–32
    HIV/AIDS statistics 478, 485–87
    HIV infection 4
    HIV infection determination 296
    lipodystrophy 189–91
    sexually transmitted diseases 395–96
Women Alive, contact information 325
"Women and AIDS Update" (Project Inform) 305n
Women Organized to Respond to Life-threatening Diseases (WORLD), contact information 326
Women's Interagency HIV Study (WHIS), defined 582
women who have sex with womens *see* homosexuality
work place
    blood exposure 53–60
    HIV infection 35–36, 399

WORLD *see* Women Organized to Respond to Life-threatening Diseases

World Health Organization (WHO)
Blood Safety Unit, Web site address 52

X

Xanax (alprazolam) 227

Y

yeast infections, treatment 10
see also candidiasis
Yin, Lillian 413–14
yoga 157
"You Can Prevent CMV (Cytomegalovirus): A Guide for People with HIV Infection" (NCHSTP) 177n
"You Can Prevent Crypto (Cryptosporisiosis): A Guide for People with HIV Infection" (NCHSTP) 171n
"You Can Prevent MAC (Mycobacterium Avium Complex Disease)" (NCHSTP) 193n
"You Can Prevent PCP: A Guide for People with HIV Infection" (NCHSTP) 197n

"You Can Prevent PCP in Children: A Guide for People with HIV Infection" (NCHSTP) 383n
"Young People at risk: HIV/AIDS among America's Youth" (NCHSTP) 489n

Z

zalcitabine (ddC) 9, 64, 127, 142, 375
ZDV *see* zidovudine
Zerit (stavudine) 9, 64, 126, 375
Ziagen (abacavir) 64, 119, 127, 142, 373
zidovudine (AZT)
    AIDS treatment 64
    drug interactions 226
    hepatitis exposure 57
    HIV infection treatment 9, 64, 124, 127, 142
    pediatric HIV infection 366, 375–76
    pregnancy 4, 11, 19, 97, 133, 136, 145, 243, 343–45, 347–48
zinc finger inhibitors, defined 582
zinc fingers, defined 582
    see also reverse transcriptase
Zithromax (azithromycin) 120, 144
Zoloft (sertraline) 231
Zovirax (acyclovir) 315
Zrivada (atazanavir) 130

Health Reference Series
COMPLETE CATALOG

Adolescent Health Sourcebook

Basic Consumer Health Information about Common Medical, Mental, and Emotional Concerns in Adolescents, Including Facts about Acne, Body Piercing, Mononucleosis, Nutrition, Eating Disorders, Stress, Depression, Behavior Problems, Peer Pressure, Violence, Gangs, Drug Use, Puberty, Sexuality, Pregnancy, Learning Disabilities, and More

Along with a Glossary of Terms and Other Resources for Further Help and Information

Edited by Chad T. Kimball. 658 pages. 2002. 0-7808-0248-9. $78.

"A good starting point for information related to common medical, mental, and emotional concerns of adolescents." — *School Library Journal, Nov '02*

"This book provides accurate information in an easy to access format. It addresses topics that parents and caregivers might not be aware of and provides practical, useable information." — *Doody's Health Sciences Book Review Journal, Sep-Oct '02*

"Recommended reference source." — *Booklist, American Library Association, Sep '02*

■

AIDS Sourcebook, 1st Edition

Basic Information about AIDS and HIV Infection, Featuring Historical and Statistical Data, Current Research, Prevention, and Other Special Topics of Interest for Persons Living with AIDS

Along with Source Listings for Further Assistance

Edited by Karen Bellenir and Peter D. Dresser. 831 pages. 1995. 0-7808-0031-1. $78.

"One strength of this book is its practical emphasis. The intended audience is the lay reader . . . useful as an educational tool for health care providers who work with AIDS patients. Recommended for public libraries as well as hospital or academic libraries that collect consumer materials." — *Bulletin of the Medical Library Association, Jan '96*

"This is the most comprehensive volume of its kind on an important medical topic. Highly recommended for all libraries." — *Reference Book Review, '96*

"Very useful reference for all libraries." — *Choice, Association of College and Research Libraries, Oct '95*

"There is a wealth of information here that can provide much educational assistance. It is a must book for all libraries and should be on the desk of each and every congressional leader. Highly recommended." — *AIDS Book Review Journal, Aug '95*

"Recommended for most collections." — *Library Journal, Jul '95*

AIDS Sourcebook, 2nd Edition

Basic Consumer Health Information about Acquired Immune Deficiency Syndrome (AIDS) and Human Immunodeficiency Virus (HIV) Infection, Featuring Updated Statistical Data, Reports on Recent Research and Prevention Initiatives, and Other Special Topics of Interest for Persons Living with AIDS, Including New Antiretroviral Treatment Options, Strategies for Combating Opportunistic Infections, Information about Clinical Trials, and More

Along with a Glossary of Important Terms and Resource Listings for Further Help and Information

Edited by Karen Bellenir. 751 pages. 1999. 0-7808-0225-X. $78.

"Highly recommended." — *American Reference Books Annual, 2000*

"Excellent sourcebook. This continues to be a highly recommended book. There is no other book that provides as much information as this book provides." — *AIDS Book Review Journal, Dec-Jan 2000*

"Recommended reference source." — *Booklist, American Library Association, Dec '99*

"A solid text for college-level health libraries." — *The Bookwatch, Aug '99*

Cited in *Reference Sources for Small and Medium-Sized Libraries, American Library Association, 1999*

■

AIDS Sourcebook, 3rd Edition

Basic Consumer Health Information about Acquired Immune Deficiency Syndrome (AIDS) and Human Immunodeficiency Virus (HIV) Infection, Including Facts about Transmission, Prevention, Diagnosis, Treatment, Opportunistic Infections, and Other Complications, with a Section for Women and Children, Including Details about Associated Gynecological Concerns, Pregnancy, and Pediatric Care

Along with Updated Statistical Information, Reports on Current Research Initiatives, a Glossary, and Directories of Internet, Hotline, and Other Resources

Edited by Dawn D. Matthews. 664 pages. 2003. 0-7808-0631-X. $78.

■

Alcoholism Sourcebook

Basic Consumer Health Information about the Physical and Mental Consequences of Alcohol Abuse, Including Liver Disease, Pancreatitis, Wernicke-Korsakoff Syndrome (Alcoholic Dementia), Fetal Alcohol Syndrome, Heart Disease, Kidney Disorders, Gastrointestinal Problems, and Immune System Compromise and Featuring Facts about Addiction, Detoxification, Alcohol Withdrawal, Recovery, and the Maintenance of Sobriety

Along with a Glossary and Directories of Resources for Further Help and Information

Edited by Karen Bellenir. 613 pages. 2000. 0-7808-0325-6. $78.

"This title is one of the few reference works on alcoholism for general readers. For some readers this will be a welcome complement to the many self-help books on the market. Recommended for collections serving general readers and consumer health collections."
— E-Streams, Mar '01

"This book is an excellent choice for public and academic libraries."
— American Reference Books Annual, 2001

"Recommended reference source."
— Booklist, American Library Association, Dec '00

"Presents a wealth of information on alcohol use and abuse and its effects on the body and mind, treatment, and prevention." — SciTech Book News, Dec '00

"Important new health guide which packs in the latest consumer information about the problems of alcoholism." — Reviewer's Bookwatch, Nov '00

SEE ALSO Drug Abuse Sourcebook, Substance Abuse Sourcebook

Allergies Sourcebook, 1st Edition

Basic Information about Major Forms and Mechanisms of Common Allergic Reactions, Sensitivities, and Intolerances, Including Anaphylaxis, Asthma, Hives and Other Dermatologic Symptoms, Rhinitis, and Sinusitis

Along with Their Usual Triggers Like Animal Fur, Chemicals, Drugs, Dust, Foods, Insects, Latex, Pollen, and Poison Ivy, Oak, and Sumac; Plus Information on Prevention, Identification, and Treatment

Edited by Allan R. Cook. 611 pages. 1997. 0-7808-0036-2. $78.

Allergies Sourcebook, 2nd Edition

Basic Consumer Health Information about Allergic Disorders, Triggers, Reactions, and Related Symptoms, Including Anaphylaxis, Rhinitis, Sinusitis, Asthma, Dermatitis, Conjunctivitis, and Multiple Chemical Sensitivity

Along with Tips on Diagnosis, Prevention, and Treatment, Statistical Data, a Glossary, and a Directory of Sources for Further Help and Information

Edited by Annemarie S. Muth. 598 pages. 2002. 0-7808-0376-0. $78.

"This second edition would be useful to laypersons with little or advanced knowledge of the subject matter. This book would also serve as a resource for nursing and other health care professions students. It would be useful in public, academic, and hospital libraries with consumer health collections." — E-Streams, Jul '02

Alternative Medicine Sourcebook, 1st Edition

Basic Consumer Health Information about Alternatives to Conventional Medicine, Including Acupressure, Acupuncture, Aromatherapy, Ayurveda, Bioelectromagnetics, Environmental Medicine, Essence Therapy, Food and Nutrition Therapy, Herbal Therapy, Homeopathy, Imaging, Massage, Naturopathy, Reflexology, Relaxation and Meditation, Sound Therapy, Vitamin and Mineral Therapy, and Yoga, and More

Edited by Allan R. Cook. 737 pages. 1999. 0-7808-0200-4. $78.

"Recommended reference source."
— Booklist, American Library Association, Feb '00

"A great addition to the reference collection of every type of library." — American Reference Books Annual, 2000

Alternative Medicine Sourcebook, 2nd Edition

Basic Consumer Health Information about Alternative and Complementary Medical Practices, Including Acupuncture, Chiropractic, Herbal Medicine, Homeopathy, Naturopathic Medicine, Mind-Body Interventions, Ayurveda, and Other Non-Western Medical Traditions

Along with Facts about such Specific Therapies as Massage Therapy, Aromatherapy, Qigong, Hypnosis, Prayer, Dance, and Art Therapies, a Glossary, and Resources for Further Information

Edited by Dawn D. Matthews. 618 pages. 2002. 0-7808-0605-0. $78.

"An important alternate health reference."
— MBR Bookwatch, Oct '02

Alzheimer's, Stroke & 29 Other Neurological Disorders Sourcebook, 1st Edition

Basic Information for the Layperson on 31 Diseases or Disorders Affecting the Brain and Nervous System, First Describing the Illness, Then Listing Symptoms, Diagnostic Methods, and Treatment Options, and Including Statistics on Incidences and Causes

Edited by Frank E. Bair. 579 pages. 1993. 1-55888-748-2. $78.

"Nontechnical reference book that provides reader-friendly information."
— Family Caregiver Alliance Update, Winter '96

"Should be included in any library's patient education section." — American Reference Books Annual, 1994

"Written in an approachable and accessible style. Recommended for patient education and consumer health collections in health science center and public libraries." — Academic Library Book Review, Dec '93

"It is very handy to have information on more than thirty neurological disorders under one cover, and there is no recent source like it." — *Reference Quarterly, American Library Association, Fall '93*

SEE ALSO Brain Disorders Sourcebook

Alzheimer's Disease Sourcebook, 2nd Edition

Basic Consumer Health Information about Alzheimer's Disease, Related Disorders, and Other Dementias, Including Multi-Infarct Dementia, AIDS-Related Dementia, Alcoholic Dementia, Huntington's Disease, Delirium, and Confusional States

Along with Reports Detailing Current Research Efforts in Prevention and Treatment, Long-Term Care Issues, and Listings of Sources for Additional Help and Information

Edited by Karen Bellenir. 524 pages. 1999. 0-7808-0223-3. $78.

"Provides a wealth of useful information not otherwise available in one place. This resource is recommended for all types of libraries."
— *American Reference Books Annual, 2000*

"Recommended reference source."
— *Booklist, American Library Association, Oct '99*

Arthritis Sourcebook

Basic Consumer Health Information about Specific Forms of Arthritis and Related Disorders, Including Rheumatoid Arthritis, Osteoarthritis, Gout, Polymyalgia Rheumatica, Psoriatic Arthritis, Spondyloarthropathies, Juvenile Rheumatoid Arthritis, and Juvenile Ankylosing Spondylitis

Along with Information about Medical, Surgical, and Alternative Treatment Options, and Including Strategies for Coping with Pain, Fatigue, and Stress

Edited by Allan R. Cook. 550 pages. 1998. 0-7808-0201-2. $78.

". . . accessible to the layperson."
— *Reference and Research Book News, Feb '99*

Asthma Sourcebook

Basic Consumer Health Information about Asthma, Including Symptoms, Traditional and Nontraditional Remedies, Treatment Advances, Quality-of-Life Aids, Medical Research Updates, and the Role of Allergies, Exercise, Age, the Environment, and Genetics in the Development of Asthma

Along with Statistical Data, a Glossary, and Directories of Support Groups, and Other Resources for Further Information

Edited by Annemarie S. Muth. 628 pages. 2000. 0-7808-0381-7. $78.

"A worthwhile reference acquisition for public libraries and academic medical libraries whose readers desire a quick introduction to the wide range of asthma information." — *Choice, Association of College & Research Libraries, Jun '01*

"Recommended reference source."
— *Booklist, American Library Association, Feb '01*

"Highly recommended." — *The Bookwatch, Jan '01*

"There is much good information for patients and their families who deal with asthma daily."
— *American Medical Writers Association Journal, Winter '01*

"This informative text is recommended for consumer health collections in public, secondary school, and community college libraries and the libraries of universities with a large undergraduate population."
— *American Reference Books Annual, 2001*

Attention Deficit Disorder Sourcebook

Basic Consumer Health Information about Attention Deficit/Hyperactivity Disorder in Children and Adults, Including Facts about Causes, Symptoms, Diagnostic Criteria, and Treatment Options Such as Medications, Behavior Therapy, Coaching, and Homeopathy

Along with Reports on Current Research Initiatives, Legal Issues, and Government Regulations, and Featuring a Glossary of Related Terms, Internet Resources, and a List of Additional Reading Material

Edited by Dawn D. Matthews. 470 pages. 2002. 0-7808-0624-7. $78.

Back & Neck Disorders Sourcebook

Basic Information about Disorders and Injuries of the Spinal Cord and Vertebrae, Including Facts on Chiropractic Treatment, Surgical Interventions, Paralysis, and Rehabilitation

Along with Advice for Preventing Back Trouble

Edited by Karen Bellenir. 548 pages. 1997. 0-7808-0202-0. $78.

"The strength of this work is its basic, easy-to-read format. Recommended."
— *Reference and User Services Quarterly, American Library Association, Winter '97*

Blood & Circulatory Disorders Sourcebook

Basic Information about Blood and Its Components, Anemias, Leukemias, Bleeding Disorders, and Circulatory Disorders, Including Aplastic Anemia, Thalassemia, Sickle-Cell Disease, Hemochromatosis, Hemophilia, Von Willebrand Disease, and Vascular Diseases

Along with a Special Section on Blood Transfusions and Blood Supply Safety, a Glossary, and Source Listings for Further Help and Information

Edited by Karen Bellenir and Linda M. Shin. 554 pages. 1998. 0-7808-0203-9. $78.

"Recommended reference source."
— *Booklist, American Library Association, Feb '99*

"An important reference sourcebook written in simple language for everyday, non-technical users. "
— *Reviewer's Bookwatch, Jan '99*

■

Brain Disorders Sourcebook

Basic Consumer Health Information about Strokes, Epilepsy, Amyotrophic Lateral Sclerosis (ALS/Lou Gehrig's Disease), Parkinson's Disease, Brain Tumors, Cerebral Palsy, Headache, Tourette Syndrome, and More

Along with Statistical Data, Treatment and Rehabilitation Options, Coping Strategies, Reports on Current Research Initiatives, a Glossary, and Resource Listings for Additional Help and Information

Edited by Karen Bellenir. 481 pages. 1999. 0-7808-0229-2. $78.

"Belongs on the shelves of any library with a consumer health collection." — *E-Streams, Mar '00*

"Recommended reference source."
— *Booklist, American Library Association, Oct '99*

SEE ALSO Alzheimer's Disease Sourcebook, 2nd Edition

■

Breast Cancer Sourcebook

Basic Consumer Health Information about Breast Cancer, Including Diagnostic Methods, Treatment Options, Alternative Therapies, Self-Help Information, Related Health Concerns, Statistical and Demographic Data, and Facts for Men with Breast Cancer

Along with Reports on Current Research Initiatives, a Glossary of Related Medical Terms, and a Directory of Sources for Further Help and Information

Edited by Edward J. Prucha and Karen Bellenir. 580 pages. 2001. 0-7808-0244-6. $78.

"Recommended reference source."
— *Booklist, American Library Association, Jan '02*

"This reference source is highly recommended. It is quite informative, comprehensive and detailed in nature, and yet it offers practical advice in easy-to-read language. It could be thought of as the 'bible' of breast cancer for the consumer." — *E-Streams, Jan '02*

"The broad range of topics covered in lay language make the *Breast Cancer Sourcebook* an excellent addition to public and consumer health library collections."
— *American Reference Books Annual 2002*

"From the pros and cons of different screening methods and results to treatment options, *Breast Cancer Sourcebook* provides the latest information on the subject."
— *Library Bookwatch, Dec '01*

"This thoroughgoing, very readable reference covers all aspects of breast health and cancer. . . . Readers will find much to consider here. Recommended for all public and patient health collections."
— *Library Journal, Sep '01*

SEE ALSO Cancer Sourcebook for Women, 1st and 2nd Editions, Women's Health Concerns Sourcebook

■

Breastfeeding Sourcebook

Basic Consumer Health Information about the Benefits of Breastmilk, Preparing to Breastfeed, Breastfeeding as a Baby Grows, Nutrition, and More, Including Information on Special Situations and Concerns Such as Mastitis, Illness, Medications, Allergies, Multiple Births, Prematurity, Special Needs, and Adoption

Along with a Glossary and Resources for Additional Help and Information

Edited by Jenni Lynn Colson. 388 pages. 2002. 0-7808-0332-9. $78.

SEE ALSO Pregnancy & Birth Sourcebook

■

Burns Sourcebook

Basic Consumer Health Information about Various Types of Burns and Scalds, Including Flame, Heat, Cold, Electrical, Chemical, and Sun Burns

Along with Information on Short-Term and Long-Term Treatments, Tissue Reconstruction, Plastic Surgery, Prevention Suggestions, and First Aid

Edited by Allan R. Cook. 604 pages. 1999. 0-7808-0204-7. $78.

"This is an exceptional addition to the series and is highly recommended for all consumer health collections, hospital libraries, and academic medical centers." — *E-Streams, Mar '00*

"This key reference guide is an invaluable addition to all health care and public libraries in confronting this ongoing health issue."
— *American Reference Books Annual, 2000*

"Recommended reference source."
— *Booklist, American Library Association, Dec '99*

SEE ALSO Skin Disorders Sourcebook

■

Cancer Sourcebook, 1st Edition

Basic Information on Cancer Types, Symptoms, Diagnostic Methods, and Treatments, Including Statistics on Cancer Occurrences Worldwide and the Risks Associated with Known Carcinogens and Activities

Edited by Frank E. Bair. 932 pages. 1990. 1-55888-888-8. $78.

Cited in *Reference Sources for Small and Medium-Sized Libraries, American Library Association, 1999*

"Written in nontechnical language. Useful for patients, their families, medical professionals, and librarians."
— *Guide to Reference Books, 1996*

"Designed with the non-medical professional in mind. Libraries and medical facilities interested in patient education should certainly consider adding the *Cancer Sourcebook* to their holdings. This compact collection of reliable information . . . is an invaluable tool for helping patients and patients' families and friends to take the first steps in coping with the many difficulties of cancer."
— *Medical Reference Services Quarterly, Winter '91*

"Specifically created for the nontechnical reader . . . an important resource for the general reader trying to understand the complexities of cancer."
— *American Reference Books Annual, 1991*

"This publication's nontechnical nature and very comprehensive format make it useful for both the general public and undergraduate students."
— *Choice, Association of College and Research Libraries, Oct '90*

New Cancer Sourcebook, 2nd Edition

Basic Information about Major Forms and Stages of Cancer, Featuring Facts about Primary and Secondary Tumors of the Respiratory, Nervous, Lymphatic, Circulatory, Skeletal, and Gastrointestinal Systems, and Specific Organs; Statistical and Demographic Data; Treatment Options; and Strategies for Coping

Edited by Allan R. Cook. 1,313 pages. 1996. 0-7808-0041-9. $78.

"An excellent resource for patients with newly diagnosed cancer and their families. The dialogue is simple, direct, and comprehensive. Highly recommended for patients and families to aid in their understanding of cancer and its treatment."
— *Booklist Health Sciences Supplement, American Library Association, Oct '97*

"The amount of factual and useful information is extensive. The writing is very clear, geared to general readers. Recommended for all levels." — *Choice, Association of College & Research Libraries, Jan '97*

Cancer Sourcebook, 3rd Edition

Basic Consumer Health Information about Major Forms and Stages of Cancer, Featuring Facts about Primary and Secondary Tumors of the Respiratory, Nervous, Lymphatic, Circulatory, Skeletal, and Gastrointestinal Systems, and Specific Organs

Along with Statistical and Demographic Data, Treatment Options, Strategies for Coping, a Glossary, and a Directory of Sources for Additional Help and Information

Edited by Edward J. Prucha. 1,069 pages. 2000. 0-7808-0227-6. $78.

"This title is recommended for health sciences and public libraries with consumer health collections."
— *E-Streams, Feb '01*

". . . can be effectively used by cancer patients and their families who are looking for answers in a language they can understand. Public and hospital libraries should have it on their shelves."
— *American Reference Books Annual, 2001*

"Recommended reference source."
— *Booklist, American Library Association, Dec '00*

Cancer Sourcebook for Women, 1st Edition

Basic Information about Specific Forms of Cancer That Affect Women, Featuring Facts about Breast Cancer, Cervical Cancer, Ovarian Cancer, Cancer of the Uterus and Uterine Sarcoma, Cancer of the Vagina, and Cancer of the Vulva; Statistical and Demographic Data; Treatments, Self-Help Management Suggestions, and Current Research Initiatives

Edited by Allan R. Cook and Peter D. Dresser. 524 pages. 1996. 0-7808-0076-1. $78.

". . . written in easily understandable, non-technical language. Recommended for public libraries or hospital and academic libraries that collect patient education or consumer health materials."
— *Medical Reference Services Quarterly, Spring '97*

"Would be of value in a consumer health library. . . . written with the health care consumer in mind. Medical jargon is at a minimum, and medical terms are explained in clear, understandable sentences."
— *Bulletin of the Medical Library Association, Oct '96*

"The availability under one cover of all these pertinent publications, grouped under cohesive headings, makes this certainly a most useful sourcebook." — *Choice, Association of College & Research Libraries, Jun '96*

"Presents a comprehensive knowledge base for general readers. Men and women both benefit from the gold mine of information nestled between the two covers of this book. Recommended."
— *Academic Library Book Review, Summer '96*

"This timely book is highly recommended for consumer health and patient education collections in all libraries."
— *Library Journal, Apr '96*

Cancer Sourcebook for Women, 2nd Edition

Basic Consumer Health Information about Gynecologic Cancers and Related Concerns, Including Cervical Cancer, Endometrial Cancer, Gestational Trophoblastic Tumor, Ovarian Cancer, Uterine Cancer, Vaginal Cancer, Vulvar Cancer, Breast Cancer, and Common Non-Cancerous Uterine Conditions, with Facts about Cancer Risk Factors, Screening and Prevention, Treatment Options, and Reports on Current Research Initiatives

Along with a Glossary of Cancer Terms and a Directory of Resources for Additional Help and Information

Edited by Karen Bellenir. 604 pages. 2002. 0-7808-0226-8. $78.

SEE ALSO *Breast Cancer Sourcebook, Women's Health Concerns Sourcebook*

Cardiovascular Diseases & Disorders Sourcebook, 1st Edition

Basic Information about Cardiovascular Diseases and Disorders, Featuring Facts about the Cardiovascular System, Demographic and Statistical Data, Descriptions of Pharmacological and Surgical Interventions, Lifestyle Modifications, and a Special Section Focusing on Heart Disorders in Children

Edited by Karen Bellenir and Peter D. Dresser. 683 pages. 1995. 0-7808-0032-X. $78.

SEE ALSO *Healthy Heart Sourcebook for Women, Heart Diseases & Disorders Sourcebook, 2nd Edition*

Caregiving Sourcebook

Basic Consumer Health Information for Caregivers, Including a Profile of Caregivers, Caregiving Responsibilities and Concerns, Tips for Specific Conditions, Care Environments, and the Effects of Caregiving

Along with Facts about Legal Issues, Financial Information, and Future Planning, a Glossary, and a Listing of Additional Resources

Edited by Joyce Brennfleck Shannon. 600 pages. 2001. 0-7808-0331-0. $78.

Childhood Diseases & Disorders Sourcebook

Basic Consumer Health Information about Medical Problems Often Encountered in Pre-Adolescent Children, Including Respiratory Tract Ailments, Ear Infections, Sore Throats, Disorders of the Skin and Scalp, Digestive and Genitourinary Diseases, Infectious Diseases, Inflammatory Disorders, Chronic Physical and Developmental Disorders, Allergies, and More

Along with Information about Diagnostic Tests, Common Childhood Surgeries, and Frequently Used Medications, with a Glossary of Important Terms and Resource Directory

Edited by Chad T. Kimball. 600 pages. 2003. 0-7808-0458-9. $78.

Colds, Flu & Other Common Ailments Sourcebook

Basic Consumer Health Information about Common Ailments and Injuries, Including Colds, Coughs, the Flu, Sinus Problems, Headaches, Fever, Nausea and Vomiting, Menstrual Cramps, Diarrhea, Constipation, Hemorrhoids, Back Pain, Dandruff, Dry and Itchy Skin, Cuts, Scrapes, Sprains, Bruises, and More

Along with Information about Prevention, Self-Care, Choosing a Doctor, Over-the-Counter Medications, Folk Remedies, and Alternative Therapies, and Including a Glossary of Important Terms and a Directory of Resources for Further Help and Information

Edited by Chad T. Kimball. 638 pages. 2001. 0-7808-0435-X. $78.

Communication Disorders Sourcebook

Basic Information about Deafness and Hearing Loss, Speech and Language Disorders, Voice Disorders, Balance and Vestibular Disorders, and Disorders of Smell, Taste, and Touch

Edited by Linda M. Ross. 533 pages. 1996. 0-7808-0077-X. $78.

Congenital Disorders Sourcebook

Basic Information about Disorders Acquired during Gestation, Including Spina Bifida, Hydrocephalus, Cerebral Palsy, Heart Defects, Craniofacial Abnormalities, Fetal Alcohol Syndrome, and More

Along with Current Treatment Options and Statistical Data

Edited by Karen Bellenir. 607 pages. 1997. 0-7808-0205-5. $78.

"Recommended reference source."
— *Booklist, American Library Association, Oct '97*

SEE ALSO Pregnancy & Birth Sourcebook

Consumer Issues in Health Care Sourcebook

Basic Information about Health Care Fundamentals and Related Consumer Issues, Including Exams and Screening Tests, Physician Specialties, Choosing a Doctor, Using Prescription and Over-the-Counter Medications Safely, Avoiding Health Scams, Managing Common Health Risks in the Home, Care Options for Chronically or Terminally Ill Patients, and a List of Resources for Obtaining Help and Further Information

Edited by Karen Bellenir. 618 pages. 1998. 0-7808-0221-7. $78.

"Both public and academic libraries will want to have a copy in their collection for readers who are interested in self-education on health issues."
— *American Reference Books Annual, 2000*

"The editor has researched the literature from government agencies and others, saving readers the time and effort of having to do the research themselves. Recommended for public libraries."
— *Reference and User Services Quarterly, American Library Association, Spring '99*

"Recommended reference source."
— *Booklist, American Library Association, Dec '98*

Contagious & Non-Contagious Infectious Diseases Sourcebook

Basic Information about Contagious Diseases like Measles, Polio, Hepatitis B, and Infectious Mononucleosis, and Non-Contagious Infectious Diseases like Tetanus and Toxic Shock Syndrome, and Diseases Occurring as Secondary Infections Such as Shingles and Reye Syndrome

Along with Vaccination, Prevention, and Treatment Information, and a Section Describing Emerging Infectious Disease Threats

Edited by Karen Bellenir and Peter D. Dresser. 566 pages. 1996. 0-7808-0075-3. $78.

Death & Dying Sourcebook

Basic Consumer Health Information for the Layperson about End-of-Life Care and Related Ethical and Legal Issues, Including Chief Causes of Death, Autopsies, Pain Management for the Terminally Ill, Life Support Systems, Insurance, Euthanasia, Assisted Suicide, Hospice Programs, Living Wills, Funeral Planning, Counseling, Mourning, Organ Donation, and Physician Training

Along with Statistical Data, a Glossary, and Listings of Sources for Further Help and Information

Edited by Annemarie S. Muth. 641 pages. 1999. 0-7808-0230-6. $78.

"Public libraries, medical libraries, and academic libraries will all find this sourcebook a useful addition to their collections."
— *American Reference Books Annual, 2001*

"An extremely useful resource for those concerned with death and dying in the United States."
— *Respiratory Care, Nov '00*

"Recommended reference source."
— *Booklist, American Library Association, Aug '00*

"This book is a definite must for all those involved in end-of-life care." — *Doody's Review Service, 2000*

Depression Sourcebook

Basic Consumer Health Information about Unipolar Depression, Bipolar Disorder, Postpartum Depression, Seasonal Affective Disorder, and Other Types of Depression in Children, Adolescents, Women, Men, the Elderly, and Other Selected Populations

Along with Facts about Causes, Risk Factors, Diagnostic Criteria, Treatment Options, Coping Strategies, Suicide Prevention, a Glossary, and a Directory of Sources for Additional Help and Information

Edited by Karen Belleni. 602 pages. 2002. 0-7808-0611-5. $78.

Diabetes Sourcebook, 1st Edition

Basic Information about Insulin-Dependent and Non-insulin-Dependent Diabetes Mellitus, Gestational Diabetes, and Diabetic Complications, Symptoms, Treatment, and Research Results, Including Statistics on Prevalence, Morbidity, and Mortality

Along with Source Listings for Further Help and Information

Edited by Karen Bellenir and Peter D. Dresser. 827 pages. 1994. 1-55888-751-2. $78.

". . . very informative and understandable for the layperson without being simplistic. It provides a comprehensive overview for laypersons who want a general understanding of the disease or who want to focus on various aspects of the disease."
— *Bulletin of the Medical Library Association, Jan '96*

Diabetes Sourcebook, 2nd Edition

Basic Consumer Health Information about Type 1 Diabetes (Insulin-Dependent or Juvenile-Onset Diabetes), Type 2 (Noninsulin-Dependent or Adult-Onset Diabetes), Gestational Diabetes, and Related Disorders, Including Diabetes Prevalence Data, Management Issues, the Role of Diet and Exercise in Controlling Diabetes, Insulin and Other Diabetes Medicines, and Complications of Diabetes Such as Eye Diseases, Periodontal Disease, Amputation, and End-Stage Renal Disease

Along with Reports on Current Research Initiatives, a Glossary, and Resource Listings for Further Help and Information

Edited by Karen Bellenir. 688 pages. 1998. 0-7808-0224-1. $78.

"An invaluable reference." — *Library Journal, May '00*

Selected as one of the 250 "Best Health Sciences Books of 1999." — *Doody's Rating Service, Mar-Apr 2000*

"This comprehensive book is an excellent addition for high school, academic, medical, and public libraries. This volume is highly recommended."
— *American Reference Books Annual, 2000*

"Provides useful information for the general public."
— *Healthlines, University of Michigan Health Management Research Center, Sep/Oct '99*

". . . provides reliable mainstream medical information . . . belongs on the shelves of any library with a consumer health collection." — *E-Streams, Sep '99*

"Recommended reference source."
— *Booklist, American Library Association, Feb '99*

Diabetes Sourcebook, 3rd Edition

Basic Consumer Health Information about Type 1 Diabetes (Insulin-Dependent or Juvenile-Onset Diabetes), Type 2 Diabetes (Noninsulin-Dependent or Adult-Onset Diabetes), Gestational Diabetes, Impaired Glucose Tolerance (IGT), and Related Complications, Such as Amputation, Eye Disease, Gum Disease, Nerve Damage, and End-Stage Renal Disease, Including Facts about Insulin, Oral Diabetes Medications, Blood Sugar Testing, and the Role of Exercise and Nutrition in the Control of Diabetes

Along with a Glossary and Resources for Further Help and Information

Edited by Dawn D. Matthews. 622 pages. 2003. 0-7808-0629-8. $78.

Diet & Nutrition Sourcebook, 1st Edition

Basic Information about Nutrition, Including the Dietary Guidelines for Americans, the Food Guide Pyramid, and Their Applications in Daily Diet, Nutritional Advice for Specific Age Groups, Current Nutritional Issues and Controversies, the New Food Label and How to Use It to Promote Healthy Eating, and Recent Developments in Nutritional Research

Edited by Dan R. Harris. 662 pages. 1996. 0-7808-0084-2. $78.

"Useful reference as a food and nutrition sourcebook for the general consumer." — *Booklist Health Sciences Supplement, American Library Association, Oct '97*

"Recommended for public libraries and medical libraries that receive general information requests on nutrition. It is readable and will appeal to those interested in learning more about healthy dietary practices."
— *Medical Reference Services Quarterly, Fall '97*

"An abundance of medical and social statistics is translated into readable information geared toward the general reader." — *Bookwatch, Mar '97*

"With dozens of questionable diet books on the market, it is so refreshing to find a reliable and factual reference book. Recommended to aspiring professionals, librarians, and others seeking and giving reliable dietary advice. An excellent compilation." — *Choice, Association of College and Research Libraries, Feb '97*

SEE ALSO *Digestive Diseases & Disorders Sourcebook, Gastrointestinal Diseases & Disorders Sourcebook*

Diet & Nutrition Sourcebook, 2nd Edition

Basic Consumer Health Information about Dietary Guidelines, Recommended Daily Intake Values, Vitamins, Minerals, Fiber, Fat, Weight Control, Dietary Supplements, and Food Additives

Along with Special Sections on Nutrition Needs throughout Life and Nutrition for People with Such Specific Medical Concerns as Allergies, High Blood Cholesterol, Hypertension, Diabetes, Celiac Disease, Seizure Disorders, Phenylketonuria (PKU), Cancer, and Eating Disorders, and Including Reports on Current Nutrition Research and Source Listings for Additional Help and Information

Edited by Karen Bellenir. 650 pages. 1999. 0-7808-0228-4. $78.

"This book is an excellent source of basic diet and nutrition information." — *Booklist Health Sciences Supplement, American Library Association, Dec '00*

"This reference document should be in any public library, but it would be a very good guide for beginning students in the health sciences. If the other books in this publisher's series are as good as this, they should all be in the health sciences collections."
— *American Reference Books Annual, 2000*

"This book is an excellent general nutrition reference for consumers who desire to take an active role in their health care for prevention. Consumers of all ages who select this book can feel confident they are receiving current and accurate information." — *Journal of Nutrition for the Elderly, Vol. 19, No. 4, '00*

"Recommended reference source."
— *Booklist, American Library Association, Dec '99*

SEE ALSO *Digestive Diseases & Disorders Sourcebook, Gastrointestinal Diseases & Disorders Sourcebook*

Digestive Diseases & Disorders Sourcebook

Basic Consumer Health Information about Diseases and Disorders that Impact the Upper and Lower Digestive System, Including Celiac Disease, Constipation, Crohn's Disease, Cyclic Vomiting Syndrome, Diarrhea, Diverticulosis and Diverticulitis, Gallstones, Heartburn, Hemorrhoids, Hernias, Indigestion (Dyspepsia), Irritable Bowel Syndrome, Lactose Intolerance, Ulcers, and More

Along with Information about Medications and Other Treatments, Tips for Maintaining a Healthy Digestive Tract, a Glossary, and Directory of Digestive Diseases Organizations

Edited by Karen Bellenir. 335 pages. 2000. 0-7808-0327-2. $78.

"This title would be an excellent addition to all public or patient-research libraries."
—*American Reference Books Annual, 2001*

"This title is recommended for public, hospital, and health sciences libraries with consumer health collections." —*E-Streams, Jul-Aug '00*

"Recommended reference source."
—*Booklist, American Library Association, May '00*

SEE ALSO *Diet & Nutrition Sourcebook, 1st and 2nd Editions, Gastrointestinal Diseases & Disorders Sourcebook*

Disabilities Sourcebook

Basic Consumer Health Information about Physical and Psychiatric Disabilities, Including Descriptions of Major Causes of Disability, Assistive and Adaptive Aids, Workplace Issues, and Accessibility Concerns

Along with Information about the Americans with Disabilities Act, a Glossary, and Resources for Additional Help and Information

Edited by Dawn D. Matthews. 616 pages. 2000. 0-7808-0389-2. $78.

"It is a must for libraries with a consumer health section." —*American Reference Books Annual 2002*

"A much needed addition to the Omnigraphics *Health Reference Series*. A current reference work to provide people with disabilities, their families, caregivers or those who work with them, a broad range of information in one volume, has not been available until now. . . . It is recommended for all public and academic library reference collections." —*E-Streams, May '01*

"An excellent source book in easy-to-read format covering many current topics; highly recommended for all libraries." —*Choice, Association of College and Research Libraries, Jan '01*

"Recommended reference source."
—*Booklist, American Library Association, Jul '00*

Domestic Violence & Child Abuse Sourcebook

Basic Consumer Health Information about Spousal/ Partner, Child, Sibling, Parent, and Elder Abuse, Covering Physical, Emotional, and Sexual Abuse, Teen Dating Violence, and Stalking; Includes Information about Hotlines, Safe Houses, Safety Plans, and Other Resources for Support and Assistance, Community Initiatives, and Reports on Current Directions in Research and Treatment

Along with a Glossary, Sources for Further Reading, and Governmental and Non-Governmental Organizations Contact Information

Edited by Helene Henderson. 1,064 pages. 2001. 0-7808-0235-7. $78.

"This is important information. The Web has many resources but this sourcebook fills an important societal need. I am not aware of any other resources of this type." —*Doody's Review Service, Sep '01*

"Recommended for all libraries, scholars, and practitioners." —*Choice, Association of College & Research Libraries, Jul '01*

"Recommended reference source."
—*Booklist, American Library Association, Apr '01*

"Important pick for college-level health reference libraries." —*The Bookwatch, Mar '01*

"Because this problem is so widespread and because this book includes a lot of issues within one volume, this work is recommended for all public libraries."
—*American Reference Books Annual, 2001*

Drug Abuse Sourcebook

Basic Consumer Health Information about Illicit Substances of Abuse and the Diversion of Prescription Medications, Including Depressants, Hallucinogens, Inhalants, Marijuana, Narcotics, Stimulants, and Anabolic Steroids

Along with Facts about Related Health Risks, Treatment Issues, and Substance Abuse Prevention Programs, a Glossary of Terms, Statistical Data, and Directories of Hotline Services, Self-Help Groups, and Organizations Able to Provide Further Information

Edited by Karen Bellenir. 629 pages. 2000. 0-7808-0242-X. $78.

"Containing a wealth of information . . . . This resource belongs in libraries that serve a lower-division undergraduate or community college clientele as well as the general public." —*Choice, Association of College and Research Libraries, Jun '01*

"Recommended reference source."
—*Booklist, American Library Association, Feb '01*

"Highly recommended." —*The Bookwatch, Jan '01*

"Even though there is a plethora of books on drug abuse, this volume is recommended for school, public, and college libraries."
—*American Reference Books Annual, 2001*

SEE ALSO *Alcoholism Sourcebook, Substance Abuse Sourcebook*

Ear, Nose & Throat Disorders Sourcebook

Basic Information about Disorders of the Ears, Nose, Sinus Cavities, Pharynx, and Larynx, Including Ear Infections, Tinnitus, Vestibular Disorders, Allergic and Non-Allergic Rhinitis, Sore Throats, Tonsillitis, and Cancers That Affect the Ears, Nose, Sinuses, and Throat

Along with Reports on Current Research Initiatives, a Glossary of Related Medical Terms, and a Directory of Sources for Further Help and Information

Edited by Karen Bellenir and Linda M. Shin. 576 pages. 1998. 0-7808-0206-3. $78.

"Overall, this sourcebook is helpful for the consumer seeking information on ENT issues. It is recommended for public libraries."
—American Reference Books Annual, 1999

"Recommended reference source."
—Booklist, American Library Association, Dec '98

■

Eating Disorders Sourcebook

Basic Consumer Health Information about Eating Disorders, Including Information about Anorexia Nervosa, Bulimia Nervosa, Binge Eating, Body Dysmorphic Disorder, Pica, Laxative Abuse, and Night Eating Syndrome

Along with Information about Causes, Adverse Effects, and Treatment and Prevention Issues, and Featuring a Section on Concerns Specific to Children and Adolescents, a Glossary, and Resources for Further Help and Information

Edited by Dawn D. Matthews. 322 pages. 2001. 0-7808-0335-3. $78.

"Recommended for health science libraries that are open to the public, as well as hospital libraries. This book is a good resource for the consumer who is concerned about eating disorders." *— E-Streams, Mar '02*

"This volume is another convenient collection of excerpted articles. Recommended for school and public library patrons; lower-division undergraduates; and two-year technical program students." *— Choice, Association of College & Research Libraries, Jan '02*

"Recommended reference source." *— Booklist, American Library Association, Oct '01*

■

Emergency Medical Services Sourcebook

Basic Consumer Health Information about Preventing, Preparing for, and Managing Emergency Situations, When and Who to Call for Help, What to Expect in the Emergency Room, the Emergency Medical Team, Patient Issues, and Current Topics in Emergency Medicine

Along with Statistical Data, a Glossary, and Sources of Additional Help and Information

Edited by Jenni Lynn Colson. 494 pages. 2002. 0-7808-0420-1. $78.

Endocrine & Metabolic Disorders Sourcebook

Basic Information for the Layperson about Pancreatic and Insulin-Related Disorders Such as Pancreatitis, Diabetes, and Hypoglycemia; Adrenal Gland Disorders Such as Cushing's Syndrome, Addison's Disease, and Congenital Adrenal Hyperplasia; Pituitary Gland Disorders Such as Growth Hormone Deficiency, Acromegaly, and Pituitary Tumors; Thyroid Disorders Such as Hypothyroidism, Graves' Disease, Hashimoto's Disease, and Goiter; Hyperparathyroidism; and Other Diseases and Syndromes of Hormone Imbalance or Metabolic Dysfunction

Along with Reports on Current Research Initiatives

Edited by Linda M. Shin. 574 pages. 1998. 0-7808-0207-1. $78.

"Omnigraphics has produced another needed resource for health information consumers."
—American Reference Books Annual, 2000

"Recommended reference source."
— Booklist, American Library Association, Dec '98

■

Environmentally Induced Disorders Sourcebook, 1st Edition

Basic Information about Diseases and Syndromes Linked to Exposure to Pollutants and Other Substances in Outdoor and Indoor Environments Such as Lead, Asbestos, Formaldehyde, Mercury, Emissions, Noise, and More

Edited by Allan R. Cook. 620 pages. 1997. 0-7808-0083-4. $78.

"Recommended reference source."
— Booklist, American Library Association, Sep '98

"This book will be a useful addition to anyone's library." *— Choice Health Sciences Supplement, Association of College and Research Libraries, May '98*

". . . a good survey of numerous environmentally induced physical disorders . . . a useful addition to anyone's library."
— Doody's Health Sciences Book Reviews, Jan '98

". . . provide[s] introductory information from the best authorities around. Since this volume covers topics that potentially affect everyone, it will surely be one of the most frequently consulted volumes in the *Health Reference Series*." *— Rettig on Reference, Nov '97*

■

Ethnic Diseases Sourcebook

Basic Consumer Health Information for Ethnic and Racial Minority Groups in the United States, Including General Health Indicators and Behaviors, Ethnic Diseases, Genetic Testing, the Impact of Chronic Diseases, Women's Health, Mental Health Issues, and Preventive Health Care Services

Along with a Glossary and a Listing of Additional Resources

Edited by Joyce Brennfleck Shannon. 664 pages. 2001. 0-7808-0336-1. $78.

"Recommended for health sciences libraries where public health programs are a priority."
— E-Streams, Jan '02

"Not many books have been written on this topic to date, and the *Ethnic Diseases Sourcebook* is a strong addition to the list. It will be an important introductory resource for health consumers, students, health care personnel, and social scientists. It is recommended for public, academic, and large hospital libraries."
— American Reference Books Annual 2002

"Recommended reference source."
— Booklist, American Library Association, Oct '01

"Will prove valuable to any library seeking to maintain a current, comprehensive reference collection of health resources. . . . An excellent source of health information about genetic disorders which affect particular ethnic and racial minorities in the U.S."
— The Bookwatch, Aug '01

Eye Care Sourcebook,
2nd Edition

Basic Consumer Health Information about Eye Care and Eye Disorders, Including Facts about the Diagnosis, Prevention, and Treatment of Common Refractive Problems Such as Myopia, Hyperopia, Astigmatism, and Presbyopia, and Eye Diseases, Including Glaucoma, Cataract, Age-Related Macular Degeneration, and Diabetic Retinopathy

Along with a Section on Vision Correction and Refractive Surgeries, Including LASIK and LASEK, a Glossary, and Directories of Resources for Additional Help and Information

Edited by Amy L. Sutton. 543 pages. 2003. 0-7808-0635-2. $78.

Family Planning Sourcebook

Basic Consumer Health Information about Planning for Pregnancy and Contraception, Including Traditional Methods, Barrier Methods, Hormonal Methods, Permanent Methods, Future Methods, Emergency Contraception, and Birth Control Choices for Women at Each Stage of Life

Along with Statistics, a Glossary, and Sources of Additional Information

Edited by Amy Marcaccio Keyzer. 520 pages. 2001. 0-7808-0379-5. $78.

"Recommended for public, health, and undergraduate libraries as part of the circulating collection."
— E-Streams, Mar '02

"Information is presented in an unbiased, readable manner, and the sourcebook will certainly be a necessary addition to those public and high school libraries where Internet access is restricted or otherwise problematic." — American Reference Books Annual 2002

"Recommended reference source."
— Booklist, American Library Association, Oct '01

"Will prove valuable to any library seeking to maintain a current, comprehensive reference collection of health resources. . . . Excellent reference."
— The Bookwatch, Aug '01

SEE ALSO *Pregnancy & Birth Sourcebook*

Fitness & Exercise Sourcebook,
1st Edition

Basic Information on Fitness and Exercise, Including Fitness Activities for Specific Age Groups, Exercise for People with Specific Medical Conditions, How to Begin a Fitness Program in Running, Walking, Swimming, Cycling, and Other Athletic Activities, and Recent Research in Fitness and Exercise

Edited by Dan R. Harris. 663 pages. 1996. 0-7808-0186-5. $78.

"A good resource for general readers." — Choice, Association of College and Research Libraries, Nov '97

"The perennial popularity of the topic . . . make this an appealing selection for public libraries."
— Rettig on Reference, Jun/Jul '97

Fitness & Exercise Sourcebook,
2nd Edition

Basic Consumer Health Information about the Fundamentals of Fitness and Exercise, Including How to Begin and Maintain a Fitness Program, Fitness as a Lifestyle, the Link between Fitness and Diet, Advice for Specific Groups of People, Exercise as It Relates to Specific Medical Conditions, and Recent Research in Fitness and Exercise

Along with a Glossary of Important Terms and Resources for Additional Help and Information

Edited by Kristen M. Gledhill. 646 pages. 2001. 0-7808-0334-5. $78.

"This work is recommended for all general reference collections."
— American Reference Books Annual 2002

"Highly recommended for public, consumer, and school grades fourth through college."
— E-Streams, Nov '01

"Recommended reference source." — Booklist, American Library Association, Oct '01

"The information appears quite comprehensive and is considered reliable. . . . This second edition is a welcomed addition to the series."
— Doody's Review Service, Sep '01

"This reference is a valuable choice for those who desire a broad source of information on exercise, fitness, and chronic-disease prevention through a healthy lifestyle." — American Medical Writers Association Journal, Fall '01

"Will prove valuable to any library seeking to maintain a current, comprehensive reference collection of health resources. . . . Excellent reference."
— The Bookwatch, Aug '01

Food & Animal Borne Diseases Sourcebook

Basic Information about Diseases That Can Be Spread to Humans through the Ingestion of Contaminated Food or Water or by Contact with Infected Animals and Insects, Such as Botulism, E. Coli, Hepatitis A, Trichinosis, Lyme Disease, and Rabies

Along with Information Regarding Prevention and Treatment Methods, and Including a Special Section for International Travelers Describing Diseases Such as Cholera, Malaria, Travelers' Diarrhea, and Yellow Fever, and Offering Recommendations for Avoiding Illness

Edited by Karen Bellenir and Peter D. Dresser. 535 pages. 1995. 0-7808-0033-8. $78.

"Targeting general readers and providing them with a single, comprehensive source of information on selected topics, this book continues, with the excellent caliber of its predecessors, to catalog topical information on health matters of general interest. Readable and thorough, this valuable resource is highly recommended for all libraries."
— *Academic Library Book Review, Summer '96*

"A comprehensive collection of authoritative information."
— *Emergency Medical Services, Oct '95*

■

Food Safety Sourcebook

Basic Consumer Health Information about the Safe Handling of Meat, Poultry, Seafood, Eggs, Fruit Juices, and Other Food Items, and Facts about Pesticides, Drinking Water, Food Safety Overseas, and the Onset, Duration, and Symptoms of Foodborne Illnesses, Including Types of Pathogenic Bacteria, Parasitic Protozoa, Worms, Viruses, and Natural Toxins

Along with the Role of the Consumer, the Food Handler, and the Government in Food Safety; a Glossary, and Resources for Additional Help and Information

Edited by Dawn D. Matthews. 339 pages. 1999. 0-7808-0326-4. $78.

"This book is recommended for public libraries and universities with home economic and food science programs."
— *E-Streams, Nov '00*

"Recommended reference source."
— *Booklist, American Library Association, May '00*

"This book takes the complex issues of food safety and foodborne pathogens and presents them in an easily understood manner. [It does] an excellent job of covering a large and often confusing topic."
— *American Reference Books Annual, 2000*

■

Forensic Medicine Sourcebook

Basic Consumer Information for the Layperson about Forensic Medicine, Including Crime Scene Investigation, Evidence Collection and Analysis, Expert Testimony, Computer-Aided Criminal Identification, Digital Imaging in the Courtroom, DNA Profiling, Accident Reconstruction, Autopsies, Ballistics, Drugs and

Explosives Detection, Latent Fingerprints, Product Tampering, and Questioned Document Examination

Along with Statistical Data, a Glossary of Forensics Terminology, and Listings of Sources for Further Help and Information

Edited by Annemarie S. Muth. 574 pages. 1999. 0-7808-0232-2. $78.

"Given the expected widespread interest in its content and its easy to read style, this book is recommended for most public and all college and university libraries."
— *E-Streams, Feb '01*

"Recommended for public libraries."
— *Reference & User Services Quarterly, American Library Association, Spring 2000*

"Recommended reference source."
— *Booklist, American Library Association, Feb '00*

"A wealth of information, useful statistics, references are up-to-date and extremely complete. This wonderful collection of data will help students who are interested in a career in any type of forensic field. It is a great resource for attorneys who need information about types of expert witnesses needed in a particular case. It also offers useful information for fiction and nonfiction writers whose work involves a crime. A fascinating compilation. All levels."
— *Choice, Association of College and Research Libraries, Jan 2000*

"There are several items that make this book attractive to consumers who are seeking certain forensic data. . . . This is a useful current source for those seeking general forensic medical answers."
— *American Reference Books Annual, 2000*

■

Gastrointestinal Diseases & Disorders Sourcebook

Basic Information about Gastroesophageal Reflux Disease (Heartburn), Ulcers, Diverticulosis, Irritable Bowel Syndrome, Crohn's Disease, Ulcerative Colitis, Diarrhea, Constipation, Lactose Intolerance, Hemorrhoids, Hepatitis, Cirrhosis, and Other Digestive Problems, Featuring Statistics, Descriptions of Symptoms, and Current Treatment Methods of Interest for Persons Living with Upper and Lower Gastrointestinal Maladies

Edited by Linda M. Ross. 413 pages. 1996. 0-7808-0078-8. $78.

". . . very readable form. The successful editorial work that brought this material together into a useful and understandable reference makes accessible to all readers information that can help them more effectively understand and obtain help for digestive tract problems."
— *Choice, Association of College & Research Libraries, Feb '97*

SEE ALSO *Diet & Nutrition Sourcebook, 1st and 2nd Editions, Digestive Diseases & Disorders*

Genetic Disorders Sourcebook, 1st Edition

Basic Information about Heritable Diseases and Disorders Such as Down Syndrome, PKU, Hemophilia, Von Willebrand Disease, Gaucher Disease, Tay-Sachs Disease, and Sickle-Cell Disease, Along with Information about Genetic Screening, Gene Therapy, Home Care, and Including Source Listings for Further Help and Information on More Than 300 Disorders

Edited by Karen Bellenir. 642 pages. 1996. 0-7808-0034-6. $78.

"Recommended for undergraduate libraries or libraries that serve the public."
— *Science & Technology Libraries, Vol. 18, No. 1, '99*

"Provides essential medical information to both the general public and those diagnosed with a serious or fatal genetic disease or disorder." —*Choice, Association of College and Research Libraries, Jan '97*

"Geared toward the lay public. It would be well placed in all public libraries and in those hospital and medical libraries in which access to genetic references is limited." —*Doody's Health Sciences Book Review, Oct '96*

Genetic Disorders Sourcebook, 2nd Edition

Basic Consumer Health Information about Hereditary Diseases and Disorders, Including Cystic Fibrosis, Down Syndrome, Hemophilia, Huntington's Disease, Sickle Cell Anemia, and More; Facts about Genes, Gene Research and Therapy, Genetic Screening, Ethics of Gene Testing, Genetic Counseling, and Advice on Coping and Caring

Along with a Glossary of Genetic Terminology and a Resource List for Help, Support, and Further Information

Edited by Kathy Massimini. 768 pages. 2001. 0-7808-0241-1. $78.

"Recommended for public libraries and medical and hospital libraries with consumer health collections."
— *E-Streams, May '01*

"Recommended reference source."
— *Booklist, American Library Association, Apr '01*

"Important pick for college-level health reference libraries." — *The Bookwatch, Mar '01*

Head Trauma Sourcebook

Basic Information for the Layperson about Open-Head and Closed-Head Injuries, Treatment Advances, Recovery, and Rehabilitation

Along with Reports on Current Research Initiatives

Edited by Karen Bellenir. 414 pages. 1997. 0-7808-0208-X. $78.

Headache Sourcebook

Basic Consumer Health Information about Migraine, Tension, Cluster, Rebound and Other Types of Headaches, with Facts about the Cause and Prevention of Headaches, the Effects of Stress and the Environment, Headaches during Pregnancy and Menopause, and Childhood Headaches

Along with a Glossary and Other Resources for Additional Help and Information

Edited by Dawn D. Matthews. 362 pages. 2002. 0-7808-0337-X. $78.

"Highly recommended for academic and medical reference collections." — *Library Bookwatch, Sep '02*

Health Insurance Sourcebook

Basic Information about Managed Care Organizations, Traditional Fee-for-Service Insurance, Insurance Portability and Pre-Existing Conditions Clauses, Medicare, Medicaid, Social Security, and Military Health Care

Along with Information about Insurance Fraud

Edited by Wendy Wilcox. 530 pages. 1997. 0-7808-0222-5. $78.

"Particularly useful because it brings much of this information together in one volume. This book will be a handy reference source in the health sciences library, hospital library, college and university library, and medium to large public library."
— *Medical Reference Services Quarterly, Fall '98*

Awarded "Books of the Year Award"
— *American Journal of Nursing, 1997*

"The layout of the book is particularly helpful as it provides easy access to reference material. A most useful addition to the vast amount of information about health insurance. The use of data from U.S. government agencies is most commendable. Useful in a library or learning center for healthcare professional students."
— *Doody's Health Sciences Book Reviews, Nov '97*

Health Reference Series Cumulative Index 1999

A Comprehensive Index to the Individual Volumes of the Health Reference Series, Including a Subject Index, Name Index, Organization Index, and Publication Index

Along with a Master List of Acronyms and Abbreviations

Edited by Edward J. Prucha, Anne Holmes, and Robert Rudnick. 990 pages. 2000. 0-7808-0382-5. $78.

"This volume will be most helpful in libraries that have a relatively complete collection of the Health Reference Series." —*American Reference Books Annual, 2001*

"Essential for collections that hold any of the numerous *Health Reference Series* titles."
— *Choice, Association of College and Research Libraries, Nov '00*

Healthy Aging Sourcebook

Basic Consumer Health Information about Maintaining Health through the Aging Process, Including Advice on Nutrition, Exercise, and Sleep, Help in Making Decisions about Midlife Issues and Retirement, and Guidance Concerning Practical and Informed Choices in Health Consumerism

Along with Data Concerning the Theories of Aging, Different Experiences in Aging by Minority Groups, and Facts about Aging Now and Aging in the Future; and Featuring a Glossary, a Guide to Consumer Help, Additional Suggested Reading, and Practical Resource Directory

Edited by Jenifer Swanson. 536 pages. 1999. 0-7808-0390-6. $78.

"Recommended reference source."
—*Booklist, American Library Association, Feb '00*

SEE ALSO *Physical & Mental Issues in Aging Sourcebook*

Healthy Heart Sourcebook for Women

Basic Consumer Health Information about Cardiac Issues Specific to Women, Including Facts about Major Risk Factors and Prevention, Treatment and Control Strategies, and Important Dietary Issues

Along with a Special Section Regarding the Pros and Cons of Hormone Replacement Therapy and Its Impact on Heart Health, and Additional Help, Including Recipes, a Glossary, and a Directory of Resources

Edited by Dawn D. Matthews. 336 pages. 2000. 0-7808-0329-9. $78.

"A good reference source and recommended for all public, academic, medical, and hospital libraries."
—*Medical Reference Services Quarterly, Summer '01*

"Because of the lack of information specific to women on this topic, this book is recommended for public libraries and consumer libraries."
—*American Reference Books Annual, 2001*

"Contains very important information about coronary artery disease that all women should know. The information is current and presented in an easy-to-read format. The book will make a good addition to any library."
—*American Medical Writers Association Journal, Summer '00*

"Important, basic reference."
—*Reviewer's Bookwatch, Jul '00*

SEE ALSO *Cardiovascular Diseases & Disorders Sourcebook, 1st Edition, Heart Diseases & Disorders Sourcebook, 2nd Edition, Women's Health Concerns Sourcebook*

Heart Diseases & Disorders Sourcebook, 2nd Edition

Basic Consumer Health Information about Heart Attacks, Angina, Rhythm Disorders, Heart Failure, Valve Disease, Congenital Heart Disorders, and More,

Including Descriptions of Surgical Procedures and Other Interventions, Medications, Cardiac Rehabilitation, Risk Identification, and Prevention Tips

Along with Statistical Data, Reports on Current Research Initiatives, a Glossary of Cardiovascular Terms, and Resource Directory

Edited by Karen Bellenir. 612 pages. 2000. 0-7808-0238-1. $78.

"This work stands out as an imminently accessible resource for the general public. It is recommended for the reference and circulating shelves of school, public, and academic libraries."
—*American Reference Books Annual, 2001*

"Recommended reference source."
—*Booklist, American Library Association, Dec '00*

"Provides comprehensive coverage of matters related to the heart. This title is recommended for health sciences and public libraries with consumer health collections."
—*E-Streams, Oct '00*

SEE ALSO *Cardiovascular Diseases & Disorders Sourcebook, 1st Edition; Healthy Heart Sourcebook for Women*

Household Safety Sourcebook

Basic Consumer Health Information about Household Safety, Including Information about Poisons, Chemicals, Fire, and Water Hazards in the Home

Along with Advice about the Safe Use of Home Maintenance Equipment, Choosing Toys and Nursery Furniture, Holiday and Recreation Safety, a Glossary, and Resources for Further Help and Information

Edited by Dawn D. Matthews. 606 pages. 2002. 0-7808-0338-8. $78.

"As a sourcebook on household safety this book meets its mark. It is encyclopedic in scope and covers a wide range of safety issues that are commonly seen in the home."
—*E-Streams, Jul '02*

Immune System Disorders Sourcebook

Basic Information about Lupus, Multiple Sclerosis, Guillain-Barré Syndrome, Chronic Granulomatous Disease, and More

Along with Statistical and Demographic Data and Reports on Current Research Initiatives

Edited by Allan R. Cook. 608 pages. 1997. 0-7808-0209-8. $78.

Infant & Toddler Health Sourcebook

Basic Consumer Health Information about the Physical and Mental Development of Newborns, Infants, and Toddlers, Including Neonatal Concerns, Nutrition Recommendations, Immunization Schedules, Common Pediatric Disorders, Assessments and Milestones, Safe-

ty Tips, and Advice for Parents and Other Caregivers

Along with a Glossary of Terms and Resource Listings for Additional Help

Edited by Jenifer Swanson. 585 pages. 2000. 0-7808-0246-2. $78.

"As a reference for the general public, this would be useful in any library." — *E-Streams, May '01*

"Recommended reference source."
— *Booklist, American Library Association, Feb '01*

"This is a good source for general use."
— *American Reference Books Annual, 2001*

■

Injury & Trauma Sourcebook

Basic Consumer Health Information about the Impact of Injury, the Diagnosis and Treatment of Common and Traumatic Injuries, Emergency Care, and Specific Injuries Related to Home, Community, Workplace, Transportation, and Recreation

Along with Guidelines for Injury Prevention, a Glossary, and a Directory of Additional Resources

Edited by Joyce Brennfleck Shannon. 696 pages. 2002. 0-7808-0421-X. $78.

"Practitioners should be aware of guides such as this in order to facilitate their use by patients and their families." — *Doody's Health Sciences Book Review Journal, Sep-Oct '02*

"Recommended reference source."
— *Booklist, American Library Association, Sep '02*

"Highly recommended for academic and medical reference collections." — *Library Bookwatch, Sep '02*

■

Kidney & Urinary Tract Diseases & Disorders Sourcebook

Basic Information about Kidney Stones, Urinary Incontinence, Bladder Disease, End Stage Renal Disease, Dialysis, and More

Along with Statistical and Demographic Data and Reports on Current Research Initiatives

Edited by Linda M. Ross. 602 pages. 1997. 0-7808-0079-6. $78.

■

Learning Disabilities Sourcebook, 1st Edition

Basic Information about Disorders Such as Dyslexia, Visual and Auditory Processing Deficits, Attention Deficit/Hyperactivity Disorder, and Autism

Along with Statistical and Demographic Data, Reports on Current Research Initiatives, an Explanation of the Assessment Process, and a Special Section for Adults with Learning Disabilities

Edited by Linda M. Shin. 579 pages. 1998. 0-7808-0210-1. $78.

Named "Outstanding Reference Book of 1999."
— *New York Public Library, Feb 2000*

"An excellent candidate for inclusion in a public library reference section. It's a great source of information. Teachers will also find the book useful. Definitely worth reading."
— *Journal of Adolescent & Adult Literacy, Feb 2000*

"Readable . . . provides a solid base of information regarding successful techniques used with individuals who have learning disabilities, as well as practical suggestions for educators and family members. Clear language, concise descriptions, and pertinent information for contacting multiple resources add to the strength of this book as a useful tool." — *Choice, Association of College and Research Libraries, Feb '99*

"Recommended reference source."
— *Booklist, American Library Association, Sep '98*

"A useful resource for libraries and for those who don't have the time to identify and locate the individual publications." — *Disability Resources Monthly, Sep '98*

■

Learning Disabilities Sourcebook, 2nd Edition

Basic Consumer Health Information about Learning Disabilities, Including Dyslexia, Developmental Speech and Language Disabilities, Non-Verbal Learning Disorders, Developmental Arithmetic Disorder, Developmental Writing Disorder, and Other Conditions That Impede Learning Such as Attention Deficit/ Hyperactivity Disorder, Brain Injury, Hearing Impairment, Klinefelter Syndrome, Dyspraxia, and Tourette Syndrome

Along with Facts about Educational Issues and Assistive Technology, Coping Strategies, a Glossary of Related Terms, and Resources for Further Help and Information

Edited by Dawn D. Matthews. 621 pages. 2003. 0-7808-0626-3. $78.

■

Liver Disorders Sourcebook

Basic Consumer Health Information about the Liver and How It Works; Liver Diseases, Including Cancer, Cirrhosis, Hepatitis, and Toxic and Drug Related Diseases; Tips for Maintaining a Healthy Liver; Laboratory Tests, Radiology Tests, and Facts about Liver Transplantation

Along with a Section on Support Groups, a Glossary, and Resource Listings

Edited by Joyce Brennfleck Shannon. 591 pages. 2000. 0-7808-0383-3. $78.

"A valuable resource."
— *American Reference Books Annual, 2001*

"This title is recommended for health sciences and public libraries with consumer health collections."
— *E-Streams, Oct '00*

"Recommended reference source."
— *Booklist, American Library Association, Jun '00*

Lung Disorders Sourcebook

Basic Consumer Health Information about Emphysema, Pneumonia, Tuberculosis, Asthma, Cystic Fibrosis, and Other Lung Disorders, Including Facts about Diagnostic Procedures, Treatment Strategies, Disease Prevention Efforts, and Such Risk Factors as Smoking, Air Pollution, and Exposure to Asbestos, Radon, and Other Agents

Along with a Glossary and Resources for Additional Help and Information

Edited by Dawn D. Matthews. 678 pages. 2002. 0-7808-0339-6. $78.

"Highly recommended for academic and medical reference collections." — *Library Bookwatch, Sep '02* [Pain SB, 2nd ed.]

"A source of valuable information. . . . This book offers help to nonmedical people who need information about pain and pain management. It is also an excellent reference for those who participate in patient education." — *Doody's Review Service, Sep '02*

"Highly recommended for academic and medical reference collections." — *Library Bookwatch, Sep '02*

Medical Tests Sourcebook

Basic Consumer Health Information about Medical Tests, Including Periodic Health Exams, General Screening Tests, Tests You Can Do at Home, Findings of the U.S. Preventive Services Task Force, X-ray and Radiology Tests, Electrical Tests, Tests of Blood and Other Body Fluids and Tissues, Scope Tests, Lung Tests, Genetic Tests, Pregnancy Tests, Newborn Screening Tests, Sexually Transmitted Disease Tests, and Computer Aided Diagnoses

Along with a Section on Paying for Medical Tests, a Glossary, and Resource Listings

Edited by Joyce Brennfleck Shannon. 691 pages. 1999. 0-7808-0243-8. $78.

"Recommended for hospital and health sciences libraries with consumer health collections." — *E-Streams, Mar '00*

"This is an overall excellent reference with a wealth of general knowledge that may aid those who are reluctant to get vital tests performed." — *Today's Librarian, Jan 2000*

"A valuable reference guide." — *American Reference Books Annual, 2000*

Men's Health Concerns Sourcebook

Basic Information about Health Issues That Affect Men, Featuring Facts about the Top Causes of Death in Men, Including Heart Disease, Stroke, Cancers, Prostate Disorders, Chronic Obstructive Pulmonary Disease, Pneumonia and Influenza, Human Immunodeficiency Virus and Acquired Immune Deficiency Syndrome, Diabetes Mellitus, Stress, Suicide, Accidents and Homicides; and Facts about Common

Concerns for Men, Including Impotence, Contraception, Circumcision, Sleep Disorders, Snoring, Hair Loss, Diet, Nutrition, Exercise, Kidney and Urological Disorders, and Backaches

Edited by Allan R. Cook. 738 pages. 1998. 0-7808-0212-8. $78.

"This comprehensive resource and the series are highly recommended." — *American Reference Books Annual, 2000*

"Recommended reference source." — *Booklist, American Library Association, Dec '98*

Mental Health Disorders Sourcebook, 1st Edition

Basic Information about Schizophrenia, Depression, Bipolar Disorder, Panic Disorder, Obsessive-Compulsive Disorder, Phobias and Other Anxiety Disorders, Paranoia and Other Personality Disorders, Eating Disorders, and Sleep Disorders

Along with Information about Treatment and Therapies

Edited by Karen Bellenir. 548 pages. 1995. 0-7808-0040-0. $78.

"This is an excellent new book . . . written in easy-to-understand language." — *Booklist Health Sciences Supplement, American Library Association, Oct '97*

". . . useful for public and academic libraries and consumer health collections." — *Medical Reference Services Quarterly, Spring '97*

"The great strengths of the book are its readability and its inclusion of places to find more information. Especially recommended." — *Reference Quarterly, American Library Association, Winter '96*

". . . a good resource for a consumer health library." — *Bulletin of the Medical Library Association, Oct '96*

"The information is data-based and couched in brief, concise language that avoids jargon. . . . a useful reference source." — *Readings, Sep '96*

"The text is well organized and adequately written for its target audience." — *Choice, Association of College and Research Libraries, Jun '96*

". . . provides information on a wide range of mental disorders, presented in nontechnical language." — *Exceptional Child Education Resources, Spring '96*

"Recommended for public and academic libraries." — *Reference Book Review, 1996*

Mental Health Disorders Sourcebook, 2nd Edition

Basic Consumer Health Information about Anxiety Disorders, Depression and Other Mood Disorders, Eating Disorders, Personality Disorders, Schizophrenia, and More, Including Disease Descriptions, Treatment Options, and Reports on Current Research Initiatives

Along with Statistical Data, Tips for Maintaining Mental Health, a Glossary, and Directory of Sources for Additional Help and Information

Edited by Karen Bellenir. 605 pages. 2000. 0-7808-0240-3. $78.

"Well organized and well written."
—American Reference Books Annual, 2001

"Recommended reference source."
—Booklist, American Library Association, Jun '00

■

Mental Retardation Sourcebook

Basic Consumer Health Information about Mental Retardation and Its Causes, Including Down Syndrome, Fetal Alcohol Syndrome, Fragile X Syndrome, Genetic Conditions, Injury, and Environmental Sources

Along with Preventive Strategies, Parenting Issues, Educational Implications, Health Care Needs, Employment and Economic Matters, Legal Issues, a Glossary, and a Resource Listing for Additional Help and Information

Edited by Joyce Brennfleck Shannon. 642 pages. 2000. 0-7808-0377-9. $78.

"Public libraries will find the book useful for reference and as a beginning research point for students, parents, and caregivers."
—American Reference Books Annual, 2001

"The strength of this work is that it compiles many basic fact sheets and addresses for further information in one volume. It is intended and suitable for the general public. This sourcebook is relevant to any collection providing health information to the general public."
—E-Streams, Nov '00

"From preventing retardation to parenting and family challenges, this covers health, social and legal issues and will prove an invaluable overview."
—Reviewer's Bookwatch, Jul '00

■

Movement Disorders Sourcebook

Basic Consumer Health Information about Neurological Movement Disorders, Including Essential Tremor, Parkinson's Disease, Dystonia, Cerebral Palsy, Huntington's Disease, Myasthenia Gravis, Multiple Sclerosis, and Other Early-Onset and Adult-Onset Movement Disorders, Their Symptoms and Causes, Diagnostic Tests, and Treatments

Along with Mobility and Assistive Technology Information, a Glossary, and a Directory of Additional Resources

Edited by Joyce Brennfleck Shannon. 655 pages. 2003. 0-7808-0628-X. $78.

■

Obesity Sourcebook

Basic Consumer Health Information about Diseases and Other Problems Associated with Obesity, and Including Facts about Risk Factors, Prevention Issues, and Management Approaches

Along with Statistical and Demographic Data, Information about Special Populations, Research Updates, a Glossary, and Source Listings for Further Help and Information

Edited by Wilma Caldwell and Chad T. Kimball. 376 pages. 2001. 0-7808-0333-7. $78.

"The book synthesizes the reliable medical literature on obesity into one easy-to-read and useful resource for the general public."
—American Reference Books Annual 2002

"This is a very useful resource book for the lay public."
—Doody's Review Service, Nov '01

"Well suited for the health reference collection of a public library or an academic health science library that serves the general population."
—E-Streams, Sep '01

"Recommended reference source."
—Booklist, American Library Association, Apr '01

" Recommended pick both for specialty health library collections and any general consumer health reference collection."
—The Bookwatch, Apr '01

■

Ophthalmic Disorders Sourcebook, 1st Edition

Basic Information about Glaucoma, Cataracts, Macular Degeneration, Strabismus, Refractive Disorders, and More

Along with Statistical and Demographic Data and Reports on Current Research Initiatives

Edited by Linda M. Ross. 631 pages. 1996. 0-7808-0081-8. $78.

SEE ALSO Eye Care Sourcebook, 2nd Edition

■

Oral Health Sourcebook, 1st Edition

Basic Information about Diseases and Conditions Affecting Oral Health, Including Cavities, Gum Disease, Dry Mouth, Oral Cancers, Fever Blisters, Canker Sores, Oral Thrush, Bad Breath, Temporomandibular Disorders, and other Craniofacial Syndromes

Along with Statistical Data on the Oral Health of Americans, Oral Hygiene, Emergency First Aid, Information on Treatment Procedures and Methods of Replacing Lost Teeth

Edited by Allan R. Cook. 558 pages. 1997. 0-7808-0082-6. $78.

"Unique source which will fill a gap in dental sources for patients and the lay public. A valuable reference tool even in a library with thousands of books on dentistry. Comprehensive, clear, inexpensive, and easy to read and use. It fills an enormous gap in the health care literature."
—Reference and User Services Quarterly, American Library Association, Summer '98

"Recommended reference source."
—Booklist, American Library Association, Dec '97

Osteoporosis Sourcebook

Basic Consumer Health Information about Primary and Secondary Osteoporosis and Juvenile Osteoporosis and Related Conditions, Including Fibrous Dysplasia, Gaucher Disease, Hyperthyroidism, Hypophosphatasia, Myeloma, Osteopetrosis, Osteogenesis Imperfecta, and Paget's Disease

Along with Information about Risk Factors, Treatments, Traditional and Non-Traditional Pain Management, a Glossary of Related Terms, and a Directory of Resources

Edited by Allan R. Cook. 584 pages. 2001. 0-7808-0239-X. $78.

"This would be a book to be kept in a staff or patient library. The targeted audience is the layperson, but the therapist who needs a quick bit of information on a particular topic will also find the book useful."
— *Physical Therapy, Jan '02*

"This resource is recommended as a great reference source for public, health, and academic libraries, and is another triumph for the editors of Omnigraphics."
— *American Reference Books Annual 2002*

"Recommended for all public libraries and general health collections, especially those supporting patient education or consumer health programs."
— *E-Streams, Nov '01*

"Will prove valuable to any library seeking to maintain a current, comprehensive reference collection of health resources. . . . From prevention to treatment and associated conditions, this provides an excellent survey."
— *The Bookwatch, Aug '01*

"Recommended reference source."
— *Booklist, American Library Association, July '01*

SEE ALSO *Women's Health Concerns Sourcebook*

Pain Sourcebook, 1st Edition

Basic Information about Specific Forms of Acute and Chronic Pain, Including Headaches, Back Pain, Muscular Pain, Neuralgia, Surgical Pain, and Cancer Pain

Along with Pain Relief Options Such as Analgesics, Narcotics, Nerve Blocks, Transcutaneous Nerve Stimulation, and Alternative Forms of Pain Control, Including Biofeedback, Imaging, Behavior Modification, and Relaxation Techniques

Edited by Allan R. Cook. 667 pages. 1997. 0-7808-0213-6. $78.

"The text is readable, easily understood, and well indexed. This excellent volume belongs in all patient education libraries, consumer health sections of public libraries, and many personal collections."
— *American Reference Books Annual, 1999*

"A beneficial reference." — *Booklist Health Sciences Supplement, American Library Association, Oct '98*

"The information is basic in terms of scholarship and is appropriate for general readers. Written in journalistic style . . . intended for non-professionals. Quite thorough in its coverage of different pain conditions and summa-

rizes the latest clinical information regarding pain treatment."
— *Choice, Association of College and Research Libraries, Jun '98*

"Recommended reference source."
— *Booklist, American Library Association, Mar '98*

Pain Sourcebook, 2nd Edition

Basic Consumer Health Information about Specific Forms of Acute and Chronic Pain, Including Muscle and Skeletal Pain, Nerve Pain, Cancer Pain, and Disorders Characterized by Pain, Such as Fibromyalgia, Shingles, Angina, Arthritis, and Headaches

Along with Information about Pain Medications and Management Techniques, Complementary and Alternative Pain Relief Options, Tips for People Living with Chronic Pain, a Glossary, and a Directory of Sources for Further Information

Edited by Karen Bellenir. 670 pages. 2002. 0-7808-0612-3. $78.

Pediatric Cancer Sourcebook

Basic Consumer Health Information about Leukemias, Brain Tumors, Sarcomas, Lymphomas, and Other Cancers in Infants, Children, and Adolescents, Including Descriptions of Cancers, Treatments, and Coping Strategies

Along with Suggestions for Parents, Caregivers, and Concerned Relatives, a Glossary of Cancer Terms, and Resource Listings

Edited by Edward J. Prucha. 587 pages. 1999. 0-7808-0245-4. $78.

"An excellent source of information. Recommended for public, hospital, and health science libraries with consumer health collections." — *E-Streams, Jun '00*

"Recommended reference source."
— *Booklist, American Library Association, Feb '00*

"A valuable addition to all libraries specializing in health services and many public libraries."
— *American Reference Books Annual, 2000*

Physical & Mental Issues in Aging Sourcebook

Basic Consumer Health Information on Physical and Mental Disorders Associated with the Aging Process, Including Concerns about Cardiovascular Disease, Pulmonary Disease, Oral Health, Digestive Disorders, Musculoskeletal and Skin Disorders, Metabolic Changes, Sexual and Reproductive Issues, and Changes in Vision, Hearing, and Other Senses

Along with Data about Longevity and Causes of Death, Information on Acute and Chronic Pain, Descriptions of Mental Concerns, a Glossary of Terms, and Resource Listings for Additional Help

Edited by Jenifer Swanson. 660 pages. 1999. 0-7808-0233-0. $78.

"This is a treasure of health information for the layperson." — *Choice Health Sciences Supplement, Association of College & Research Libraries, May 2000*

"Recommended for public libraries."
—American Reference Books Annual, 2000

"Recommended reference source."
—Booklist, American Library Association, Oct '99

SEE ALSO Healthy Aging Sourcebook

■

Podiatry Sourcebook

Basic Consumer Health Information about Foot Conditions, Diseases, and Injuries, Including Bunions, Corns, Calluses, Athlete's Foot, Plantar Warts, Hammertoes and Clawtoes, Clubfoot, Heel Pain, Gout, and More

Along with Facts about Foot Care, Disease Prevention, Foot Safety, Choosing a Foot Care Specialist, a Glossary of Terms, and Resource Listings for Additional Information

Edited by M. Lisa Weatherford. 380 pages. 2001. 0-7808-0215-2. $78.

"Recommended reference source."
— Booklist, American Library Association, Feb '02

"There is a lot of information presented here on a topic that is usually only covered sparingly in most larger comprehensive medical encyclopedias."
— American Reference Books Annual 2002

■

Pregnancy & Birth Sourcebook

Basic Information about Planning for Pregnancy, Maternal Health, Fetal Growth and Development, Labor and Delivery, Postpartum and Perinatal Care, Pregnancy in Mothers with Special Concerns, and Disorders of Pregnancy, Including Genetic Counseling, Nutrition and Exercise, Obstetrical Tests, Pregnancy Discomfort, Multiple Births, Cesarean Sections, Medical Testing of Newborns, Breastfeeding, Gestational Diabetes, and Ectopic Pregnancy

Edited by Heather E. Aldred. 737 pages. 1997. 0-7808-0216-0. $78.

"A well-organized handbook. Recommended."
— Choice, Association of College and Research Libraries, Apr '98

"Recommended reference source."
— Booklist, American Library Association, Mar '98

"Recommended for public libraries."
—American Reference Books Annual, 1998

SEE ALSO Congenital Disorders Sourcebook, Family Planning Sourcebook

■

Prostate Cancer Sourcebook

Basic Consumer Health Information about Prostate Cancer, Including Information about the Associated Risk Factors, Detection, Diagnosis, and Treatment of Prostate Cancer

Along with Information on Non-Malignant Prostate Conditions, and Featuring a Section Listing Support and Treatment Centers and a Glossary of Related Terms

Edited by Dawn D. Matthews. 358 pages. 2001. 0-7808-0324-8. $78.

"Recommended reference source."
— Booklist, American Library Association, Jan '02

"A valuable resource for health care consumers seeking information on the subject. . . .All text is written in a clear, easy-to-understand language that avoids technical jargon. Any library that collects consumer health resources would strengthen their collection with the addition of the *Prostate Cancer Sourcebook*."
—American Reference Books Annual 2002

■

Public Health Sourcebook

Basic Information about Government Health Agencies, Including National Health Statistics and Trends, Healthy People 2000 Program Goals and Objectives, the Centers for Disease Control and Prevention, the Food and Drug Administration, and the National Institutes of Health

Along with Full Contact Information for Each Agency

Edited by Wendy Wilcox. 698 pages. 1998. 0-7808-0220-9. $78.

"Recommended reference source."
— Booklist, American Library Association, Sep '98

"This consumer guide provides welcome assistance in navigating the maze of federal health agencies and their data on public health concerns."
—SciTech Book News, Sep '98

■

Reconstructive & Cosmetic Surgery Sourcebook

Basic Consumer Health Information on Cosmetic and Reconstructive Plastic Surgery, Including Statistical Information about Different Surgical Procedures, Things to Consider Prior to Surgery, Plastic Surgery Techniques and Tools, Emotional and Psychological Considerations, and Procedure-Specific Information

Along with a Glossary of Terms and a Listing of Resources for Additional Help and Information

Edited by M. Lisa Weatherford. 374 pages. 2001. 0-7808-0214-4. $78.

"An excellent reference that addresses cosmetic and medically necessary reconstructive surgeries. . . . The style of the prose is calm and reassuring, discussing the many positive outcomes now available due to advances in surgical techniques."
— American Reference Books Annual 2002

"Recommended for health science libraries that are open to the public, as well as hospital libraries that are open to the patients. This book is a good resource for the consumer interested in plastic surgery."
—E-Streams, Dec '01

"Recommended reference source."
—Booklist, American Library Association, July '01

Rehabilitation Sourcebook

Basic Consumer Health Information about Rehabilitation for People Recovering from Heart Surgery, Spinal Cord Injury, Stroke, Orthopedic Impairments, Amputation, Pulmonary Impairments, Traumatic Injury, and More, Including Physical Therapy, Occupational Therapy, Speech/ Language Therapy, Massage Therapy, Dance Therapy, Art Therapy, and Recreational Therapy

Along with Information on Assistive and Adaptive Devices, a Glossary, and Resources for Additional Help and Information

Edited by Dawn D. Matthews. 531 pages. 1999. 0-7808-0236-5. $78.

"This is an excellent resource for public library reference and health collections."
—American Reference Books Annual, 2001

"Recommended reference source."
— Booklist, American Library Association, May '00

▓

Respiratory Diseases & Disorders Sourcebook

Basic Information about Respiratory Diseases and Disorders, Including Asthma, Cystic Fibrosis, Pneumonia, the Common Cold, Influenza, and Others, Featuring Facts about the Respiratory System, Statistical and Demographic Data, Treatments, Self-Help Management Suggestions, and Current Research Initiatives

Edited by Allan R. Cook and Peter D. Dresser. 771 pages. 1995. 0-7808-0037-0. $78.

"Designed for the layperson and for patients and their families coping with respiratory illness. . . . an extensive array of information on diagnosis, treatment, management, and prevention of respiratory illnesses for the general reader."
— Choice, Association of College and Research Libraries, Jun '96

"A highly recommended text for all collections. It is a comforting reminder of the power of knowledge that good books carry between their covers."
— Academic Library Book Review, Spring '96

"A comprehensive collection of authoritative information presented in a nontechnical, humanitarian style for patients, families, and caregivers."
—Association of Operating Room Nurses, Sep/Oct '95

▓

Sexually Transmitted Diseases Sourcebook, 1st Edition

Basic Information about Herpes, Chlamydia, Gonorrhea, Hepatitis, Nongonoccocal Urethritis, Pelvic Inflammatory Disease, Syphilis, AIDS, and More

Along with Current Data on Treatments and Preventions

Edited by Linda M. Ross. 550 pages. 1997. 0-7808-0217-9. $78.

Sexually Transmitted Diseases Sourcebook, 2nd Edition

Basic Consumer Health Information about Sexually Transmitted Diseases, Including Information on the Diagnosis and Treatment of Chlamydia, Gonorrhea, Hepatitis, Herpes, HIV, Mononucleosis, Syphilis, and Others

Along with Information on Prevention, Such as Condom Use, Vaccines, and STD Education; And Featuring a Section on Issues Related to Youth and Adolescents, a Glossary, and Resources for Additional Help and Information

Edited by Dawn D. Matthews. 538 pages. 2001. 0-7808-0249-7. $78.

"Recommended for consumer health collections in public libraries, and secondary school and community college libraries."
— American Reference Books Annual 2002

"Every school and public library should have a copy of this comprehensive and user-friendly reference book."
— Choice, Association of College & Research Libraries, Sep '01

"This is a highly recommended book. This is an especially important book for all school and public libraries." *— AIDS Book Review Journal, Jul-Aug '01*

"Recommended reference source."
— Booklist, American Library Association, Apr '01

"Recommended pick both for specialty health library collections and any general consumer health reference collection." *— The Bookwatch, Apr '01*

▓

Skin Disorders Sourcebook

Basic Information about Common Skin and Scalp Conditions Caused by Aging, Allergies, Immune Reactions, Sun Exposure, Infectious Organisms, Parasites, Cosmetics, and Skin Traumas, Including Abrasions, Cuts, and Pressure Sores

Along with Information on Prevention and Treatment

Edited by Allan R. Cook. 647 pages. 1997. 0-7808-0080-X. $78.

". . . comprehensive, easily read reference book."
— Doody's Health Sciences Book Reviews, Oct '97

SEE ALSO Burns Sourcebook

▓

Sleep Disorders Sourcebook

Basic Consumer Health Information about Sleep and Its Disorders, Including Insomnia, Sleepwalking, Sleep Apnea, Restless Leg Syndrome, and Narcolepsy

Along with Data about Shiftwork and Its Effects, Information on the Societal Costs of Sleep Deprivation, Descriptions of Treatment Options, a Glossary of Terms, and Resource Listings for Additional Help

Edited by Jenifer Swanson. 439 pages. 1998. 0-7808-0234-9. $78.

"This text will complement any home or medical library. It is user-friendly and ideal for the adult reader."
—American Reference Books Annual, 2000

Sports Injuries Sourcebook, 1st Edition

Basic Consumer Health Information about Common Sports Injuries, Prevention of Injury in Specific Sports, Tips for Training, and Rehabilitation from Injury

Along with Information about Special Concerns for Children, Young Girls in Athletic Training Programs, Senior Athletes, and Women Athletes, and a Directory of Resources for Further Help and Information

Edited by Heather E. Aldred. 624 pages. 1999. 0-7808-0218-7. $78.

Sports Injuries Sourcebook, 2nd Edition

Basic Consumer Health Information about the Diagnosis, Treatment, and Rehabilitation of Common Sports-Related Injuries in Children and Adults

Along with Suggestions for Conditioning and Training, Information and Prevention Tips for Injuries Frequently Associated with Specific Sports and Special Populations, a Glossary, and a Directory of Additional Resources

Edited by Joyce Brennfleck Shannon. 614 pages. 2002. 0-7808-0604-2. $78.

Stress-Related Disorders Sourcebook

Basic Consumer Health Information about Stress and Stress-Related Disorders, Including Stress Origins and Signals, Environmental Stress at Work and Home, Mental and Emotional Stress Associated with Depression, Post-Traumatic Stress Disorder, Panic Disorder, Suicide, and the Physical Effects of Stress on the Cardiovascular, Immune, and Nervous Systems

Along with Stress Management Techniques, a Glossary, and a Listing of Additional Resources

Edited by Joyce Brennfleck Shannon. 610 pages. 2002. 0-7808-0560-7. $78.

Stroke Sourcebook

Basic Consumer Health Information about Stroke, Including Ischemic, Hemorrhagic, Transient Ischemic Attack (TIA), and Pediatric Stroke, Stroke Triggers and Risks, Diagnostic Tests, Treatments, and Rehabilitation Information

Along with Stroke Prevention Guidelines, Legal and Financial Information, a Glossary, and a Directory of Additional Resources

Edited by Joyce Brennfleck Shannon. 606 pages. 2003. 0-7808-0630-1. $78.

Substance Abuse Sourcebook

Basic Health-Related Information about the Abuse of Legal and Illegal Substances Such as Alcohol, Tobacco, Prescription Drugs, Marijuana, Cocaine, and Heroin; and Including Facts about Substance Abuse Prevention Strategies, Intervention Methods, Treatment and Recovery Programs, and a Section Addressing the Special Problems Related to Substance Abuse during Pregnancy

Edited by Karen Bellenir. 573 pages. 1996. 0-7808-0038-9. $78.

SEE ALSO Alcoholism Sourcebook, Drug Abuse Sourcebook

Surgery Sourcebook

Basic Consumer Health Information about Inpatient and Outpatient Surgeries, Including Cardiac, Vascular, Orthopedic, Ocular, Reconstructive, Cosmetic, Gynecologic, and Ear, Nose, and Throat Procedures and More

Along with Information about Operating Room Policies and Instruments, Laser Surgery Techniques, Hospital Errors, Statistical Data, a Glossary, and Listings of Sources for Further Help and Information

Edited by Annemarie S. Muth and Karen Bellenir. 596 pages. 2002. 0-7808-0380-9. $78.

Transplantation Sourcebook

Basic Consumer Health Information about Organ and Tissue Transplantation, Including Physical and Financial Preparations, Procedures and Issues Relating to Specific Solid Organ and Tissue Transplants, Rehabilitation, Pediatric Transplant Information, the Future of Transplantation, and Organ and Tissue Donation

Along with a Glossary and Listings of Additional Resources

Edited by Joyce Brennfleck Shannon. 628 pages. 2002. 0-7808-0322-1. $78.

"Recommended for libraries with an interest in offering consumer health information." — *E-Streams, Jul '02*

"This is a unique and valuable resource for patients facing transplantation and their families."
— *Doody's Review Service, Jun '02*

∎

Traveler's Health Sourcebook

Basic Consumer Health Information for Travelers, Including Physical and Medical Preparations, Transportation Health and Safety, Essential Information about Food and Water, Sun Exposure, Insect and Snake Bites, Camping and Wilderness Medicine, and Travel with Physical or Medical Disabilities

Along with International Travel Tips, Vaccination Recommendations, Geographical Health Issues, Disease Risks, a Glossary, and a Listing of Additional Resources

Edited by Joyce Brennfleck Shannon. 613 pages. 2000. 0-7808-0384-1. $78.

"Recommended reference source."
— *Booklist, American Library Association, Feb '01*

"This book is recommended for any public library, any travel collection, and especially any collection for the physically disabled."
— *American Reference Books Annual, 2001*

∎

Vegetarian Sourcebook

Basic Consumer Health Information about Vegetarian Diets, Lifestyle, and Philosophy, Including Definitions of Vegetarianism and Veganism, Tips about Adopting Vegetarianism, Creating a Vegetarian Pantry, and Meeting Nutritional Needs of Vegetarians, with Facts Regarding Vegetarianism's Effect on Pregnant and Lactating Women, Children, Athletes, and Senior Citizens

Along with a Glossary of Commonly Used Vegetarian Terms and Resources for Additional Help and Information

Edited by Chad T. Kimball. 360 pages. 2002. 0-7808-0439-2. $78.

Women's Health Concerns Sourcebook

Basic Information about Health Issues That Affect Women, Featuring Facts about Menstruation and Other Gynecological Concerns, Including Endometriosis, Fibroids, Menopause, and Vaginitis; Reproductive Concerns, Including Birth Control, Infertility, and Abortion; and Facts about Additional Physical, Emotional, and Mental Health Concerns Prevalent among Women Such as Osteoporosis, Urinary Tract Disorders, Eating Disorders, and Depression

Along with Tips for Maintaining a Healthy Lifestyle

Edited by Heather E. Aldred. 567 pages. 1997. 0-7808-0219-5. $78.

"Handy compilation. There is an impressive range of diseases, devices, disorders, procedures, and other physical and emotional issues covered . . . well organized, illustrated, and indexed." — *Choice, Association of College and Research Libraries, Jan '98*

SEE ALSO *Breast Cancer Sourcebook, Cancer Sourcebook for Women, 1st and 2nd Editions, Healthy Heart Sourcebook for Women, Osteoporosis Sourcebook*

∎

Workplace Health & Safety Sourcebook

Basic Consumer Health Information about Workplace Health and Safety, Including the Effect of Workplace Hazards on the Lungs, Skin, Heart, Ears, Eyes, Brain, Reproductive Organs, Musculoskeletal System, and Other Organs and Body Parts

Along with Information about Occupational Cancer, Personal Protective Equipment, Toxic and Hazardous Chemicals, Child Labor, Stress, and Workplace Violence

Edited by Chad T. Kimball. 626 pages. 2000. 0-7808-0231-4. $78.

"As a reference for the general public, this would be useful in any library." — *E-Streams, Jun '01*

"Provides helpful information for primary care physicians and other caregivers interested in occupational medicine. . . . General readers; professionals."
— *Choice, Association of College & Research Libraries, May '01*

"Recommended reference source."
— *Booklist, American Library Association, Feb '01*

"Highly recommended." — *The Bookwatch, Jan '01*

∎

Worldwide Health Sourcebook

Basic Information about Global Health Issues, Including Malnutrition, Reproductive Health, Disease Dispersion and Prevention, Emerging Diseases, Risky Health Behaviors, and the Leading Causes of Death

Along with Global Health Concerns for Children, Women, and the Elderly, Mental Health Issues, Research and Technology Advancements, and Economic, Environmental, and Political Health Implications, a

Glossary, and a Resource Listing for Additional Help and Information

Edited by Joyce Brennfleck Shannon. 614 pages. 2001. 0-7808-0330-2. $78.

"Named an Outstanding Academic Title."
> *—Choice, Association of College & Research Libraries, Jan '02*

"Yet another handy but also unique compilation in the extensive Health Reference Series, this is a useful work because many of the international publications reprinted or excerpted are not readily available. Highly recommended." *—Choice, Association of College & Research Libraries, Nov '01*

"Recommended reference source."
> *—Booklist, American Library Association, Oct '01*

Teen Health Series

Helping Young Adults Understand, Manage, and Avoid Serious Illness

Diet Information for Teens
Health Tips about Diet and Nutrition

Including Facts about Nutrients, Dietary Guidelines, Breakfasts, School Lunches, Snacks, Party Food, Weight Control, Eating Disorders, and More

Edited by Karen Bellenir. 399 pages. 2001. 0-7808-0441-4. $58.

"Full of helpful insights and facts throughout the book. ... An excellent resource to be placed in public libraries or even in personal collections."
— *American Reference Books Annual 2002*

"Recommended for middle and high school libraries and media centers as well as academic libraries that educate future teachers of teenagers. It is also a suitable addition to health science libraries that serve patrons who are interested in teen health promotion and education." — *E-Streams, Oct '01*

"This comprehensive book would be beneficial to collections that need information about nutrition, dietary guidelines, meal planning, and weight control. ... This reference is so easy to use that its purchase is recommended." — *The Book Report, Sep-Oct '01*

"This book is written in an easy to understand format describing issues that many teens face every day, and then provides thoughtful explanations so that teens can make informed decisions. This is an interesting book that provides important facts and information for today's teens." — *Doody's Health Sciences Book Review Journal, Jul-Aug '01*

"A comprehensive compendium of diet and nutrition. The information is presented in a straightforward, plain-spoken manner. This title will be useful to those working on reports on a variety of topics, as well as to general readers concerned about their dietary health."
— *School Library Journal, Jun '01*

Drug Information for Teens
Health Tips about the Physical and Mental Effects of Substance Abuse

Including Facts about Alcohol, Anabolic Steroids, Club Drugs, Cocaine, Depressants, Hallucinogens, Herbal Products, Inhalants, Marijuana, Narcotics, Stimulants, Tobacco, and More

Edited by Karen Bellenir. 452 pages. 2002. 0-7808-0444-9. $58.

"This is an excellent resource for teens and their parents. Education about drugs and substances is key to discouraging teen drug abuse and this book provides this much needed information in a way that is interesting and factual." — *Doody's Review Service, Dec '02*

Mental Health Information for Teens
Health Tips about Mental Health and Mental Illness

Including Facts about Anxiety, Depression, Suicide, Eating Disorders, Obsessive-Compulsive Disorders, Panic Attacks, Phobias, Schizophrenia, and More

Edited by Karen Bellenir. 406 pages. 2001. 0-7808-0442-2. $58.

"In both language and approach, this user-friendly entry in the *Teen Health Series* is on target for teens needing information on mental health concerns." — *Booklist, American Library Association, Jan '02*

"Readers will find the material accessible and informative, with the shaded notes, facts, and embedded glossary insets adding appropriately to the already interesting and succinct presentation."
— *School Library Journal, Jan '02*

"This title is highly recommended for any library that serves adolescents and parents/caregivers of adolescents." — *E-Streams, Jan '02*

"Recommended for high school libraries and young adult collections in public libraries. Both health professionals and teenagers will find this book useful."
— *American Reference Books Annual 2002*

"This is a nice book written to enlighten the society, primarily teenagers, about common teen mental health issues. It is highly recommended to teachers and parents as well as adolescents."
— *Doody's Review Service, Dec '01*

Sexual Health Information for Teens
Health Tips about Sexual Development, Human Reproduction, and Sexually Transmitted Diseases

Including Facts about Puberty, Reproductive Health, Chlamydia, Human Papillomavirus, Pelvic Inflammatory Disease, Herpes, AIDS, Contraception, Pregnancy, and More

Edited by Deborah A. Stanley. 400 pages. 2003. 0-7808-0445-7. $58.

Health Reference Series

Adolescent Health Sourcebook

AIDS Sourcebook, 1st Edition

AIDS Sourcebook, 2nd Edition

AIDS Sourcebook, 3rd Edition

Alcoholism Sourcebook

Allergies Sourcebook, 1st Edition

Allergies Sourcebook, 2nd Edition

Alternative Medicine Sourcebook, 1st Edition

Alternative Medicine Sourcebook, 2nd Edition

Alzheimer's, Stroke & 29 Other Neurological Disorders Sourcebook, 1st Edition

Alzheimer's Disease Sourcebook, 2nd Edition

Arthritis Sourcebook

Asthma Sourcebook

Attention Deficit Disorder Sourcebook

Back & Neck Disorders Sourcebook

Blood & Circulatory Disorders Sourcebook

Brain Disorders Sourcebook

Breast Cancer Sourcebook

Breastfeeding Sourcebook

Burns Sourcebook

Cancer Sourcebook, 1st Edition

Cancer Sourcebook (New), 2nd Edition

Cancer Sourcebook, 3rd Edition

Cancer Sourcebook for Women, 1st Edition

Cancer Sourcebook for Women, 2nd Edition

Cardiovascular Diseases & Disorders Sourcebook, 1st Edition

Caregiving Sourcebook

Childhood Diseases & Disorders Sourcebook

Colds, Flu & Other Common Ailments Sourcebook

Communication Disorders Sourcebook

Congenital Disorders Sourcebook

Consumer Issues in Health Care Sourcebook

Contagious & Non-Contagious Infectious Diseases Sourcebook

Death & Dying Sourcebook

Depression Sourcebook

Diabetes Sourcebook, 1st Edition

Diabetes Sourcebook, 2nd Edition

Diabetes Sourcebook, 3rd Edition

Diet & Nutrition Sourcebook, 1st Edition

Diet & Nutrition Sourcebook, 2nd Edition

Digestive Diseases & Disorder Sourcebook

Disabilities Sourcebook

Domestic Violence & Child Abuse Sourcebook

Drug Abuse Sourcebook

Ear, Nose & Throat Disorders Sourcebook

Eating Disorders Sourcebook

Emergency Medical Services Sourcebook

Endocrine & Metabolic Disorders Sourcebook

Environmentally Induced Disorders Sourcebook

Ethnic Diseases Sourcebook

Eye Care Sourcebook, 2nd Edition

Family Planning Sourcebook

Fitness & Exercise Sourcebook, 1st Edition

Fitness & Exercise Sourcebook, 2nd Edition

Food & Animal Borne Diseases Sourcebook

Food Safety Sourcebook

Forensic Medicine Sourcebook

Gastrointestinal Diseases & Disorders Sourcebook